Conversations with Nora

a family's journey with Alzheimer's

A NOVEL BY

ELAINE LOHRMAN

ISBN: 978-1468058987

Heartfelt thanks to the many friends who encouraged me to write this story, and in particular to those who gave of their time, gifts and hearts to make it possible…

Ellen Bachman
Martha Lipscomb
Linda Makinson
Carlyn Moyer

…and with the greatest of love and admiration for my husband, who completes me.

Bill Lohrman
"I appreciate you."

*Lovingly dedicated to
all those who suffer from dementia,
to their families and friends,
and to my own beloved Mother.*

Prologue

The table was set for eight. Two hungry children hovered over the preparations as the three older women busied themselves in the kitchen. The eldest was the matriarch of the family and presided at all holiday gatherings with ease, directing the flow of steaming dishes from the kitchen to the table, which was always perfectly set with her finest linens, wedding china, and fresh flowers.

Nodding approval at the table and pausing long enough to straighten the crystal gravy boat on its tray, she wiped her hands on her crisp white apron before giving her gangly granddaughter a warm hug. Charlotte, affectionately called Char by her family and elementary school classmates, responded with a quick smile full of braces and offered to take drink orders with the help of her younger brother.

Untying her apron and placing it in the laundry room, the vibrant grandmother smoothed her linen dress with her hands before glancing in the hallway mirror to check the hemline for signs of a lace slip peeking out. After tidying her hair and applying lipstick, the slender brunette walked into the living room where her husband and two sons-in-law were setting up the 8mm movie projector and portable screen in anticipation of family movie night. The screen was not being cooperative, and her newest son-in-law, Thomas Babstock, wrestled with it for a few moments before triumphantly convincing it to stand upright on three spindly legs. Holding her hands gracefully in front of her, she watched the men with great pride and then, smiling warmly, announced that dinner was ready.

The candles were lighted by Charles, the youngest member of the family, an inquisitive boy with freckles and a strong resemblance to his grandfather after whom he was named. The golden brown turkey was ceremoniously brought in to a round of applause on a white platter surrounded by roasted carrots and potatoes. Heads bowed and the elder Charles seated at the head of the table offered thanks for another Christmas where all were safe, healthy and happy. The couple's younger son-in-law, Matthew Butler, a master wrought iron craftsman, was elected to carve the turkey, and rose from the table to take the prized bird back into the kitchen. Matt was tall and muscular and used to working with his hands, which were large enough to pick up the heavily laden platter in one hand. With Grandmother proudly overseeing the feast, the rest of the family set about passing the dishes of sweet potatoes, green beans, stuffing, ambrosia salad and dinner rolls.

Imogene Adams was happiest when organizing gatherings, which she planned weeks in advance before finally orchestrating the details. A gracious hostess, she taught the finer points of etiquette by example, and Amanda Allison, her eldest daughter, and Louisa, two and a half years younger, were eager students with families and homes of their own.

Christmas dinner was traditionally followed by a viewing of home movies where her husband acted as cinematographer extraordinaire, painstakingly threading the old movie projector with reels and reels of black and white 8mm films starring two little girls primly showing off their perfect Easter finery, offset by squabbles over bicycles as they learned to ride without training wheels. Snuggled down in the huge sofa, on the floor, and draped over easy chairs in the living room, aided by bowls of popcorn and trail mix, three generations laughed at the fashions and hair styles from twenty years ago, recalled the Oklahoma camping trip spoiled by a thunder and lightning storm, and relived the trip to New York City where they got lost on the Henry Hudson Parkway. The next few reels gave the history of the girls' teenage years as the scenes clicked through Girl Scout outings, family fishing and canoeing trips, and the churning of homemade peppermint ice cream in the kitchen sink. The show continued with each of the daughters' weddings and the birth of two grandchildren, at which point the film magically turned to color. The jerky movements of the film and familiar click-click-whirr of the old projector created a feeling of tradition and belonging which provided a place of intimacy for the eight individuals gathered together in the cozy living room.

After the leftovers were put away, and the dishes cleaned and placed in the racks to dry, Grandmother joined the moviegoers and allowed herself to sink back in an armchair to enjoy the laughter and chatter of her family 'round about.   With her granddaughter seated at her feet and Amanda Allison's hand resting on her arm, Imogene was happier than anytime she could remember.   She looked around at the family pictures lavishly displayed on the walls and the end tables, serenely recalling many such happy times.   This was her finest hour, relaxing in the afterglow of a family dinner in the warmth of the home that she and Charles had lovingly created.   Little did anyone in the room that night foresee that in a few years she would not remember any of them at all.

Chapter 1

"*A*llison, growing old is a gift," her soft voice floated across the table, and even in the midst of the crowded and noisy sandwich shop, the quiet intensity of her words struck me in a place I had not ventured to go before.

As one facing that time in my own life when I, too, would be "old" - or at least by the definition of my niece and nephew – the thought of growing into oldness had an all too poignant meaning. Growing toward one's end seemed like an oxymoron and caused my heart to ache, not just for myself as I pondered what I had done with the last five decades of my life, but rather for my mother who faced growing old with dementia. Her journey would be a struggle for both of us as we rediscovered and redefined our relationship, one that had never been an easy path to begin with.

"Well, growing old beats the alternative," I lamely replied, and Nora and I laughed short little laughs that I had hoped would change the subject.

Nora, the dear friend that she was, however, would not let me be sidetracked and kept coming back with the voice of someone who had traveled down the same path which Mother and I now reluctantly walked. Nora and I had met for dinner to talk about her experiences and thoughts after the passing of her own mother in the hope that she could guide me through the myriad of emotions and difficulties that dementia doles out to the adult child of a parent who is fading away. At first I felt guilty asking her to relive the pain of those last years, when surely all she wanted was to turn off those difficult images. However, true to her helping nature, Nora willingly took on the role of guide and comforter and readily agreed to meet for dinner on a regular basis.

Mother had just been diagnosed with the early stages of

dementia a few weeks before, and I had already begun poring over information online in search of clues as to why her memories were leaving her and why this loving and devoted parent had suddenly turned on me with such animosity and suspicion. My ordinarily warm and supportive parent had changed into someone that, if she had not been my mother, I would have avoided on the sidewalk or in the grocery store. Her sparkling and loving personality had simply vanished. I suppose that if we had lived in the same town as she, my sister Louisa and I would have noticed the changes, but in our phone conversations across the miles, we had only detected that she was easily irritated and very forgetful – something neither of us mentioned, chalking it up to just growing old.

"Mom is not just growing old," I suddenly said to Nora with a new realization of my mother's metamorphosis.

I stopped spreading butter on my roll, and putting down the knife, tearfully looked my friend in the eyes and slowly repeated, "Mom is not just growing old. This illness has completely taken hold of her and reversed time. She does things a child might do. We took her on a dinner cruise one night last fall when she came to visit us here in Upstate New York and she took her shoes off and put them on top of the table."

I continued excitedly, "When the waiter came over to refill our water glasses, he found her shoes sitting on the white tablecloth right next to the bread basket."

Nora smiled, recalling a time when her mother had done similar things. She patted my arm and assured me that Mother's actions made her "normal." She was behaving exactly as a dementia patient is expected to behave.

"Well, I suppose it's nice to know that Mom is normal," I chirped and we laughed, this time with the balm of real laughter.

Our conversations became dotted with laughter after that. In the face of simply not being able to comprehend the quirkiness, if you will, of dementia, Nora and I found the healing powers of laughter. In confronting memory loss head on, not allowing it to overwhelm us, and laughing at the all too infrequent opportunities for lightness, we found a way to disengage ourselves from the heartbreaking reality of watching an elderly parent grow away from us.

Nora and I had much in common; the one whose mother had already journeyed this way and had obtained the end, and the other whose mother had just stepped onto the pathway. Only two such people who understood the cavernous depth of the experience could know the value of laughter.

"Growing old is a gift," Nora reiterated, "but not one that we always know what to do with."

It was my turn to respond, and I confessed quite unwillingly that I had done a poor job of accepting my mother's illness and had, perhaps, even made it worse for her in my initial misunderstanding of the disease. There is a common misconception, and I, too, had fallen prey to the idea that dementia only affects one's ability to remember. Dementia touches all parts of a person's life. As Mother and I moved along this path with great uncertainty, I was quickly learning that the disease attacks not only the individual's short and long-term memory, but also their ability to use good judgment, to follow conversations, to read a newspaper article and comprehend it, and eventually even how to hold a spoon or how to swallow. All inhibitions are stripped away, leaving the individual with a diminished sense of right and wrong. One's cognitive abilities, social functionality, financial management, language skills, personality, and physical capabilities are all compromised the shrinking and misfiring of the brain.

"How do we deal with that kind of reality? How is growing old a good thing when faced with this kind of prognosis? Where is God's benevolence in this?" I asked.

I lost interest in my salad and did not really expect my friend to answer the somewhat rhetorical question, hoping my outburst was not noticed by others enjoying their meals around us. Nora sensed my anger - my anger with God, my anger with my mother, and my anger with a disease that I wanted so desperately to understand and to control, if not to completely remove from our lives.

My anger was, in fact, the beginning of the entire family's journey. My sister and I had each wondered for some time the reasons behind Mother's forgetfulness and had been reluctant to mention it to one another until a few days before Christmas when she could not remember where she had spent Thanksgiving. Those kinds of things you don't forget easily - not in a family that ritualistically alternated holidays between the homes of family members. My sister warned me that I would notice a profound difference in Mother's memory when they all flew up from Texas to spend Christmas with Tom and me in Upstate New York.

True to Louisa's prediction, over the first few days that my family was with us for the holiday, it quickly became evident that alarming changes had occurred in Mother since last I saw her. Ordinarily eager to jump in and help with the cooking, she sat motionless in a chair and watched us from behind dull eyes and a furrowed brow. Usually easy to talk to and quick to ask about our hobbies and interests, her words centered exclusively on herself, taking strange turns between fact and fantasy and containing coarse language that surprised us all. Her suitcase, usually meticulously organized, was in complete disarray, and her clothing was rumpled and mismatched. Medication bottles and loose pills littered her room. She was easily disoriented in the house, repeatedly opening the coat closet door in search of the bathroom. Mother was not the woman I remembered as the warm and gracious head of our family.

One morning at breakfast, she ceremoniously plopped several prescription bottles and a pill sorter onto the table in front of us, as if to impress upon us the fact that she methodically took her medications at precise hours every day. This had been a common display on her part, and we always smiled about it - but this time I noticed that many of the compartments were missing pills, while other compartments had duplications. After we finished breakfast and the dishes were cleared, she was still sitting alone at the table pushing the pill sorter around in front of her. I paused from washing the dishes and sat down next to her to visit and to ask her about the various medications. My intentions were to find out why a woman known for her meticulous manner of doing things would have such an unusual jumble of medications in front of her.

While Mother may be known for her organizational skills, I am not known for my ability to cover my intentions or to show much patience. Perhaps it is in my tone of voice or poorly chosen words that she has always been able to tell when I am about to question her actions; and in response to my offensive approach, no matter how well-intentioned, Mother immediately goes into defensive overdrive.   Our exchange at the breakfast table that morning proved to be no exception, and, what I thought was an innocent and simple inquiry, was met with hostility. She could not tell me why there were three blue pills in Monday's breakfast slot and none in Tuesday's, or why last night's compartment was still full of pills. The names and purposes of many of her medications had completely escaped her.

Learning that she was unable to recall what medications she had taken a few minutes prior, I launched into what I hoped was a gently-delivered reminder of the dangers of overdosing and mismanaging medications.   As I should have predicted, Mother's natural defense mechanism kicked into overdrive, and after several minutes of garbled explanations that she had already told me twice in the same conversation, she could go no further with her confused thoughts and suddenly blurted out, "You are a dictatorial daughter!"

My eyes stung and my heart burned as I grabbed several of the many sleeping pills out of her hands and forcefully threw them in the trashcan a few yards away with an accuracy that impressed my teenage nephew Charlie.

"...and you are a stubborn old woman who doesn't listen," was my parting retort, and I left the room with the rest of the family as incredulous witnesses to both of our outbursts.

Mother found her way back to bed, and I sought refuge at the computer. I had no idea what had come over my mother to make her turn on me with such vicious words, and I was equally ashamed that my patience with her had run its course and had turned into anger.

A caregiver I am not. Perhaps it is God's blessing to me that I was never able to have children, because the gifts of loving kindness and patience fall second to those of organizing and directing. Mother was right in some sense – I love to formulate and direct a plan of action. My forte is diagnosing a problem, researching solutions, and then executing the steps toward a conclusion. I am a person of great focus and am driven to direct and orchestrate multiple projects - valuable skills in the corporate world, but ineffectual in a world where cognition, emotions, and memories are fading - for this is the world of an Alzheimer's patient.

Nora listened intently to my dismay at Mother's inability to comprehend the danger in taking triple doses of blood pressure pills in one day and none for the next two days.

"Why can't she understand and accept that she isn't able to safely handle her medications anymore?" I asked.

My voice was full of frustration. Knowing all too well the futility of trying to reason with a person in the depths of Alzheimer's, Nora assured me that her mother, too, had lost the ability to follow simple and logical thought processes.

"You can't reason with her. If she says the sky is green, it is best to go with it. Nothing will convince her otherwise," she said firmly.

"There is such a huge difference, though, in harmlessly agreeing that the sky is green compared to applauding her for taking three kinds of sleeping aids," I protested.

"Sadly, she is not capable of understanding that logic. Her mind is working on the level of a child," Nora gently told me.

Her words struck me hard, and I realized for the first time that I was becoming the parent, and my parent was becoming the child - something I had read about and witnessed in others, but unrealistically thought my family would be immune to such a dark reality.

The Christmas holiday wore on in slow motion. Mother spent most of the time in bed claiming that she was too weak to join us for meals or family games. One afternoon when everyone else had gone to the movies, I went into her bedroom with the offer of refreshment, and she startled me by asking if the young man in the hallway had left yet. I quickly turned to look and was relieved to see an empty hallway. Yet, she insisted there was a stranger standing in my house leering at her... and it was then that I knew my mother was, indeed, seriously ill. As I spent the next few hours sitting on the bed next to her, my anger and impatience melted away. Lying there motionless between the bed sheets she seemed so small and vulnerable.

Over the course of that afternoon there were brief moments when we really connected. She apologized for calling me dictatorial, and I in turn admitted that I had become impatient. For a few precious hours we talked intimately about mother-daughter things, interspersed with periods when she traveled into some unknown world full of hallucinations and wild stories of worms living in her dishwasher and a man trying to break in through her back door. She had no realization that she was living in two different worlds, as they were both equally real to her. My frustration with a stubborn and eccentric old woman began to evolve into compassion, an emotion I did not know I possessed.

Mother emerged from her bedroom on Christmas morning for the exchange of gifts, but lost interest in family activities soon afterward and retreated back to her bed leaving the rest of us to prepare dinner. This was a relief in some ways, as she was not known for her cooking abilities. We were glad we did not have to keep shooing her around the kitchen from station to station before finally assigning her napkin-folding duties. For several of the last holiday meals it had hurt her feelings greatly when none of us embraced her request to make a dish for the festivities. We prayed she never discovered how we really felt about her watered-down soups, steaks as tough as shoe leather, and mysterious gelatinous concoctions passed off as dessert. In order to avoid a dinner of turkey franks and watery potato soup, the arrival time for a visit to our parents' house was always crucial, and we carefully calculated the driving time to reach their front door well after mealtime.

In Mother's defense, she worked miracles in sticking to a very tight budget as Louisa and I were growing up, and her frugal efforts to substitute less costly ingredients in order to put a meal on the table served us well through tough economic times. We never lacked for something to eat, albeit it fat-free, sugar-free, and taste-free, in keeping with my father's efforts to lose weight and control his cholesterol. Dad's weight and health issues were always foremost in his wife's mind. She was a devoted student of low-fat and heart healthy cookbooks and most likely was to be thanked for Dad's success in fighting heart disease until well into his seventies.

Mother's devotion to our father was deeply rooted not only in her love for him, but also in her strong belief that the man is the head of the household and a wife's duty is to maintain a well-run household. We never doubted that they loved each other fervently, and I can only recall one time that they ever fought in our presence

– a heated discussion over the inequity of time spent with the two sides of the family at Christmas.

"What is it about the holidays that bring out the worst in families?" I asked.

I was not sure that Nora concurred with the sentiment behind my question. I had met her daughter and granddaughter, and there could not have been two more cheerful people on Earth. It was doubtful that Nora's family ever had many cross words for each other, and I wondered if she understood the aching and longing I felt for a peaceful, if not joyful holiday with my family.

On Christmas evening all seven of us sat down to a candlelight dinner of maple ham, spiced apples, sweet potato casserole, and homemade rolls. Mother had surprised us by getting out of bed, dressing, and ceremoniously joining us in the dining room. We all relaxed into the familiar customs of enjoying Christmas dinner together - until Mother declared the ham too rich and spent the rest of the meal eating only French onion dip. The sweet moments the two of us had shared the day before quickly dissolved, and it would be many months before my mother embraced me again with kind words.

That night she began throwing up, and for the next three days refused to eat anything, not even French onion dip. She became so weak I had to lift her on and off the toilet.

"Nothing we tried perked her up or enticed her to eat. She stayed in the darkness of the bedroom while most of the family went to church, played cards and dominos, and went out to eat. Those used to be things she wouldn't have missed for anything," I said emphatically.

Nora responded, "Avoidance of social gatherings is part of the mystery of Alzheimer's behavior. They just aren't interested in being a part of activities any longer. My mother just simply stopped going out. That is very common. More interaction and stimulation is what they actually need, but more and more they become loners. It's a sad paradox."

I thought back over my mother's life in the preceding months. She no longer participated in water aerobics, had withdrawn from leadership of the church travel group, and had not attended worship services, gone to the theater, or taken in a single symphony concert this season. My brow furrowed as I realized that Mother had, in fact, become a social hermit without any of us realizing it. I wondered what she did with herself all day alone in her cottage.

My father had passed away eight years before, and two years later she made the decision to move into a cottage in a progressive care community for seniors called Waverly Place. Louisa and I were grateful that Mother had made this decision on her own, although navigating the sale of the house by herself had proven to be a strain on everyone. Adamantly refusing to seek guidance from her children, who had bought and sold numerous houses between them, she prematurely cashed in several investment funds to make the down payment at Waverly Place, a mistake from which she never financially recovered.

Mother was very protective of her financial affairs. She prided herself on her lists of accounts. On the rare occasions when she allowed me to see her checkbook ledger, the checks were all neatly recorded, but that is where her skills ended – no balances, no deposits, no reconciliation marks – just a list of checks. Her questions regarding investment planning were superficial and only addressed which institutions had the highest interest rates and how quickly she could get to her money. She had no understanding of market variables or risk, and any mathematical equations involving more than simple addition or subtraction were simply lost on her. All attempts on the part of her family to offer guidance resulted in the entrenched belief that, "You are just trying to steal my money." My warnings against less-than scrupulous brokers went unheeded, and she subsequently lost many tens of thousands of dollars simply because of her fear of admitting that she needed counsel.

"Her scorn and fear of me is just dumbfounding, Nora. She not only refuses to listen, but will deliberately do the opposite out of the mistaken belief that I am trying to trick her…," I said tearfully, shaking my head.

My words faded away as Nora reached out for my arm and said, "That isn't your mother. That is the disease."

My first realizations that Alzheimer's robs one of a loved one, even while they are yet alive, left me in a state of prolonged sadness. It was time to say goodbye to the kind and loving mother of my youth. The face full of smiles and the beautiful words of praise and encouragement which had often crossed her lips were replaced by cold unfamiliar eyes, a constant frown, and harsh words of rebuff to my every word. Nothing I could say pleased her. Everything was mistaken as a threat.

Sadly, her world was also shrinking, and she was no longer able to visualize life outside of her little town of San Angelo. Just a short time before we had shared stories about our world travels, talked intimately about our lives, and delighted in each other's hobbies interests. Topics of conversation had dwindled down to the weather forecast for the dry, hot prairies of West Texas, a place as barren as our conversations.

The occasional accounting of events which Mother did tell nowadays caught me quite by surprise. Once full of joyful family stories, weddings and births, her accounts were now full of strange events and unknown persons, all of which I knew were far from factual. Mother's life stories had become fairy tales and products of her own imaginings.

"She just makes things up, and the stories are always something dark and horrible," I told Nora.

I just could not understand why Mother repeatedly told me about murders in her back yard, about gangs of teenagers roaming her neighborhood, or about a suspect plotting to bomb the sports stadium near her house. The bomb plot story was in response to my account of Tom and me watching a baseball game in the corporate suite at the new stadium across the river.

"I have better things to do than watch baseball," she scornfully retorted when my recounting of the team's new pitching phenom failed to draw any interest from her. Nothing seemed to draw a positive response. Over the course of several months, I had tried many different topics in which to engage her; topics that at one time would have spurred an animated exchange, but instead, now drew comments like "he's a jackass" and "you're full of crap." I was bewildered at her use of language that no one in our family had ever used before.

Louisa claims that Mother never tells her these stories, but I suspect that my sister does not really listen. She naively filters out the many indicators pointing toward Mother's failing mind. I applaud her for her ability to see the positive in any situation and love her dearly for continually lifting the flagging spirit, but Louisa's encouraging words and optimistic attitude about life can be both refreshing and infuriating at the same time. The fact that Mother repeats the same stories of fantasy over and over does not daunt my sister, and until disproven, she believes all tales woven by our mother, no matter how unusual or outlandish they may be.

"These events that your mother tells you about are now her reality," Nora pointed out. "What she can't remember precisely, she fills in with snippets of news stories or things a neighbor may have recently told her. Her mind puts together whatever things it can find in its shrinking memory bank.

I wondered to myself, *"Why in the world does Mom feel the need to tell me these terrible stories?"*

As if reading my mind, Nora put down her sandwich and continued, "Maybe she is trying to impress you. Mothers always have the desire to be needed. She may be feeling the loss of her identity as your parent as much as you are grieving the loss of her mothering. Making up or weaving stories together to impress you may be her way of trying to regain her status as the parent who is looked up to by her daughter. She still wants to be important to you."

Nora's comments suddenly rang true in my head, and I was overwhelmed again with feelings of compassion. In spite of her struggle to function in a world that she could not quite grasp, Mother still clung to that instinct to love and care for someone else. I had deprived her of that role through my own self-centered need to be justified by her. I sought her words of praise and signs of interest in my life, while she was desperately trying to regain her footing as my mother, the one who had given me birth and raised me into adulthood.

We both desired the same thing – to be justified in each other's sight. She needed me to ask her opinion on a topic, to value her contributions to a conversation, to acknowledge her life as meaningful; while I wanted her to give me some little word that she was proud of me, that she was pleased at the things I had accomplished in my life, and that she loved me.

The shift in her personality was actually first pointed out by

Louisa, who uncharacteristically acknowledged that a change was taking place in Mother. Usually the undying singer of praise, Louisa surprised me with the observation, "Mom only talks about herself now." Perhaps, my sister was beginning to feel the lack of affirmation as keenly as I was. It was as if Mother's personality had faded, and she was not capable of digging herself out of the darkness and emerging back into the sunlight of what used to be a life full of joyful activity. Her days were now spent in front of the television with its never-ceasing drone of bad news, illicit soap operas, and horrific weather reports. "Horrible" had become one of her favorite words. My niece Charlotte laughingly pointed out that there always seemed to be a "horrible, horrible dust storm" in Grandmother's life, a comment which had more truth than she realized.

A knowing smile had come across Nora's face in one of our soup and sandwich conversations as she told me about her mother's struggle to identify with an ever-shrinking world and to discern fact from fantasy. Mommie was often convinced that the reports of hurricanes in the Atlantic were happening right there at her retirement home located far away in the desert. Terrified of the danger, she would tell Nora about the rising water and the flooded businesses along Main Street, even though the town had not seen a tropical storm cross its city limits since the mid 1920's. After many harrowing nights fighting hurricanes, hail, and tornados located hundreds of miles away, Nora and her twin sister finally activated parental controls on their mother's television, and she soon settled into a happy routine of watching cartoons, the only shows which put a smile on her troubled face.

Louisa and I had chuckled together over the same idea. Putting parental controls on Mother's television actually sounded like a good idea. Prompted by reports of a prowler on the opposite side of town, Mother pressed her emergency button and reported to the security guard of her gated community that a man was peering in the window at her and another was trying to break through her back door. Such a powerful fear overcame her that she broke the deadbolt on the back door in an effort to secure it from the imagined intruder. Whether flamed by news reports of crimes in town or created in the mind of someone prone to hallucinations, the television was a constant source of difficulty for Mother.

The entrance of a television into our parent's house had actually been a huge shock to all of us when Dad passed away and a small television set suddenly appeared in Mother's den. It should not have surprised us that she wanted companionship and the sound of another human voice, even in the form of a "boob tube," another term we had never heard her use before. She quickly became addicted to tabloid news and soap operas.

Our family had never owned a television, except for one week in November of 1963. How well I recall the presence of my grandmother's television set in our living room. We had Nana's set on loan while her house was being remodeled. I was looking forward to coming home after school and watching cartoons or *"Andy of Mayberry"* and *"Lassie."* To my dismay, however, President Kennedy was assassinated that very day, and my visions of Daffy Duck and Mickey Mouse turned into a front row seat for the rolling caissons of a presidential funeral parade. The television went back to my grandmother's after that dismal week was ended, and we never saw another set in its place – until after my father died thirty-seven years later.

"Nora, last night Mom told me her set was broken, that she could only get four channels, and she did not like to watch television any more. She said the television made her 'hear voices in her head.' So, Mom disconnected the set from the wall and tried to take it out to the curb for trash pickup the next morning."

We giggled at the image of my elderly mother wrestling a bulky piece of electronics out to the street. She got no further than the dining room and decided to put it back for her teenage grandson Charlie to carry out the next time he was there. It suddenly hit me how frightening Mother's world had become if she was mistaking television actors as real people in her living room. Maybe throwing out the set was not such a bad idea after all. Louisa naively disagreed and convinced her that perhaps the difficulty was not the set, but that she didn't know how to work the remote. At first Mother rebuffed her for insinuating that she did not know how to operate the control, but my sister recalled that our mother's typical technique for using the remote was to point it at the ceiling and punch any number of buttons until the screen either finally glowed with life or remained stubbornly dark. After many distressed phone calls between the two of them, Louisa finally convinced her to keep the television and wait for Charlie's next visit to reprogram the remote and attempt to teach her how to use it - again.

Having become a television junkie herself, my sister contends that we grew up like everyone else and led very normal lives. I shake my head in disagreement. Everyone on the block, except us, had a television. Growing up without this modern marvel taking up a large portion of the living room was considered backwards. Never-the-less, Louisa becomes indignant when I mention that its absence was but one indication of how different our lives were from other children. She is the one blessed with an overly optimistic rose-colored view of the world, while I was given the more realistic, slightly bluer view of things.

If normalcy is defined as learning to play the piano, joining the Girl Scouts, and playing on the Slip-n-Slide, then we did, indeed, grow up as any average American girl in the 1950's. But, if one considers that we didn't have a television in our home, rarely read a newspaper, never owned a poodle skirt, and could not carry on a conversation beyond what piano piece we were learning to play, then life was simple for us, shielded from the events of the outside world. We were protected from the worldliness of violence, political issues, social happenings, and harsh language. Sex was a forbidden topic of conversation, music was limited to the easy listening choices of our parents, and phone calls were monitored. Alcohol was not allowed in our house, and our parents only attended the occasional church or Boy Scout social function, the organization for which my father worked. Mother set dinner on the table promptly at six o'clock every evening, and we all sat down to grace, identical plates of salad and meatloaf, and small talk about our respective days.

My first day in a college dorm was my own personal emancipation day, and I was more than ready to learn about the rest of the world and what I had missed in the first seventeen years of my life. My mother later told me that she was hurt when I seemed so happy to be going off to college and leaving her protective arms behind. Now, thinking back on it, my mother may have been a little jealous of her eldest child venturing so far from home to pursue a college degree. I suppose I should have cried a bit to convince her that I would miss our quiet little life together, but from that day on I was all too happy to be free of our *"Father Knows Best"* meets *"Leave it to Beaver"* home, although I had never seen a single episode of either show.

In retrospect, my mother had created what in her mind was the perfect home, and in many ways it was. On a very small budget, she and my father had purchased a house and a car, raised two girls, and put us through college. I was the first of twelve cousins to go to college. Two years behind me, my sister was the second. We never had much money – the monthly fifteen-cent hamburger day was a big event. Mother made most of our clothes herself and cut our hair using a ruler across our foreheads as a guide for the bangs. I learned to swim in the portable pool in our backyard, and my parents rented a piano so I could learn to play. We went on family vacations, hauling our aluminum tent trailer behind us, taking in sights stretching from the east coast to the west. No fancy restaurants on the road – just pimento loaf, or when spared that dubious delicacy, bologna sandwiches fresh out of the cooler under Mother's feet in the front floorboard of the car.

She and Dad were both leaders in the church, taught Sunday school and served on various church boards and committees. The four of us faithfully attended worship every Sunday, a practice which I continued through college and into my adult life. It hurt me to hear her now say that she was completely disinterested in church and could not be bothered to get up on Sunday mornings, dress, and drive to services. In retrospect, that should have been one of our first clues that something was terribly wrong.

Mother had also been active with the local genealogical society, as family research had been a passion of hers. Family ties meant everything to her, although after I was ten years old we never lived close to either side of the family again. Dad's career with the Boy Scouts moved us all over the state of Texas. Going to Nacogdoches to visit relatives always involved ten to twelve-hour car rides across the state, and was the venue for the only parental squabble we ever witnessed. The topic – the percentage of time allocated to visit the two different sides of the family. Dad was an only child, but Mother's family of siblings, in-laws and nieces and nephews had grown to over forty relatives. She maintained that it was not fair for Dad to spend two days with his one Adams relative, while she had two days to visit with forty-plus Hickson relatives. I do not recall the outcome of the argument, but the number of days we spent in Nacogdoches remained the same.

Hickson family get-togethers were punctuated by noisy birthday parties and happy outings to each other's houses. I recall spirited board games, piñata parties, and volleyball in my cousin's backyard. We loved the freedom of romping through the woods or picnicking by a pond out in the countryside where the cousins lived. As the self-appointed family genealogist, Mother kept up with every individual's birthday, faithfully sending cards to each niece or nephew on their special day, as well as in celebration of weddings, births, baptisms, and graduations. Mother kept up with them all. Upon the death of her parents, she became grande dame of the family and spearheaded many a Hickson family reunion. She led the relatives in rousing campfire songs, followed by watermelon seed spitting contests and domino tournaments.

In contrast to our many cousins, my sister and I led very protected lives when back in our own home, nurtured by our parents in a quiet atmosphere, much like our father's childhood. Our relationship with Nana Adams and visits to her house in the northern suburbs of Nacogdoches were characterized by a stillness which seemed to communicate that there was an expected and proper way to behave. We were happy there, but activities always followed an unspoken sense of orderliness. My memories of Nana revolved around her huge claw foot bathtub, the birdbath in the backyard, picking sweet peas and pansies from her garden, and the occasional trip to the zoo. My favorite memory is of two Christmas presents which I still have – a china doll and a tiny little rocking chair just right for a three-year-old. Christmas was celebrated around a perfectly decorated tree and presents were systematically distributed to the five of us, unwrapped and carefully examined and approved one at a time before the next family member in the circle could open their presents for all to admire. Nana loved those few precious days that we spent with her every year, and I found pleasure in the beauty around her home and in her company.

I can't say that Mother shared those same feelings of peace when in my grandmother's presence. Nana Adams had apparently made it clear that my mother was not an acceptable choice in a wife for my father. In spite of his mother's strong wishes, though, Dad married the girl of his dreams. After a very short courtship, primarily across the secretarial desk at the First Baptist Church where the slender beauty worked, Dad popped the question on their first date. By his accounting it took her three dates to say yes, and they were married a few months later in the fellowship hall of the church. In photographs, the smile on my father's face was as wide as the corresponding frown on Nana's face. Mother, a shy, uncertain girl when away from the familiar laid-back ways of East Texas, never felt comfortable in her presence and labored under Nana's close supervision to provide her only son with a proper home and well-behaved children.

Looking back, I now realize the heartache my mother felt during the years she spent under the close scrutiny of her overbearing mother-in-law. Mother carried that burden with dignity and never caved in under the pressure of becoming the perfect homemaker and wife. My sister angrily recalls the disfavor Nana dealt our mother with her critical eye and harsh words. She tearfully told me that I reminded Mother of Nana Adams, which had prompted Mother to burst out with the unforgettable and hurtful words, "You are a dictatorial daughter." Mother's uncharacteristic explosion of emotions when trying to explain herself in whatever way made sense to her failing memory must have been agonizing for my mother, for she finally voiced out loud that her eldest daughter reminded her of the one woman in the world that she despised.

"Nora, I simply didn't know what to say. Am I really such a bad person that my own mother despises me?" I choked back sobs and let the full impact wash over me like the tide pounding the shoreline. I had long since lost my appetite and, with a soggy napkin in my hand, I continued to tell my friend about the blow I had been dealt.

That Christmas visit where Mother's feelings erupted to the surface like a bubbling volcano seemed as though it would never end. She was too weak to get on the plane the morning they were to all fly back home to Texas. She had not eaten anything substantial in days and could not get in and out of bed without assistance. Louisa and I made the decision that Mother should stay on with Tom and me until she had regained her strength. The following day I took her to see my primary care physician who gave her something to calm her stomach and kindly encouraged her to eat. She loved the attention he gave her and responded to his gentle ways. I took note of that and tired to emulate his soft and attentive approach, for I suspected that her strange behaviors were due in part to a need for attention.

I worried and doted over my mother the next few days, but saw little progress in her condition. Occasionally, when she smiled and sweetly said thank you, I saw glimpses of her former personality peaking out of the darkness. However, in spite of the lavish attention, the strange behaviors continued. She continued to see "that young man lurking in the hallway" and told me the same dark stories over and over as if I had never heard them before. The biggest battle continued to be over her medications. Mother sorely tried my patience with her reluctance to acknowledge that she needed help taking her medications.

"There is nothing wrong with my memory. I can take my own medications," she angrily declared, gathering up all the loose pills on her bedside table and popping a few in her mouth as if they were candy.

Finally, on the third day, when I had to lift her on and off the toilet and she was still unable to eat and keep anything of substance down, I called my doctor again. He recommended that she be put in the hospital and treated for dehydration, and while she was there to be tested for dementia. I told Mother what he suggested, without mentioning the tests for dementia, and she eagerly found her shoes among the items strewn about her room, and we headed for the emergency room. It was curious how quickly she perked up when a trip to the emergency room was mentioned. In some strange way she always found that exciting and seemed to look upon it as some sort of field trip.

I stayed by her hospital bed as much as my patience would allow. Whatever was wrong with my mother's memory and her declining abilities to function wore heavily on me, for I was not accustomed to hearing the same story repeated three times in the same conversation. Nor was I forgiving of her unexpected criticisms of the "negro in the White House" and the "big fat slob of a man" that my cousin had married. To my dismay, my mother was uttering words that would have earned me a spanking when I was a child. I needed a break from her outbursts and wild stories. I needed to breathe fresh air and was grateful that I had to report to work for at least part of each day.

It was hospital policy that if a family member could not be with a dementia patient around-the-clock, they were to be assigned a sitter to be at their bedside to prevent them from wandering and becoming lost in the labyrinth of corridors. Some weeks later I overheard Mother describe the person quietly reading a book in the corner of her hospital room as an "armed guard who grabbed my wrist and would not let go." No amount of explaining could convince her otherwise, and at times she was certain that she had been strapped to the bed and secretly moved into another room in the middle of the night. Perhaps she mistook the IV and all the leads and wires of the EEG as straps which constrained her movement, and in her dehydrated and demented fog, could not remember the care and concern she received from every person who entered her room.

Each test run on her was done in the gentlest manner and with great respect for her elderly state. An MRI, cognitive skills exams, an EEG, interviews, and lab work all pointed in the same direction. After four days of tests and treatment for dehydration, the neurologist arrived for his final visit and to deliver his diagnosis.

He looked my mother in the eyes and stated very simply, "You have dementia."

He then turned and looked at me and emphasized, "It will only get worse."

The meaning behind his words escaped me, for at the time I knew very little about dementia and its relentless progression through one's life. However, his diagnosis should not have surprised me in the least, for just in the week that she had been with us, I knew something was seriously wrong and that this was not something we could just ignore. A bevy of questions ran through my head.

"*What would this mean for her? How would she adjust and how could we help her? When she went back home alone, what happens then?*"

In her determination to be the perfect mother who did not need to rely on a daughter's assistance, Mother would have none of my offers to help her explore the diagnosis and what it might mean for her future. She refused to talk about her experience in the hospital or the diagnosis that the neurologist had so easily conferred upon her, but instead, she seemed to have gathered up a new resolve to be as cold as stone towards me. She had regained her strength, but still refused to eat very little if anything that I prepared for her, spitting it back out in the kitchen sink. Tom's offer of a bowl of cereal was a big hit, though, and I suppose that should have given me a hint that she was not only angry with me, but was terrified of me, as well.

Hoping to boost her spirits and curry favor once again, I presented her with a new pill organizer to replace the one that was missing four days of the week. She received the gift with an expressionless face, but undaunted, I continued on. We sat together while I reviewed the days of the week and the four slots for her breakfast, noontime, dinnertime, and bedtime pills. The sweetness I had seen in her a few days prior was gone, and she reverted back to a sullen and disinterested attitude. She tossed the organizer on the table and said it was confusing. With only a slight understanding of her diminished ability to learn something new, I begged her to try it again.

"It's very simple, Mom. Here are the days of the week plainly spelled out and the four compartments...," and I held my head in utter disbelief that something as ordinary as the days of the week were beyond her. She felt my frustration, countered with her own chilly silence, and retired early to pack for the flight home.

Her plane was due to leave mid-morning the next day, and as we were heading out the door, she decided that she would need a sweater which was packed in her suitcase. Tom hoisted the suitcase onto the table and we dug into it searching for her sweater. Usually a textbook example of a perfectly packed bag, her suitcase was instead a jumble of toiletries, medications, Christmas presents and undergarments - but no outer clothing.

"Mom, where are your clothes?" I asked.

She didn't know. I raced downstairs after glancing at the clock which showed our travel time to the airport ticking away.

"Allison, you must have been frantic," Nora interjected.

Upon hearing about my frustrations with Mother's lack of travel preparation, a sad little smile had crossed Nora's face as she recalled the last travels her mother was able to make.

"We wouldn't tell Mommie until the day before that she was going somewhere. She stressed out over anything out of her usual routine. We basically packed for her, but let her put the items in the suitcase so that she had a feeling of having done her own packing."

I nodded at my friend, empathetic with the strangeness of watching our parents struggle so with everyday living.

My story continued, "When I got downstairs, Mom's clothes were all still hanging in the open closet."

I yanked them off the hangars and ran back upstairs to look for room in her suitcase.

"Those aren't mine," she said gruffly, and began closing up the suitcase again.

"Mom, how can you not recognize your own clothes? They *are* yours." I yelled at her before shifting into overdrive, yanking Christmas presents out of her suitcase, throwing away more bottles of sleeping pills, and quickly folding clothes to fit back into the rolling bag.

Mother shuffled off into the family room in silence and sat down in tom's easy chair glaring at me. Once again, she took affront to my straightforward no-nonsense way of handling things. The Christmas visit, traditionally a time for celebration and joy, ended with a wall of defiance between us.

Had I known that my sweet mother's unusual behavior was not driven by a desire to defy me, but by an illness which had changed her very persona, I would have dug deeper to find the patience to deal with her actions and attitudes. At that point I had so much to learn, but had probably damaged our relationship beyond reconciliation, as Mother had already reached the stage where reasoning and logical thinking were no longer within her grasp. Much like my departure to college, she boarded the waiting airplane without looking back, and I cried unashamedly on my husband's shoulder in the middle of the concourse until I could no longer see the plane as it taxied down the runway.

My mother had begun a voyage that no one chooses to embark upon, but dementia shows no prejudice in whose lives it resides. Some families confront this challenge head on through family conferences, frank discussions, and by joint planning for the future; while others whisper among themselves, avoid talking about it with their loved one, and attempt to go about their daily lives in the hope that the diagnosis will go away. While I chose a course which sought out knowledge with which to understand the disease, my sister and my mother chose denial, a reaction very common when first realizing that one's memory is slipping away. Mother was intelligent enough in her genealogical research to know that Alzheimer's ran in her family. Although the disease was not readily given a name at the time of her ancestors, we all knew that the failing memory and loss of cognitive abilities in the Hickson lineage was a sign of a demented mind, whether it be Alzheimer's or one of the other myriad forms and causes of memory loss.

"A demented mind – what a terrible term," Louisa had mentioned.

I agreed. Nobody wants to be called demented. In my mother's generation a faltering memory was considered a personal shortcoming, and she referred to her friends that had dementia in the most pitiable terms. She herself, of course, could not have this disease. The fear of being "locked up in the loony bin" where "they only give you two diapers a day" was inconceivable.

We had no real clue where she got the idea that the residents of the two memory support units in Waverly Place were only given two diapers a day, but we suspected that her ninety-year-old neighbor Imelda was the purveyor of many of the misguided ideas she has adopted. Imelda seemed pleasant enough when Louisa and I met her one afternoon at the cottage - until Mother began complaining about her answering machine and the twenty messages that she could not retrieve from it. Imelda commiserated with her and urged her to call the phone company to complain. Mother exclaimed excitedly that she had already called the phone company to register a complaint about the answering machine and that they told her they could not help her, which incensed her even more. The well-meaning neighbor, completely oblivious to the fact that her friend could no longer operate the intricacies of an answering machine, and that phone companies had long since stopped dealing with in-house equipment issues, suggested that Mother not pay the next month's phone bill.

The hair on the back of my neck bristled and I quickly jumped into the conversation by correcting Mother in front of her neighbor - a mistake which certainly did nothing to endear me to her - and reminded her that Louisa had managed to retrieve the one or two messages that were, in fact, on the machine and everything was fine.   I advised her that she should pay her phone bill next month.   Mother rolled her eyes at me and gave Imelda a look which said, "You see what I mean?"

Louisa believed, and probably quite accurately, that the two friends sat and talked about their insidious relatives and how they were plotting to move them into the Big House, where they envisioned the residents sitting in their own filth and staring blankly into antiseptic white walls.   Mother's fears were perpetuated by the sight of the residents at the Waverly Place beauty shop, carrying dolls and repeatedly shouting that no one loved them.

"Mom lives in fear, Nora. Her perceptions of the care levels at Waverly Place are formed in part by a crazy neighbor whom she chooses to believe over her own daughters. She is in constant fear that she will be taken from her little cottage and left in the loony bin. It sounds like some kind of horror show where the residents are treated like inmates, and…" My words had a hollow, empty ring to them because I know I am one of the people of whom my mother is most afraid.

"Paranoia is part of the Alzheimer's footprint," Nora said reassuringly. "They often fear the people they love the most."

"Interesting you should say that, because my sister told me the same thing a few days ago when she was trying to console me. That does not lessen the hurt," I said, gathering up the cups and napkins and heading toward the trashcan, mostly because I had to be busy for fear of having a public meltdown.

Returning to the table a bit calmer, having worked out a small part of my frustration by clearing the table, I continued, "All I did was to see that Mom had medical attention, and suddenly I become her worst enemy. I cannot wrap my mind around the thought that I am no longer welcome in my mother's arms or heart."

Nora could do little to ease my pain, and so we parted with only a promise to talk on the phone in a few days. I focused on gathering as much information as possible on the subject of dementia, and began a search for literature that would explain my mother's strange actions and release her from the repeated nightmares of her relatives marching down the street armed with hoes and broomsticks to take her away. I hoped to read that these symptoms were temporary, that after a change in medication and some rest, she would be back to normal - laughing and participating in social and family activities with her usual fervor. It was not to be. All the material I read indicated that this was permanent...and it would only get worse. Where had I heard those words before?

The neurologist had pinpointed the diagnosis so quickly. No doubt he had seen a familiar pattern in Mother and recognized that she had all the warning signs for Alzheimer's. As we drove out of the hospital parking lot, questions flew around in my mind like a tornado.

"Could Dr. Cohen follow up with further testing if he suggested that she stay on with us for another few weeks? Would he be able to give us clues on how to slow the inevitable... how to live with this new reality?"

Staying here with Tom and me, however, could not have been further from Mother's mind. She was so anxious to leave that it may very well have been impossible to keep her from calling a taxi and taking herself to the airport. She was determined to escape back to her safe little house on the prairie where no one suggested that she was anything but a gentle, sweet widow who wished to live out her days as she pleased, far away from her daughter's meddling. Mother and I were deeply entrenched in a battle between her desire to maintain her independence and my desire for her to remain safe and healthy.

"Which is more important, Nora, her need to live her own life or her need for health and safety? It's sort of like raising a stubborn teenager," I laughed.

It had become our weekly ritual to spend a few minutes in a sort of emotional debriefing, and Nora had been able to slowly draw me out of a constant feeling of foreboding.

"Where do we draw the line between dignity and safety?" I asked.

"What do you mean by safety?" Nora's queried.

Her questions were never meant to make me uncomfortable, but rather to guide me into deeper thought. Perhaps these were some of the same questions she herself had pondered before me. Her mother's passing was still new, but Nora never shed a tear in my presence. She knew the pain of the journey and quietly rejoiced that her mother was now beyond that pain. Nora had a sense of calm and acceptance regarding her mother's death, and I prayed that my family's journey would be as peaceful in the end.

She continued with her line of thought, asking "Is it your mother's mental state of mind, her physical person, or her financial well-being and safety that you are most worried about, or...," and she paused. "...do you have a deeper desire to be in control?"

I squirmed and didn't answer because my first fleeting thought was, *"I can fix this, if Mom will just listen to me."*

I wanted to help Mother overcome this deficit, and I wanted to be the one to diagnose the problem, come up with a plan, and execute the healing. How ridiculously uncaring and mechanical that sounded. She was not some math problem on the chalkboard that needed solving. She was a scared elderly woman who wanted to hear the words "I love you" without any attempts to mold her into the perfect wife and mother.

"Oh, God, I am my grandmother all over again," and the realization sent a bolt of electricity through me. "I have done this to my mother. I have made her feel judged and criticized when all she wants to be is loved."

Although my first response to Mom's passage through the darkness of Alzheimer's had been one of anger and frustration, I suddenly felt great compassion for her – an emotion that I last felt in the quietness of her bedroom on Christmas day.

Compassion takes time to mature, and I am not a patient person. Mother's journey was teaching me how to love with greater understanding, with no strings attached. To deeply and genuinely love another requires the ability to give up one's own interests and desires in favor of the other. Alzheimer's tests the depth of one's love. It measures one's patience and the thickness of one's skin. I had much to learn about myself... and about my mother.

❖

Chapter 2

*M*other's life was beginning a slow journey to the center of her soul, where still resided the desire to be strong. As the outer layers of her sparkling personality grew faint, every thought and sentence became a hard fought battle for recognition and survival. Once my teacher and guide, she now struggled to retain those roles, for the parent had become the child.

"Nora, it feels so, almost unholy, to be grieving for someone while they are still alive. I have glimpses of her old vivaciousness every now and then, and I jump to grab hold of her before she fades off somewhere else again."

We had reunited at the sandwich shop to catch up with the events in each others' lives. Steaming bowls of clam chowder and slices of buttered bread awaited us, as did rejuvenating food for the soul.

"Yesterday she told me about her next door neighbor's Lamborghini," I said with amusement.

"Is that the ninety-year-old neighbor? What is she doing driving a Lamborghini?"

I laughed before answering, "Well, you have to remember that is Mom's description. It could actually be a station wagon. Two sentences later she told me about it all over again, as if she had never mentioned it before. It's like instant replay, word for word."

Nora grinned and shook her perfectly white bobbed hair and said, "Just wait until she forgets what she is talking about in the middle of a sentence. The first part of Mommies' sentences might be about her cat and the second part about the motorcycle going down the street. The next thing you know the motorcycle has climbed a tree. I had the most difficult time acting like she had not said anything out of the ordinary."

"Mom gets extremely agitated and defiant if I confront her on anything, but, I just can't let her go on making mistakes like that," I protested.

Nora quickly interrupted me, "But, you *have* to. She really doesn't know that she has uttered anything odd at all. She is like a preschooler trying to learn to make conversation, except in reverse. Her mind can't get all the facts together to carry through with a complete thought, and she fills in with whatever makes sense in her mind."

Nora concluded by putting her hand on my arm and saying, "It's actually more damaging to reprimand her."

"But, she's wrong," I insisted, laughing at myself over the absurdity of my statement. "I feel compelled to correct her."

Pausing to reflect, I continued more seriously, "It truly bothers me to hear her just out and out lie, and I hesitate to use that term now that you have said she doesn't really know what she is saying. Lying implies that someone willingly tells an untruth to accomplish an end; and in one sense, I believe that Mom wants to impress me – to tell me something important that will make me gasp. She came from a poverty-stricken village buried deep in the piney woods of East Texas, where she had an outhouse and milked a cow - a very hard way of life, and very removed from my own life with its marble bathrooms and six choices of organic milk."

Nora smiled at the comparison, and we took advantage of the break in conversation to concentrate on the dessert menu and then spent the rest of the time together talking about Mother's return home. Louisa and I quickly made the decision to visit her in hopes of helping her recover from her ordeal and to begin dealing with the diagnosis that had changed her life forever.

"I should forewarn you, Mom is really mad at you, Allison," my sister hesitantly told me a few days after Mother had returned home. "She told me about being tied to the bed and guarded by two armed policemen."

"And you believed her?" I asked incredulously. "You know that I would never allow that to happen."

I was quick to point out that Louisa had not been there to witness Mother's odd behavior and had not heard the doctor deliver his diagnosis. She was caught between a mother ranting and raving about mistreatment and a sister who was certain that their mother had Alzheimer's. Louisa felt obligated to be the communication conduit between us. I detected a questioning note in her voice, as if she wasn't sure whom to believe, a pattern which was to repeat itself many times over the coming months. While she remained certain that Mother was indeed ill, she was equally unsure of the right path to take in dealing with her recovery, if that was at all possible. Looking at Mother through rose-colored glasses, my sister was convinced that "whatever-this-is" could be fixed and that we would all soon return to our happy lives as a loving family.

I arrived in Houston two weeks after Christmas to drive Louisa and I to San Angelo for our visit with Mother. We set out along the highway with great optimism, quickly leaving the city skyline behind us, heading west with determination in our hearts. On the six-hour drive across the state we compared notes, separately ticking off items on a mental health checklist before determining that we both had observed the same changes in Mom over the past six months. Like parents discussing their young adolescent's schooling and immunization records, Louisa and I laid out a plan for the next four days – the one of us looking for a way to deal with an uncertain future of lost memories and abilities, and the other seeking ways to disprove it.

We set the wheels in motion by convincing Mother to make a follow-up appointment with her primary care doctor. The struggle to get her to consent to make the appointment was fierce, and we were never really sure up until the moment we walked into the examining room whether she would keep the appointment. Not wishing to embarrass or aggravate her in front of the doctor, Louisa and I had prefaced the appointment with a letter to Dr. Zachariah, detailing the changes and behaviors we had noted in her patient. Our primary goal was to either confirm or dispute the diagnosis and to help her plan for the future. While I was in an information-gathering and action mode, Mother was still very firmly entrenched in a denial mode, while Louisa straddled the line between us.

For those of my mother's generation, dementia was considered to be a personal failure. Those of her friends who had gone down this road before her were always described in the most despairing of terms and became the subject of much tongue wagging. Dementia was not a disease for a proper Southern lady like my mother - as if she had a choice in selecting which geriatric discomforts would strike her.

Not only was there the denial that dementia can strike anyone as early their mid-fifties, Mother did not understand that dementia is an umbrella term describing dozens of memory and cognitive impairing disorders and diseases, Alzheimer's being only one of them. Incorrect administration of medications alone could account for memory problems. Her tendency to overdose and under dose on prescription and over-the-counter drugs might very well have been the cause of her memory lapses, as well as the hallucinations that were becoming more and more frequent. She was not willing, however, to listen to any of these explanations and remained recalcitrant, refusing to discuss the topic. The need to seek medical follow-up was essential.

"I just don't understand her stubborn determination to ignore this, Nora. She usually rushes home from a doctor's appointment to look up whatever diagnosis has been delivered. Dad had this huge drug dictionary, and they pored over it to glean whatever additional facts they could."

Searching for answers was one of my father's strengths. He believed that the constant push for knowledge was a key to success in life, and I admired his thirst to constantly know more. Dad enjoyed filling his mind with interesting tidbits, and it gave him a wide perspective from which to approach life's problems. A diagnosis of such magnitude would have sent him running to the library for information on the disease; its symptoms; the cause; and, finally, the prognosis. He would have prepared himself for the task, fully armed with the emotional tools of how to continue living through every stage. Fortified with a brave spirit, he faced arthritis, leukemia, and congestive heart failure – the final challenge in his well-lived life.

Mother typically conducted her search for facts with a different goal in mind, only wanting to know the symptoms and the prognosis. Then she sprang into action curing the fever, fluffing the pillows, and serving the soup and crackers. Mother only needed to know what she could do with her hands and feet to manage the symptoms and make her patient feel better – but, this time she was the patient.

I reached out to Nora, "That's why it is so surprising that she doesn't want to know the symptoms and the prognosis. She is choosing to remain aloof."

Nora responded with reassuring words, "That is a normal reaction. By ignoring it, she is hoping it will go away. To this point, the symptoms of dementia are more abstract for her, harder to understand and deal with on an emotional level because there are no real physical issues right now that can be easily identified. It isn't like a broken arm. This is not fixable with a splint, and she probably knows that."

I thought about Nora's words as Louisa and I drove along a long stretch of highway. A sense of sadness overcame me as I realized the range of emotions Mother must be feeling as our arrival drew nearer. After Christmas, she had returned to the solitude of her cottage in hopes of leaving behind the words the neurologist had uttered at the foot of her hospital bed; but her daughters would not let it end there. They were coming to put the word "dementia" back in front of her, to force her to acknowledge that she was not of sound mind, to dictate changes…

To put our visit in a more pleasant light and to give mother a reason to look forward to our coming, I offered to sing a concert for her and her friends in the church sanctuary that Louisa and I had grown up in. Mother, herself, loved to sing around the house and would spontaneously burst into a chorus of "Daisy, Daisy, give me your answer true." She had always been supportive of my own interest in music, and she and Dad faithfully attended my college recitals and were proud of my master's degrees in music and education. In years past Mother insisted that I sing for worship services each time I went home for a visit. Louisa was certain that the prospect of hearing a vocal concert especially selected for her would please her. We envisioned Mother sitting front and center, beaming with pride that her daughter wished to honor her with a musical treat while surrounded by her friends. I had contacted the church in advance, secured the church sanctuary for later that week, and invited the pastor, who was also a concert pianist, to accompany me. Pastor Art, whom Mother adored, was thrilled with the idea, and I sent him a packet of music by overnight courier.

Turning to the church for help was a natural choice. Louisa and I had been raised in a Christian home, and while we were not an evangelical family, we chose to follow the example of our parents. We had all been leaders in our respective areas – Louisa and I in the youth activities, Mother in the women's mission group, and Dad in the administrative functioning of the church. Seeking Pastor Art's counsel as our mother faced a difficult time seemed not only right, but essential, and we made an appointment with him for that afternoon prior to arriving at her cottage.

On the way into town we phoned ahead to confirm the appointment, only to find out that the pastor would be unavoidably detained. He had been called away to an emergency with a church member. As we pulled into the church parking lot, we sat in the car contemplating our next step. Should we go on to Mother's house or wait for him to return? The church secretary saw us sitting in the parking lot and came out to talk to us. She tentatively walked toward the car. There was something very hesitant in her approach and she was wringing her hands. After introducing herself, she paused and then took a big breath, as if having made a decision.

"Art is at the hospital with your mother," she almost apologetically exclaimed.

The world stopped and a thousand thoughts rushed through our minds. We were shocked and pressed her for details.

"I didn't really know whether I should tell you or not. I'm sorry, but I don't have any details about why she is there," she said apologetically. "Imogene doesn't want you to know."

We assured her that we understood completely and resisted the urge to rush to the hospital. I closed my eyes to keep the attentive secretary from seeing the tears welling up as she invited us into the church office to wait for Art. I was shaking, in part because of the cold January day, but mostly because of the uncertainties that lay before us.

"Nora, the pastor has known Mother for many years. He was hired by the church shortly before Dad died, and in fact, my father's funeral may have been one of the first he performed at the church. He knows Mom very well. When he finally arrived, he took us into his office to tell us that she would be fine. She had awakened that morning with pain in her neck and shoulder and asked a neighbor to take her to the emergency room. Her muscles were so tight with tension that she could not turn her head."

"She was dreading your visit so much that she went to the emergency room?" Nora was amazed and put down her soup spoon.

"Yes, apparently so. Art thought Mom was anxious about our impending arrival. He called an elder of the church, a woman that she knows, who met them at the emergency room and together they took her back home. We asked him if she would even receive us, and after a moment of contemplation, he thought she would. He couldn't share with us any specifics, but he had noticed a marked change in just the last few months," I explained. "He said he missed her sparkle and enthusiasm."

We learned that Mother had not been attending church for close to three months, something which surprised us greatly; contrary to what she had led us to believe, she had not been deserted by the church. Every Sunday afternoon a church member had called and offered to serve Communion in her home, and according to Pastor Art, she had been receiving these visits and had been held close in the prayers and hearts of the congregation. I wondered momentarily why she had told us the opposite.

Having seen the packet of music on his desk and eager to set up a practice for Friday's concert, I asked Art when it would be convenient for him to rehearse. He slowly took off his glasses, and looking down at his hands, said, "Allison, she doesn't feel up to having you sing for her. I'm sorry. Maybe on your next visit she will change her mind."

For the second time that day, my heart plummeted, but this time it did not rise again. A great sense of sadness overcame me as I realized my mother did not wish to hear my voice. Singing is such a personal expression of myself, and I could think of no other gift that might have broken down the wall between us. As the suspicious and paranoid person she had become, Mother was not emotionally well enough to accept my gift.

"Nora, the refusal to hear me sing placed an ache in my heart that does not go away. I must have said something in reply to him, but I don't remember how the appointment ended. I just felt numb," my voice had dropped to a whisper.

Nora and I sat silently over dessert for a few minutes. She, too, was a member of the church choir. We had not only shared our deepest and most secret thoughts about our mothers, but we had experienced a bond that comes only through blending voices together in song.

"I am so sorry," she said with empathy in every word. She knew the depth of my hurt.

Louisa and I left Art's office bolstered by his last words, "Be gentle with her." Encouraged a bit by his openness, we headed toward Waverly Park where Mother waited for us in fear and pain. Before finding her street, we stopped at the front office to introduce ourselves to the social worker for independent residents. Our purpose was two-fold: to assure that our names and phone numbers were listed in the emergency contacts records, and to seek the social worker's help in executing powers of attorney. Mother had a will and a medical directive, but needed the additional security of indicating her desires for financial and medical decisions made on her behalf.

Louisa and I agreed on the long drive into town that she should be the spokesperson for accomplishing these things because Mother responded so affirmatively to her patient and non-accusatory ways as opposed to my matter-of-fact no-nonsense approach. I was resigned to maintaining a low profile.

"Do you know how hard that was for me to just sit and not be able to put in my two cents worth?" I jokingly asked Nora.

Nora and I laughed easily over the somewhat rhetorical question. We had talked our way through soup, sandwich, and dessert before lingering over coffee and tea.

"I did, though. I let my sister do most of the talking those four awful days, and we made a bit of progress," I was pleased to say.

Deborah Barnes greeted us with a warm smile and handshake as we sat down at her conference table to discuss the situation. Mother was well-known to the administrative offices, having regularly called security, the EMTs, and the staff for a variety of real and imagined issues. Louisa presented our dilemma to Deborah, who, experienced in working with senior adults and their families, immediately understood our objective and the delicacy of the situation. She took the blank documents which I had brought with us, and, placing them in a file, promised to bring them out at the appropriate moment in a pre-arranged meeting with Mother, Louisa, and me.

It bothered me that we were resorting to subterfuge to accomplish this end. However, in the mountains of literature I had read in the two short weeks between the diagnosis and our trip to see her, there were many accounts and bits of advice from professional counselors who all concurred that when dealing with a dementia patient, it is necessary to use whatever means available to accomplish goals for their well-being. This well-documented advice relieved my feeling of guilt only slightly. Somehow such manipulation seemed dishonorable and went against everything I had been taught as the daughter of a Scout Executive.

"Dad would be so distressed to see this happening to Mom," I told Louisa as we headed back to the car for the short drive over to the cottage.

We didn't voice it, but I am sure that we both felt a sense of relief that our father had been spared the heartbreak of seeing his life's love struggling so.

As I guided the car into the short driveway, Louisa did voice another concern, "I wonder if she will even open the door for us."

In our brief meeting with Deborah, the social worker shared with us that Mother had called the security guard that morning with the license plate number and description of the car we were driving. She instructed him not to let her son-in-law through the gate. Deborah assured us that they do not stop relatives from coming in, but she did wonder why Mrs. Adams had mentioned a son-in-law, as she saw no evidence of either of our husbands. This puzzled us, as well, and we all surmised that she was overwrought with worry, so much so that she had apparently called her neighbor to drive her to the emergency room that morning. That was news to Deborah, who immediately made a note in the bulging file, only one of many about Mrs. Adams' self-imposed trips to the emergency room.

We stood on the front porch in hopeful anticipation of the door opening. Louisa rang the bell again and the door finally opened to reveal Mother standing in her flannel pajamas, hair disheveled, and a foam neck brace wrapped securely under her chin. She seemed so forlorn with drooping shoulders and uncertainty on her face. Louisa cried out, "What happened to you?" and threw her arms around her. Mother simply patted my arm without looking me in the eyes, and then turned away to tell Louisa about the pain in her neck. Louisa and I knowingly locked eyes over her shoulder, silently agreeing that we would never mention that we had seen Pastor Art. We made small talk the rest of the day, avoiding any discussion of the elephant in the room, and retired early, exhausted by the events of the day.

By the next day, Mother had enough strength to dress, but still sported the neck brace like a badge. The brace completely swallowed her collarbones and neck and forced her chin upwards at an exaggerated angle. She complained that it was rubbing against her face and chest, and I suggested that perhaps she did not need to wear it any longer.

"Nora, she ignored me and went on fussing with it, complaining the whole time. I think she wanted the attention it afforded her," I said.

The tone in my voice must have told Nora that I was a bit disgusted with my mother's display, and she countered with, "Your mother lives alone without much contact with anyone else. She probably *does* need the attention, and you have to find a way to fill that need in a positive way."

My face turned red. All my years of teaching elementary school, and in particular working with emotionally disturbed children, had taught me that the most basic of human need above that of physical security and contact, is that of acknowledgement. While quick to praise honest achievement and hard work, I did not readily award praise just for the sake of stroking a child's self esteem. Perhaps my viewpoint is a bit hardened, and Nora sensed that I recoiled from heaping what I considered to be unwarranted attention and accolades on my mother.

"You have never had a pet, have you?" Nora observed, trying a different approach to my recalcitrance.

"Well, do fish count?" I replied.

She smiled and her eyes twinkled before continuing.

"A dog will gladly take any amount of attention and love you can give it. They are like sponges when it comes to head pats and belly scratches. The response you get from them is nothing short of joyful."

I smiled at the vision of my sister's two dogs receiving a scratch behind their ears and seeing their tail ends wagging with abandon.

"That is love - unrestrained, freely given, and joyfully received," she said; and I remorsefully knew her words to be true.

I wished that I had heard Nora's eloquent, yet simple explanation before Louisa and I went to San Angelo. It would have helped me view things from the right perspective while tending to Mother that week. While childlike in her craving for attention, and as difficult as it was for me to give it, she was as equally hesitant to receive it from me. Whatever fears held her back, they manifested themselves in strange ways, as we learned during lunch that first day.

Finding refuge from chit-chat that was so difficult to carry on with someone who did not wish to communicate, I took over the daily preparation of meals, not only to free myself from having to visit with my sullen and stone faced mother, but also because I love to cook. Mother had not regained her strength completely from being so dehydrated over Christmas and said she preferred not to cook, and I jumped at the chance to relieve her of that burden. An immediate challenge of preparing a meal in her kitchen presented itself, however, as I searched for a knife. There didn't seem to be one of any kind, even a butter knife, anywhere in Mother's little galley kitchen.

"Mom, where would I find a knife to cut up this chicken?" I called out to her.

"Oh, uh... We've had trouble with one of the maids," she sputtered. "She was stealing things. She has been fired, but she still has my house key, so I hid the knives from her."

"If she still has your house key, then security needs to change your locks," I said, eyebrows raised in a quizzical look.

She made no reply, and puzzled, I went back to trying to cut up the chicken armed with a box of plastic knives I managed to find in the picnic supplies, breaking several in the process. Preparations finally completed, I set the table and served a piping hot chicken-a-la-king over noodles with pear compote for dessert. The three of us sat down at the table, and Louisa, who had not heard the previous exchange, soon jumped up to search for a knife.

"Mom, where are the knives?" she innocently asked, pulling open several drawers in a futile search.

Mother got up and slowly made her way into the kitchen. She whispered something in Louisa's ear. A look of understanding crossed Louisa's face and she replied, "Oh, gotcha," before sitting back down at the table. We started the meal with grace, as was our custom, and then an eerie silence fell over us, until we stumbled on the topic everyone was the most comfortable with – the weather, which had turned as cold as the atmosphere at the table.

When the meal was mercifully over and Louisa and I were alone in the kitchen cleaning up, I quietly asked, "What was that all about with the knives?"

"Mom thinks that you will get angry, so she hid the knives in the trunk of the car..." she whispered back, "along with all of her important documents."

"Nora, I was completely speechless," I said with a tone of utter disbelief. Not only had my mother acted so irrationally out of an imagined fear, but my sister gave her approval and did not come to my defense."

It was difficult to keep my voice down in the crowded restaurant. Nora paused just long enough for me to know that what she was about to say would be difficult for me to hear.

"Your sister is stuck in the middle of the two of you. Stopping to argue the point with your mother about the knives would not have accomplished anything because your mother is not capable of thinking soundly. She is driven purely by emotion, and the emotion foremost in her mind is fear. Louisa knows that between you and your mother, you are now the emotionally whole person, and perhaps she thought that you would be able to handle her taking sides at that moment better than your mother would have."

Nora's admonition stayed with me the rest of the evening and into the morning as I tried to push my ill feelings aside. I began to realize that there was a very real certainty that dementia would not only affect the life of my mother, but could potentially tear my family apart. Nora encouraged me to seek ways to put aside the hurt and to deal with Mother's emotional incapacity with an equal maturity of my own.

"You have to learn to put blinders on your heart, and stay focused on the fact that you love your mother regardless of the blows her illness delivers," she said.

Louisa and I finished the dishes in silence, and I went for a brisk walk while the two of them took naps. My feet took me down several blocks to an open field in front of a gazebo, and I sat down on a bench to contemplate the prior twenty-four hours. Noticing that the view across the grounds took in the high-rise apartment building which housed the dementia unit on the bottom floor, I wondered what it was about that place that gave my mother such fear. The cold January wind blew through the gazebo and I drew my jacket collar up tight around my neck, but it did little to warm my spirits.

In my head I knew that my mother was lonely and craved assurance as a person worthy of her daughter's affection. Mother was a child crying for my attention. I felt remorse for my own insensitivity and sought freedom from my judgmental attitude. As I meditated in the emptiness of the gazebo, the compassionate words of St. Francis crossed my lips.

> *Lord, make me an instrument of your peace…*
> *where there is hatred, let me sow love…*
> *where there is injury, pardon…*
> *where there is doubt, faith…*
> *where there is despair, hope…*
> *where there is darkness, light…*
> *where there is sadness, joy.*
>
> *O Divine Master,*
> *Grant that I may not so much seek to be consoled,*
> *As to console;*
> *To be understood, as to understand;*
> *To be loved, as to love.*
> *For it is in giving that we receive,*

It is in pardoning that we are pardoned,
And it is in dying that we are born to Eternal Life.
Amen.

I hoped that my plaintiff prayer for Mother and me would be heard. As I retraced my steps back down the sidewalk, past the koi pond and the mailboxes, I prayed that my mother would find peace for her troubled mind - and that I would find the maturity to love her more completely... and to forgive my sister.

Upon my return to the cottage some hours later, both were in better moods, and Louisa and I talked Mother into going out for dinner. Helping her organize to leave the house took some time, for going out meant putting on sturdy shoes and warm socks, several layers of clothing that she could peel off depending on the temperature in the restaurant, coat and gloves, wrap-around sunglasses, and a head scarf. I wondered if she had not been experiencing dementia for some time because I recalled as a pre-teen being dressed by her to go outside and play in the snow one winter. The layers of clothing were many and my arms stuck straight out from my sides because of the many layers under my coat.

When I was a rebellious teenager, many mother-daughter arguments centered upon choosing my own level of appropriate clothing, and I rarely left the house without a comment from her about how hot or cold I would be. Mother was adamant that, while I was not going to be a candidate for the best dressed senior at homecoming, I would be warm in the pantsuit she painstakingly made for me.

With the task of dressing completed, Mother negotiated her walker through the back hallway, into the garage, and into the trunk of the car next to the knives which I pretended not to see, and then several minutes later off we drove to her favorite country restaurant that served a "nice fat-free vegetable plate." We enjoyed the distraction of playing tic-tac-toe on the paper tablecloth while waiting for the vegetable medley and mashed succotash to reach our table. In keeping with her duties as a hostess, Mother offered to pay for dinner, and I guided her to the checkout and supervised the selection of a credit card and the completion of the transaction. She left the checkout counter without adding a tip to the bill, and I quietly returned to the table to place a few dollars under the salt shaker. We reached home a bit tired from the outing - Mother and Louisa from the physical exertion of going out and me from the weighty feeling of responsibility that had descended upon my shoulders. The complexities of caring for an individual who did not acknowledge her need for help was a difficult balancing act. I felt much like the parent of a four-year-old who insists on tying her own shoelaces, but then wonders why her shoes won't stay on her feet.

The night was rounded out by watching the evening news, to which Mother made nonsensical political commentary and Louisa chimed in with her opinion of the candidates for governor. I asked them each to explain their viewpoints and neither could do so, not that it really mattered to me as I had not lived in the Lone Star State for over ten years. The conversation that I soon wished I had not started at all ended with Mother telling me to mind my own business. I stopped talking as the weather report thankfully flashed across the screen. After hearing a forecast of more cold and wind, we turned out the lights and all headed for bed. The emotions of the day overcame me, and I cried into my pillow deep tears of grief for the family I felt I was losing.

The next morning brought the warmth of the West Texas sun streaming into the cottage, and I hoped that this day would be better, for this was the day of two vital appointments – one with Deborah to execute the financial and medical powers of attorney and the other with Mother's doctor. We made quick work of our morning routines, and feigning the desire to take a tour of the office complex, I drove the three of us over to the administrative offices. We slowly made our way from the first handicap parking space into the well-appointed office where Mother easily made the introductions. Louisa, Deborah, and I acted as though it was the first time we had met, and the four of us sat down around the conference table to visit.

After the obligatory small talk, Deborah suggested that she get out Mother's file to be sure everything was up to date. Seeing the medical directive in the file gave Louisa the perfect opportunity to ask Mother if she had a financial and medical power of attorney.

Louisa very slowly and simply described the documents, their purpose, and the benefits Mother would derive from designating powers of attorney. Deborah chimed in at the appropriate moment, saying that she thought there were some blank forms in her office and that there was a notary in the office that could witness everything. I sat quietly in my chair, only nodding my head at suitable intervals. After a few questions, Mother assigned Louisa as the first power of attorney and me as the backup. The notary affixed her seal, Deborah made copies, and after thanking her for her assistance, we gathered the documents, and continued with the tour of the front offices.

Louisa and I, not daring to look at the other, each breathed a sigh of relief, having overcome another challenge to seeing Mother smoothly started on her journey.

"Bravo," Nora said. "We did not have to opportunity to do that with Mommie. She was already in a nursing home by the time we realized we had to begin making decisions for her. The only option at that point was a guardianship, which was costly to put into place. You are so fortunate."

I listened with interest while Nora talked about the transition of her mother's medical and financial independence into a guardianship arrangement. While the ease with which Mother agreed to the powers of attorney had surprised me, I was grateful that it was accomplished and we were spared the inconveniences of hiring an attorney and going to court.

Perhaps it was in the formality of designating her proxies that Mother became more assured that we had not come to dislodge her from her cozy cottage and deposit her into a dementia unit, for lunchtime seemed to be a bit more relaxed. She was talkative about her house plants, as well as, that "darned" lawn service that repeatedly skipped over her yard when mowing the lawns.

"I know it's because I reported them for not fixing the sprinkler heads so they don't spray my windows. They're getting back at me by not mowing my lawn," she sputtered repeatedly. We heard the same story several times during the course of lunch, and each time we reacted with dismay at the "unmitigated gall" of the workers.

Lunch consisted of a box of rice pilaf I found tucked away in the back corner of the pantry layered with chunk tuna and cheese, and liberally sprinkled with dried parsley flakes which had expired three years prior. None-the-less, we were all hungry and gave our steaming plates our full attention. Before long, I noticed that Mother was carefully separating out the long grains of brown rice and pushing them off to one side of her plate.

"Mom, you don't care for rice pilaf?"

"Well, Daughter – a term of endearment that she used when emphatically pressing a point with me – we have been having such a problem with these bugs," she said, all the while carefully excommunicating all but the whitest grains of rice to a corner of her plate. "I just don't know how to get rid of them except to use my fork and push them along."

My eyes quickly met Louisa's, imploring her to say something, sure that I would lose control and burst out laughing. The consummate professional in these situations, she mumbled a few words about how good pest control is hard to find these days and went on eating as if Mother had not done anything out of the ordinary.

Unsure whether Mother had forgotten about the looming doctor's appointment, we hurriedly finished clearing the lunch dishes and encouraged her to get ready to go, giving a ten-minute departure time. She shuffled into her bathroom without question - presumably to brush her teeth - and emerged a few minutes later to gather her walker, coat, scarf, gloves, sunglasses, purse, keys, garage door opener, and hospital records; all of which took several minutes to locate and organize, particularly when she repeatedly put them down, forgot where she had placed them and had to search all over again. We let her go through this process for several minutes before stepping in and gently assisting in locating the wayward items.

Finally underway, the car was filled with chatter about Mother's need for a permanent wave and what a slob Cousin Zelda's husband had become. My own husband always thought my family was entertaining, and he would have found the conversation interesting, if not comical.

The receptionist greeted us very cordially before informing Mother that she was several hours early for the appointment and that she was welcome to wait or to come back at the appointed time. Mother was incensed that "they have the time wrong" and grumbled profusely as we all made our way back to the car with coats, scarves and gloves not quite as well organized as when we left the cottage, but with Mother clutching the records packet as if it would suddenly fly out of her hands. We carefully placed our feet to avoid the patches of ice on the parking lot, but moments before reaching the car, we heard a voice from behind and turned to see the receptionist motioning for us to come back in. Mother's doctor of many years had overheard the conversation and kindly decided that she could work Mother into the schedule a few hours early.

The wait was not long, but in keeping with the signage "As a courtesy to others, please turn off your cell phone," we also kept our voices just above a whisper adding to the tension in the room. The magazines invited various comments as we browsed through them, but questions hung in the air.

"Would the doctor see the same things Louisa and I had observed in the past few weeks?   Was she a physician who readily included family in the treatment of her elderly patients, and had she received our letter? Would she even allow us in the examining room?"

Mother's name was called and, gathering up all the winter outerwear that we had shed, the three of us followed the nurse into a very small examining room. By arranging ourselves carefully on the table and two chairs with a slight space for the doctor to perch on her stool, we all fit snugly into the small space like a jigsaw puzzle to wait again, this time in complete silence.   Dr. Gail Zachariah entered the room and easily greeted her patient. She was a pleasant-looking woman in her late fifties with an easy smile, and commanding air about her. She smiled patiently at us as Mother fumbled with the introductions, and it was easy to see why Mother was so endeared to her.

Dr. Gail, as patients referred to her, had looked after not only local residents for many years, but also had a personal interest in serving the medical needs of an indigenous tribe of people who lived on the western plains. Several times a month she traveled into the adjoining state to spend time treating families that still lived in adobe houses built by their ancestors. This charitable heart carried over into her practice at home, but often took her away when

Mother was in need of her gentle touch.

The easy-going doctor started the visit with a simple question, "Tell me what brings you in today," but soon interrupted her patient's first few sentences to ask, "May I discuss your medical treatment with your daughters, since I see they are here to support you today?"

Mrs. Adams quickly answered "Yes, of course" before proceeding with her version of her illness over Christmas. I suspected that she truly would rather have said, "No, Allison must leave," but rather than make a scene, she acquiesced and gave us both equal rights to her medical information.

Louisa did not move in the chair next to me. We both could have won Oscars for the covert role we had just played in getting information to Dr. Zachariah, information that could help pinpoint the cause of Mother's lapses in memory, her strange behavior, and unexplainable personality changes.

"I got sick on Christmas Day," Mother began with a completely lifeless expression. "… and, uh, couldn't stop throwing up. My legs were so weak I couldn't stand and my head was just swimming. My eldest daughter put me in the hospital."

Without looking my way she motioned over in the general vicinity of where Louisa and I were sitting. I wanted to jump in and correct her, *"I did not put you in the hospital. My doctor admitted you."* Mother seemed intent on incriminating me as the cause of her memory problems, and I was equally intent on defending myself. However, rather than making a comment which was sure to start an ugly conversation and only serve to emphasize the widening gulf between us, I held my tongue and pressed my lips together so hard that they turned white.

Dr. Zachariah flipped through the packet of documents which Mother had handed to her, and smiling, said, "You look good now. How are you feeling?"

She replied, "Well…I still feel weak and my head swims. The doctor gave me a prescription for a pain patch."

"No, Mom, it is not a pain patch. It is a medication for your memory," I silently shouted out at her. *"Why can you not accept this?"*

Mother handed the prescription to the doctor who glanced at it and, leaning toward her elderly patient, quietly asked, "Do you recall what the doctor, let's see... his name is Dr. Cohen, a neurologist... told you when you were released from the hospital?"

The furrows in Mother's brow deepened and she sat up very straight on the table before speaking with great indignation, "Nothing. He said I was fine and that my biggest problem was my family."

I froze in my seat. The coat and scarves suddenly became very heavy in my lap - as if the very weight of her words were pulling them down to bury me. Knowing the futility in convincing her otherwise, and realizing that she either could not remember or chose to deny her condition, I said nothing, as did my sister.

The doctor gently continued, "Let's put this aside and I will write you a prescription for a patch which should help you." She didn't say in what way it would help, but I recognized the name of the drug as one used to treat Alzheimer's. The heaviness in my heart lifted a bit as I silently thanked God for giving insight to this woman who seemed to look into my mother's heart and, while knowing the anxiety she must be feeling, gently redirected the pent up anger which Mother had finally unleashed on me. She did not correct Mother's misconception that the prescription was a pain medication.

Treating her patient with dignity and offering nothing but encouragement and understanding, the white-haired doctor continued, "I would like for you to take a little memory test, just to rule out some things."

Perhaps, she hoped that Mother would agree to the test if it was presented as something designed to verify her account of the neurologist's report that her family was her only problem rather than a disease which the elderly feared above all others. Mother jumped at the opportunity to prove the point and quickly agreed to the test.

As the doctor left the room in search of her nurse, Mother turned to me, and with a tone that would have broken stone said, "I bet you're glad that..." She stopped cold.

"Glad about what, Mom?" My tone matched hers in its defensiveness.

"No, I won't say it," she haughtily replied, turning her face away from me and staring at a smudge on the wall.

Tension started to rise as did the volume of my retort, "You obviously have something to say to me about this, so go ahead."

Louisa jumped in with, "This is not the time or place for this," as a nurse entered the room and asked Mother to accompany her.

Glad to be on her way to proving that the only thing out of place with her was her daughter's meddling, she stumped out of the room striking her walker hard against the floor. Louisa and I were left alone in the room.

My sister broke the silence first, "At least we know Dr. Zachariah got our letter. I'm so relieved that she understands."

"Do you think Mom really believes that the neurologist told her that nothing was wrong, or is that a story that she has made up as a defense mechanism?"

"It's possible," Louisa replied. "But, I wasn't there, so I just don't know."

There it was again – that little hint of doubt and questioning in my sister's mind. Suddenly, it hit me that Louisa might, in fact, not believe or be ready to accept the diagnosis. We had made this trip with the specific intention of obtaining a definite diagnostic result from Mother's own doctor, but our end objectives may not have been the same. I was fully convinced that she was in the early stages of Alzheimer's, while Louisa was hoping for a diagnosis far less malignant, such as a medication overdose or a hormone imbalance. We were not at cross purposes, but not exactly on the same page, and there was a palpable awkwardness between us.

Louisa's relationship with our mother was close, and now that Louisa was a mother herself, the two of them enjoyed talking intimately about raising children, a topic I could only observe from the sidelines, not having had children. Mother and Louisa saw each every few months when one or the other would travel to one another's homes. Unlike me, Louisa was quick to lavish praise on her, whether justified or not. Mother fell into a comfortable rhythm of reciprocal sentiments, and the two were like schoolgirls walking arm in arm, sharing secrets and giggling. Louisa was proud of what Mother had accomplished in her life, having lived on her own quite happily and successfully until now. Mother responded to the love and respect Louisa showed her.

Mother and I were more like rivals, vying for each other's attention and approval, for even in the midst of her illness, I valued her opinion of me. Rather than holding me close and whispering how much she loved me, she had fallen into a dark mire of punishing words. The things she said to me now were more likely meant to attack and tear down than to build up. My own desire to be justified in my mother's sight caused me heartache because it seemed that all she was capable of giving me was dismissive criticism.

I was aroused from my troubled thoughts as the door opened and Mother came back into the room declaring with a toss of her head that she passed the test with flying colors. Louisa helped her back up onto the examining table and rejoiced with her over her triumph.

"That's wonderful, Mom. See, I knew you could do it," she exclaimed.

I smiled and waited for the doctor to give an official report before I would allow myself to join in the celebration. Dr. Zachariah came in shortly thereafter and while perched lightly on her stool, she silently read the test results. The room stood still as we waited for her to speak.

"Mrs. Adams, the test shows that you have mild memory impairment," she said, putting down the file. Pausing to take off her glasses and look Mrs. Adams in the eyes with compassion and warmth, she continued. "This is something different from normal aging. Have you had any trouble when driving, remembering where you are going or how to get there?"

Mother sat motionless, arms hanging at her side, staring at the doctor, quite unable to comprehend what she was hearing.

Regaining her speech, she blurted out, "No. I have only gotten lost once on the way back from the airport. I couldn't find the exit from the airport."

Louisa took her arm and assured her that everything was fine, that airports can be very confusing.

"This is San Angelo," I said to myself. *"There are only four gates at the airport and one exit. How hard can it be? Stop defending her and open your eyes, little sister."*

The doctor nodded her head in agreement and continued,

"Yes, it can, but I want you to limit your driving to daytime hours only. I am also recommending that, if you want to remain living alone in your house, that you have a home healthcare aide to help you with things like medications. You don't need to be constantly opening bottles and sorting medications."

Upon hearing these words, my spirits suddenly lifted for the first time in days. Mother was now on a journey that had a name and a plan of care was being written that would help her adjust and cope with fading memories and abilities. This was, indeed, a reason to rejoice and only then did I allow myself to break out into a heartfelt smile.

"I would like to see you back in three months. Do you have any questions for me?"

None of the three of us had any that we were willing to voice at the time, although I wish that we had, for the opportunity for all of us to be present with this kind physician would never come again. We began gathering up the winter wraps as Dr. Zachariah bid us goodbye. I went ahead to warm up the car as Louisa and Mother made their way to the reception desk to check out. A sharp feeling of envy overcame me as I saw the two of them walking arm in arm and chattering away as they approached the desk. How thankful I was, though, that they shared such closeness. With Dad gone, Mother needed someone that she felt safe with; someone she felt she could confide in; someone who loved her unconditionally – a type of love that I was only beginning to understand.

On the drive back to Waverly Place, the warmth of the car was in sharp contrast to the frosty discussion among its occupants. Mother, who had *not* passed the memory test with flying colors, blurted out, "I don't want someone in my house. I want my privacy and I don't need anyone to help me."

"It's just a home healthcare aide who would be there only a few hours every day. She won't get in your way and will be a big help to you," I offered from the driver's seat.

Mother was in the back seat and I could see her face in the rear view mirror, and it was obvious that my words were not received well. She set her jaw and stared unseeingly out the window.

Louisa tried to smooth things over by saying, "You would be her employer and she would do whatever you ask. You would have control and decide what time of day she comes and how long she would stay."

...and then I played the trump card, "This is what you have to do if you want to keep living alone in your cottage."

"I probably should not have said that, Nora, but it was all I could think of that would either convince her or force her to accept help," I bemoaned. "There is only so much we could do because she is still an adult, even though her thinking is more like an elementary student at this point. She looks so confused. Just in those few days we were there, I watched her wander from room to room looking for something, but she could never tell me what was lost. It's so sad. She must know that things aren't right."

"That is probably what scares her the most. She knows the world looks different and unfamiliar, but doesn't know why," observed Nora. "What's more, she doesn't know how to fix it."

The conversation in the car dwindled away until we reached the Waverly Place administrative offices where I pulled into a handicap parking space and put the car into park.

"How about we start by asking Deborah for a list of healthcare agencies that you could contact," I suggested with a spritely expectation in my voice, catching Louisa's eye in the rearview mirror.

She quickly took the cue and offered to go in and ask about such a list. To fill the cavernous silence in the car after Louisa climbed out, I commented on one of Mother's favorite plants in the winter landscape - a pyracantha bush with its bright red berries next to the sidewalk - anything to take her mind out of defensive mode and into a more positive frame of mind. My efforts were to no avail and the car was filled with one-way chatter about the landscaping and the squirrels and how nice the paint color on the buildings looked.

Louisa came back with a piece of paper in her hand about the time I ran out of mindless topics to expound upon and, climbing into the back seat, she excitedly said, "Deborah had the perfect person to suggest and thinks that she might be available for a few hours a week. When we get to your house, Mom, we can call her to come over for an interview, if you want."

She replied with a halfhearted, "Sure," continuing to stare out the window, barely noticing when we backtracked to the pharmacy to fill the prescription for the memory patch. When we reached the cottage, Louisa called the perspective employee to set up the appointment for the next morning, while I set about the task of preparing yet another meal without the aid of a knife. I was becoming quite good at using whatever resources were on hand, including dental floss to slice the brownies and a hacksaw which I found in the garage to cut up the chicken. I was determined not to let Mother see me sweat over her little escapade with the knives, but she had long since retreated into her bedroom and slammed the door shut. Neither Louisa nor I ventured to disturb her and left her alone to consider all that had happened that day.

Dinner that evening consisted of fresh tomato soup and chicken breaded in cornflakes, which Mother raved about, forgetting that she was giving me the cold shoulder. She asked me what was in the soup recipe and we exchanged ideas on the best way to blanch fresh tomatoes. I couldn't remember the amounts of oregano and basil that I had dashed into the simmering chicken broth – was it two shakes of the herb jar or one each - and I stopped eating to give it more thought, grateful that my mother had finally broken the icy silence that she had imposed upon us since leaving Dr. Zachariah's office.

"See," she almost shouted as she pounced on my inability to recall the recipe. "We all forget things now and then. I'm nearly eighty-years-old and I can be expected to forget things now and then."

Mother folded her arms across her chest and smiled triumphantly over at me, and the three of us gathered around the table spontaneously erupted into laughter. For fear of making matters worse by protesting that she did, indeed, have a memory problem beyond that of normal aging, I began to clear the table to make way for brownies a-la-mode. Louisa reached out for both of Mother's hands and repeated the doctor's orders that she should have a helper with her every day. The lightheartedness of the brief few moments before suddenly dissolved and Mother's haughtiness returned.

"I don't think I need someone, and certainly not every day," Mother huffed.

Louisa tried another approach. "It would make Allison and me feel better to know that you were not here alone all day."

"Then *you* can foot the bill for it," she retorted. "I can't afford to pay someone to come in and push me around."

After much cajoling and gentle persuasion on Louisa's part and a silent, but strong presence at the table on my part, Mother became resigned to the fact that the condition for remaining in the cottage was that she hire someone to help her with daily living skills. We went to bed with that idea firmly entrenched in her mind, and she woke up the next morning in a more receptive mood and ready to conduct an interview with the candidate.

I wrote out a list of items that she might want to ask. Mother seemed relieved to have the list, which greatly surprised and pleased me that she would accept this small offering of assistance, and I slowly reviewed each question with her. Arriving right on time, the candidate, Elena Diaz, was a cheerful Latin woman in her late fifties with bright eyes and a quick smile. Shorter than her would-be employer by a good four inches, she immediately put Mother at ease and lavished her full attention on her, while assuring that privacy and confidentiality would always be maintained. Elena treated Mother with respect, and near the conclusion of the interview I noticed that the edginess in Mother's voice and demeanor suddenly relaxed under Elena's soft and encouraging hand.

Mother had made a decision – this petite Latin woman, who always addressed her as Mrs. Adams and said "Yes, Ma'am" and "No, Ma'am," would be her aide. My agenda was that Mother should have assistance every day for the bulk of the morning through lunch time, in order to cover morning and noontime medications, as well as to ensure that she was remembering to eat. The plan was laid out simply and quietly on a paper that I laid on the table before her, but she immediately balked at this idea and, digging in her heels, crossed her arms and shook her head. The scowl on her face and look of anger towards me could not possibly have been more pronounced when Louisa literally stepped between us to take over the negotiations. She slid the paper off the table and handed it to me behind her back before sweetly suggesting that Elena come three days a week for two hours each time, an idea which quickly met with Mother's approval. A time schedule and fees were agreed upon and Mrs. Adams graciously ushered her new home healthcare aide to the door.

The interview between Mother and Elena concluded, Louisa followed Elena out onto the porch in the pretense of saying goodbye, but in fact to exchange phone numbers and to set up weekly calls with updates on how our mother was faring.

"I like her, Mom," I ventured to say as she and I began clearing the tea cups and glasses. "Do you feel better now?"

To my utter surprise, my mother began sobbing and laid her head on my shoulder. I wrapped my arms around her gently, for she seemed so frail at that moment. We held on to each other in a genuine embrace filled with both grief and compassion. She allowed me to console her, and for those few brief moments we were at peace with who we were as two women in need of each other.

The moment was broken as she pulled away when Louisa re-entered the room.

"What's wrong, Mom?" she asked, seeing Mother's weepy face.

"It's just not a good time for me. This is so hard."

Louisa comforted her, saying, "It will get easier."

I flinched at those words, for I knew them to be untrue. Mother's journey was just beginning and it would be many, many months before the path leveled out again.

We pulled the trembling woman into the busy task of helping us rinse and load the dishwasher. We soon discovered that all three of us had very distinct viewpoints on the proper way to load a dishwasher. Louisa had adopted the theory that utensils would become clean only if like utensils were kept separate with only one of each kind per compartment. We kibitzed back and forth about what happened when there were not equal numbers of utensils to equal number of compartments and began giggling over the infinite number of ways a dishwasher could be loaded. Mother broke out of her gloomy mood and began to describe her unique method of loading a dishwasher, to which Louisa and I paid mock attention. She firmly stated that first the utensils had to be scrubbed with a brush, sorted by type, and then placed with the "business end" of the tines, scoops, and blades pointing up – as many as could be stuffed into one compartment. Exaggerating the motions with great flare and sending spurts of soap bubbles everywhere, she sent us into peals of laughter with the animated demonstration, the first truly joyful moments we had shared in some time. Louisa and Mother linked rubber gloved hands together dripping soapy dishwater on the floor and, turning to me, asked how I load my dishwasher.

I was laughing so hard that I could barely speak, and could only manage to say, "I don't remember." Mother immediately reached a soapy glove over on the kitchen counter and, holding up the new box of medication, asked, "Do you want to borrow one of my memory patches?"

There was a slight twinkle in her eye and a softening of her face as she made the effort to come to some uneasy truce between us. That was the closest she ever came to admitting to me that she had dementia.

Not wanting to wait until our next dinner engagement to tell Nora about the hiring of an aide for Mother, I cornered her on the way to choir rehearsal the next Sunday morning.

"I don't really know why that whole interview process bothered me, Nora. Those brief moments depicted a complicated network of relationships between the four of us," I said, disheartened by a victory I viewed as only half achieved. "Six hours out of a one-hundred-sixty-eight hours a week is just a mere gesture toward significant help. Mom does not know how to sort her medications and take them properly. How are six hours going to make a difference?"

Nora directed us into the church library where we settled into the deep musty cushions of two armchairs in the children's section, surrounded by stories about David and Goliath, the great grasshopper plague, and the rainbow in the sky.

"I agree, Allison. It seems like your mother needs more than just a few hours every few days. She is an adult, though, and still has the right to make decisions for herself, even if those decisions seem wrong or misdirected," Nora said while leaning in toward me to emphasize her point. "Loving someone does not mean holding their hand every step of the way. Some of those steps they have to take by themselves."

I paused and smiled a bit before commenting, "It is funny that we are sitting in the children's section of the library. Your metaphor works equally well for the child learning to cross the street alone, for the teenager going out on a first date, and for an elderly parent driving herself to the store. They are all dangerous activities on some level and my first instinct is to protect each of them as much as I can. Why am I being punished for wanting this?"

My question was not to be answered just then, for choir members began passing by the door on their way to rehearsal. We put a temporary hold on the conversation to gather our things before heading up the stairs into the choir room. As the grand piano began the familiar run of notes up and down its length, Nora gave my hand a squeeze and promised to meet me for dinner the next week. As we scurried around the choir room searching for hymnals, folders and sharpened pencils, I felt a fresh assurance that one day all would be well for my mother.

Chapter 3

*L*ouisa and I returned home with one of us fully satisfied that our parent would now be living a safer and happier life and the other of us believing that her issues would not simply drift away, but grow painfully deeper like a foggy night enveloping a shoreline.

I missed my mother none-the-less and continued to reach for her somewhere in that fog. The days passed and my phone calls to her became more difficult until one evening I lost my patience.

"Mom, you have told me that same story now three times in the last ten minutes," I sharply said over the phone.

I was irritated, almost as much with Mother as with myself. My vow to treat her more gently and with respect due her as my mother had lasted only a few weeks. We had ventured into dangerous territory again - although the subject had been presented by Mother, I mistakenly thought that made it a safe topic for discussion. Usually our twice weekly phone calls were rather sparse in nature, but she surprised me this time and said that she had been to visit her insurance agent to make sure her car coverage was up-to-date. A letter from the carrier stating that her coverage might be inadequate had prompted her to call her agent – the same unscrupulous agent who had previously sold her numerous and ill-advised insurance products. Refusing to believe that the generic form letter was anything more than a polite request to pull her into the agent's office, Mother dutifully made an appointment and went to see him.

"I was so appreciative of his attention. He told me about ways I could invest my money and increase my monthly income," she said proudly, not realizing that, as a senior citizen, she may have been targeted as an easy sale.

I slowly and calmly followed up with, "Mr. Fitz is a

salesperson. He does not really care about your well-being, Mom. All he wants to do is sell you something so that he can make a sales commission."

In spite of the gentle delivery, I could almost hear her resolve hardening over the phone as my comments were met with steely silence.

In spite of the warning signs, I continued, "Why do you insist on listening to other people rather than your own family?"

What I really wanted to ask was why she specifically listened to men rather than to her own daughter, but that would have been opening up a whole new battleground which I did not have the energy to pursue at that moment. Louisa and I had often compared notes on Mother's tendency to follow the advice of whatever male figure she last encountered, regardless of the credibility of that individual. Her obsession with authoritative figures based solely on their gender annoyed both Louisa and I. Her generation of women grew up with the *Good Housekeeping* and *Ladies Home Journal* image of the happy housewife dutifully washing, cooking, and ironing to provide a serene home for the working man who made all the major decisions on behalf of the family. Combined with the fact that Mother grew up in a Southern Baptist home that emphasized the man as the head of the household, she had no understanding of the modern couple, each with a career, who equally shared the childrearing and household responsibilities. My father could not boil an egg and my mother could not balance a checkbook. Their two worlds were as far apart as the east and the west, and her perception of the alpha male providing a safe undergirding for her life carried over into all her decisions after my father had passed on.

Purely for the fact that the insurance agent was a male and a very persuasive salesman, she decided to cash in several CDs at her bank and purchase one larger CD through the insurance company, believing that the slightly higher interest rate would gain a higher profit.

"There are penalties for cashing in your CDs which far exceed the tiny amount you will gain from the higher interest rate with Mr. Fitz. This is not a good investment move, Mom," I insisted after consulting my husband for his opinion.

Tom verified my suspicions and calculated that she would suffer a loss of several thousand dollars. "She would lose more money than she would gain in addition to the increased risk of an investment not backed by the FDIC," he advised.

She ignored us both and a few days later visited her bank to complete the transaction.

"Nora, a year ago Mother would have gladly received our advice and thanked us for helping her make a sound financial decision, but that was before her mind became such a tangle," I declared, making no attempt to hide my frustration. "Something happened last summer that marked the beginning of a decline in her ability to think. She just can't make reasonable decisions anymore, and the weirdest part is that she refuses to act on my advice. She asks for it, and then does the opposite. Why does she even bother asking me?"

I dropped my fist onto the table in frustration. A long weary week had gone by since my friend and I had said goodnight after choir practice. We found two seats in the crowded sandwich shop and had barely placed our trays down before beginning a review of the week. Nora's new kitchen cabinets were an inch too long and my car needed a new muffler after hitting one of the city's legendary potholes. However, my story about Mother's tires trumped all other accounts of the week.

"It was really nice to hear Mom asking for my advice regarding her tires. But no sooner had I listened to her describe the wobbling and shaking of the car when she drove it on the highway out to the airport – an image that sent shivers down my spine – she changed her mind about asking for my advice and very sweetly said, 'Only a man can do some things, dear. I'm going to call S.T. about my tires.'"

Nora nearly choked on her broccoli chicken soup, no doubt remembering similar conversations with her mother.

"It's a generational thing, Allison," she said, finally grabbing enough breath to speak. "Women were far less liberated to claim their own intelligence and many had to fight for the right to, well... to have a brain. She is stuck in the era where men handled certain jobs and women handled others."

"...and making decisions about tires is a man's job," I said with a halfhearted smile.

Mother was not likely to change her viewpoint on women's lib, nor admit that her eldest daughter did indeed have a head on her shoulders. My knowledge about uneven wear on tires, and the solution found in every Powder Puff Mechanics 101 class to balance and rotate said tires, once again fell on deaf ears, and sometime later that week she called S.T., a longtime family friend. He gladly went over to her house, examined the tires, and declared that they needed to be rotated. When I reminded my mother that had been my exact suggestion a week ago, she retorted, "You don't know what you are talking about," and changed the subject to a lively report on the hailstorm that had just come through. My mother firmly believed that some jobs were meant for men and some for women and one should not stray between the two. My advice about the tires was, therefore, discarded as "bologna," leaving me wondering why she had even asked me in the first place.

"Allison," Nora compassionately pointed out once again, "Your mother is ill. Let go of your pride and desire to be right. It's getting in your way."

Going over her parting words consumed the better part of my evening and I fell asleep asking to be released from my stubborn ways, no matter how honestly I may have come to have them.

Perhaps due to the curative nature of prayer and contemplation, I was blessed with a restful sleep that night and awoke to marvelous memories of traveling to far off places with my parents and little sister. While many of my elementary classmates had never ventured outside the state, the four of us merrily set out every summer for unknown adventures. We visited exciting places from Texas to Maine to Oregon and every state in between, hauling our tent trailer behind the beloved wood-paneled station wagon. There were no cell phones, personal tablets, or dropdown screens playing our favorite DVDs to entertain us – had not even been invented, yet – and we eagerly looked forward to spotting license plates from far-away places, watching the distant purple mountains grow closer and closer until we could see that they were, in fact, golden green with aspen trees. Family vacations were a time of exploration outside the confinement of our strict home life and gave us the opportunity to stretch our eyes and our minds.

As Louisa and I grew older and gradually left home and began adventures of our own, Mother and Dad began traveling by themselves in a somewhat more sophisticated fashion as members of pre-arranged tour groups. No country or place was off limits, and they took in sights from Alaska to Beijing and from the Vatican to the Tower of London. After my father's passing, Mother gathered a group of friends around her who called themselves the Seniors-on-the-Go travel group. She set about recruiting members, researching interesting places to visit, booking the reservations, arranging for transfers, and generally acting as tour organizer for an intrepid group of senior citizens who gladly followed her lead around the world.

I explained to Nora, "Mom was the lifeblood of this group for several years, but with each passing tour she forgot more and more details, until a cruise through the Panama Canal had to be cancelled because she lost all of the group's passports."

Nora gasped, "Did she ever locate them? You know, it is not unusual for things to turn up in strange places or for dementia patients to accuse others of having taken them."

"Yes, they were in her suitcase, but she didn't discover them until a few weeks later, and the trip had already been cancelled. She was terribly embarrassed that she let her friends down so dreadfully," I said, feeling badly for my mother. "Most of them have not spoken to her since."

We sat in silence for a while, working on our salads. The mood at the table was somber, and Nora was unusually quiet. She had also experienced a difficult week with the unexpected passing of her brother-in-law. Nora and her husband, Mark, had known each other since they were thirteen and were the best of friends. Their two families had been entwined for over fifty years. The loss of a brother-in-law was keenly felt in a close-knit family such as theirs.

I realized that my friend needed a soothing balm for her own heart, but before I could think of the words to reach out to her, Nora pushed aside her thoughts and commented, "Alzheimer's takes away so much. Your mother's world will become smaller and smaller as her abilities to maintain friendships diminishes. In your conversations with her it is important not to place too much emphasis on her friendships. They will slowly begin to implode and disappear."

I recalled how the past summer Mother had begun complaining about her closest friend, Sylvia Walker, for not spending more time with her. Yet by the same token, Mother admitted that she had forgotten concerts and dinner dates and stood Sylvia up on more than one occasion. With disdain in her voice, she claimed that her friend would simply show up at her house for a luncheon date which Mother is certain she had not made, and consequently, their friendship had become very tenuous over the past year.

"I guess the excuses are her way of covering up for her increasing forgetfulness. It's sort of funny, Nora, that Sylvia gave her a calendar for Christmas," I smiled as I recalled how proud she was of the beautiful Monet prints at the top of each month. "She can't seem to keep track of appointments, though, even with the calendar. It must be hard to be a good friend when you can't remember to keep in touch."

Mother was one of three sisters who did manage to stay in touch even though several hundred miles of prairie, hill country and coastal plains separated them. The eldest of the trio, Mother faithfully kept the phone lines open, and she and Aunt Minnie and Aunt Goldy shared a close relationship, keeping each other updated on their lives and that of their children. With ten children between the three of them, the sisters chatted over the years about the many marriages, births, graduations, anniversaries, and job promotions - never running out of joyful things to share. In recent years, however, it seems that Mother's reminiscing was becoming more on the dark side involving stories of who had lost their job, who was drinking too much, and who had cheated on their spouse. Louisa and I were appalled that Mother had become such a gossip.

All three of the sisters were now widowed, which brought them closer together through the bond of communal grief. Growing older came more gracefully to Aunt Goldy and Aunt Minnie, who accepted illnesses, strokes, and arthritis somewhat more in stride than Mother, who provided drama enough for them all. The spring following that terrible Christmas, she called me at work one afternoon, which she rarely did, and tearfully told me that Aunt

Goldy had a "massive infection and was not going to make it" through a hip replacement. Checking in with my closest cousin, the infection and hip surgery were indeed true, but the dying was another of Mother's dramatic statements either intended to draw attention and sympathy, or simply because she did not understand her sister's condition. Yet, true to her desire to be helpful in whatever small way, Mother hastily boarded a commuter plane, and with Aunt Minnie in tow, she rushed to her sister's side. Mother's loving concern brought comfort to Aunt Goldy, and in spite of the histrionics, Aunt Goldy did not die, after all.

The days wore on with Mother uncharacteristically complaining about one thing or another, forgetting both her sons-in-laws' birthdays, and completely losing track of when and where she was supposed to be for Thanksgiving and Christmas. She repeatedly confused the two holidays, until finally she arrived at Louisa's house for the pre-appointed Thanksgiving visit – a full day early. Louisa was peeved as her preparations for the holiday had not been completed, and Mother, in spite of her desire to help, slowed things down to a snail's pace. Other than her unexpected early arrival, the thing that struck Louisa the most was how poor Mother's short term memory had become, even to the point of repeating herself several times in the same conversation.

"I have read, Nora, that the ability to carry on a conversation is one of the last things that a person loses, but if you really listen to the words, they don't quite make sense," I commented. "The pleasantries may still be there, but the content is off a bit. I am afraid that is where I lose my patience and want to jump in to challenge Mom the most."

"And that is a mistake, right?" Nora smiled and then became much more serious as she spoke her next words with measured care. "Talk with her while you still can. The ability to hear her voice while she still knows who you are is something to be treasured. At some point she will not be able to use a phone, and that connection with her will be gone."

The sandwich shop had become alive with noise as the constant foot traffic of hungry patrons sought after-work energy from hot coffee and pastries. A group of young soccer players streamed in through the doors along with their mothers who tried in vain to organize them into an orderly line at the counter. We watched the energetic little girls, who were more interested in each other's shoes than in selecting a sandwich, and marveled that the women were able to get the whole mass of constantly moving bodies from the order counter to the pick-up counter and into adjoining booths in less than ten minutes.

People-watching was actually a nice reprieve from having to think about my friend's sobering words. I did not want my mother to lose the ability to communicate. As much as Mother and I disagreed on just about every conceivable topic we broached, my heart did not want her to fall silent.

How I wished that I had recalled Nora's words as a few days later. Mother and I began a conversation with the hallmark pattern of every conversation of late – warm greeting, review of the weather forecast for each of us, catching up on Louisa and her family. This time was no different and the phone call began with how much we had missed each other, how cold it was where we lived and how hot it was where she lived, how well my sister and her family were doing, and finally with Mother seeking my approval on her latest financial decisions. What began as a genuine exchange of love and affection turned into an argument over her purchase of a CD at a kiosk in the mall. I was appalled at the transaction and berated her for having made the purchase. Our conversation ended abruptly when she vehemently told me to leave her alone, that she knew what she was doing, and that I was interfering with her life. Although I did not know it at the time, "I don't want to talk to you," were the last words I would hear from her for quite some time.

Nora listened with her heart as much as her ears, and I found myself pouring my heart out to her in the now almost deserted restaurant. We had long since finished our meals and had nothing before us except for cups of steaming tea and coffee.

"Nora, she was like a child throwing a tantrum. She just cut off the conversation and hung up," I said, not wanting to believe that my mother was acting like the squirmy, loud little girls we had just seen.

From my readings I knew that Alzheimer's reverses a person's aging back to and even beyond a point in childhood when abstract thinking skills are not well developed and emotional outbursts are common ways to communicate. It pained me to think that Mother's journey was taking her back full circle to her beginnings – a retrogenesis in behavior and thinking.

Nora smiled faintly at the image of a willful child trying to defend her actions in a way that made sense to her still young mind. As one who had witnessed this before, Nora explained, "It's easier for your mother to throw a tantrum than to try and explain something beyond her abilities. She doesn't know what to say, doesn't even know what questions to ask to get a handle on her life. It's her way of covering up the fact that she is no longer capable of managing her own affairs. She is hurting, Allison."

I inhaled deeply, slowly taking in this new thought. The idea that Mother knew her abilities were failing was disturbing. On the one hand she knew in the dimness of her mind that she needed guidance, but on the other hand believed that someone was threatening her autonomy and, therefore, refused to accept their guidance. How frightening it must be for an individual to realize that they can no longer keep up with their lives, as if the merry-go-round was spinning wildly out of control. Those of us on the outside want a sense of normalcy to return - to see our loved one restored to wholeness - but certainly no less than the individual wishes for themselves. Fear and uncertainty moves in where confidence used to live.

As Mother's paranoia deepened, so too did her fear of me. In spite of my good intentions and willingness to be available for her in the years following Dad's death, she saw me as a threat, in part motivated by her natural avoidance of a daughter who overwhelmed her, and in part as a result of her illness. "They are just trying to get my money" became a theme often voiced to my sister. My husband and I could only watch as she made one poor decision after another, eating away at the careful investments my father had made over a lifetime of hard work and planning. There were no more phone conversations about financial planning... or anything else for that matter... as my calls now went unanswered.

"She won't take my phone calls anymore, Nora. She told my sister that she was taking a break from our relationship and refuses to talk to me. It's as though I have been fired," I bemused, although there was no real amusement in my voice. "You know, she fired Dr. Zachariah the week after we left."

"She did what?" Nora was startled and stopped short on her way over to the drink counter with cups in hand. "I thought she liked her doctor."

We made our way through the crowd to a table next to the window, and setting down our trays, searched for another chair to pull up. It seemed that our quiet out-of-the-way sandwich shop had suddenly gained in popularity with its newly found fame as one of the countryside's finest bistros, according to a New York food critic. Nora and I had known this for some time and had hoped that it would remain a well kept secret, but it looked like we might have to begin widening our choice of venues for our weekly dinner and conversation.

"Mom told Louisa that she was not going to keep her appointment with Dr. Zachariah and had written her a letter firing her," I said, raising my voice to be heard above the din.

Nora leaned in to hear me better.

"She seems to be in a mode of pushing everyone away that has even hinted at the slipping of her memory. I suppose that is natural as someone would tend to go into a fight or flight stance, but she is running away from the people who can help her the most," I bemoaned.

"Does she have a doctor at all now to follow up on her issues?"

"She made an appointment with a cardiologist that her medical buddy Sylvia knew about, but she won't tell us his name. I think Mom believes that we had too much influence with Dr. Zachariah and were in 'cahoots with her'."

"Cahoots! It's been a long time since I've heard that word," Nora said, laughing out loud.

I smiled and said, "Mom is just fighting this so hard. It would be amusing, if it weren't so difficult to see her go through it. Elena said that there have been a lot of lawyers coming and going at the cottage lately."

My thoughts over the next few weeks were constantly on my mother. There were few moments that I did not feel the heavy burden of guilt and grief. Although it appeared that her reactions were perfectly normal for an Alzheimer's person, but my heart bore a feeling of responsibility for her angst - as if by my insistence that she listen to me and my constant pushing her to accept my guidance, I had driven her to this dark place.

"Allison, please do not think for an instant that you are the cause of your mother's reaction," Nora implored. "This is to be expected, in fact. This is what they do. They single someone out on whom to place blame and to identify as the main suspect in causing all their difficulties. You did not create this terrible thing. The hurt you are feeling is a measure of your love for your mother."

Nora's ever-present words of reassurance sustained me over the coming weeks as Mother's hatred intensified. The sweetness of Nora's face every Thursday night at choir rehearsal warmed my spirit and acted as a counter-balance to the pain I felt. We never spoke of our relationship when with others, but the kinship of having shared the path that all Alzheimer's families walk quietly bolstered me for the journey.

Louisa called late one night to check on me. I thought it was sweet that she was concerned about how I might be taking Mother's self-imposed blackout on my phone calls. Thanks to the caller ID feature that Louisa had added to the phone service in the hope that Mother would be able to avoid unsolicited sales calls, not only had she refused to answer my calls, but she was also ignoring my husband's calls, a fact that he found very perplexing and troubling. Tom and his mother-in-law had a very unique relationship in that they were train buddies. Every few days he would call her from the commuter train on his way home from work. They would joyfully exchange stories of their days and had quite a happy time of it, until Tom's cell phone number was added to her mental "Do Not Answer" list. Quite innocently, he was thrown into the same category as I - persona non grata.

My sister played the role of mediator as best she could. Mother's fears morphed into full blown paranoia and she became quite agitated at the mention of Tom and me. Ignoring the edict that Alzheimer's persons cannot be reasoned with, Louisa continually reminded Mother of how much we did indeed care for her. While she chose to believe that Mother heard and espoused her words, Louisa's assurances continued to fall on deaf ears.

"Tom loves my mother, Nora. He finds her truly enjoyable and entertaining. His patience with her is limitless, and he truly doesn't mind listening to the same stories day after day. However, in her anger and distrust of me, she also screens her phone for his cell number. He's really hurt by it even though he knows that he has done nothing to deserve this kind of treatment."

"Tom is such a sweet, gentle person. He must be very troubled by that," Nora said, looking equally perplexed.

"He is and he isn't. I don't think he is surprised, however, having had a grandfather who was institutionalized for trying to burn down his parents' house. Tom knows it isn't anything that he did, but just that Mom's mind isn't firing on all cylinders. It's very sad."

By Louisa's account, Mother and her caregiver seemed to have settled into a routine of Tuesday-Thursday-Saturday mornings consisting of applying Mother's memory patch - which she refers to as her pain patch - and running errands around town. She did not want the neighbors, probably most specifically her closest neighbor Imelda, to know that she had anybody coming to help her, for it would be a blight on her character to admit that she was not fully capable of taking care of herself when her much older neighbor enjoys complete freedom and "drives a Lamborghini." She insisted that Elena park her car around the corner near the alley where it could not be seen and that they run about town in Mother's car with the elder woman at the wheel. I cringed at this arrangement, whereas my sister continued to applaud Mother's independence.

In the weekly phone conversations with Louisa and I about how the caregivers' relationships and Mother's care was progressing, Elena recounted the many near misses with other cars and the many circuitous routes to the grocery store and post office, places Mother had been frequenting for close to forty years. A longtime resident of San Angelo herself, Elena knew that Mother was losing her sense of direction and was easily confused when trying to drive somewhere. Nevertheless, Elena was the ever cheerful companion and helper, and the two began to form an uneasy bond. Gradually over the weeks Mother confided more and more in Elena about a frightening - albeit completely imagined - hidden life of which Louisa and I were not aware.

"Elena tells us that Mom is seeing a 'Negro man' outside her windows peering in at her. She is so scared that she has covered all the windows in the house with newspaper."

Nora gasped as I told her about the fear which pervaded my mother's life.

"Elena convinced Mom that the newspaper didn't look good, and would in fact draw more attention from the neighbors. So, she helped Mom take it all back down... except for the garage windows. It is still a mystery why she refuses to take down the garage papers. They agreed that, if anyone asked, the garage was very hot and the newspaper helped keep the sun out."

"Does the patch seem to be helping her?" Nora asked as I got up briefly to get more napkins to clean up the soup I had just spilled.

When I returned to the table, I answered her question, "Louisa seems to think so, but I am not so sure. Her memory lapses are still puzzling and her moods swing back and forth between her natural bubbly self and periods of agitation and fear. Elena can have normal conversations with her for several days and then something sets her off and she falls back into confusion and moodiness. It's a constant struggle for her. Elena told me that Mom often talks to herself and says things like, 'Imogene, you are acting crazy.'"

"Perhaps your mother needs a psychiatrist, as well as a neurologist," Nora ventured to say while adjusting her chair to avoid the rays of the setting sun.

"That sounds like the most logical step to take, Nora, but Mom is now seeing a cardiologist rather than a primary care physician, and he does not seem to have any indication of her dementia. He is sending her to a gastroenterologist for a pain in her abdomen. Personally," I conjectured, "she has these imaginary ailments and actually relishes going to a doctor or, even better, the emergency room. She is her own worst enemy, though, because of her denial about the real issues."

As much as it disturbed me that my mother would not pick up my calls, I stuck to my routine of phoning her every three or four days. I knew that she did not know how to retrieve my messages from her answering machine, but hoped that as she was screening the calls, she would hear the cheer I struggled to interject into my voice. Louisa, however, continued to receive the brunt of Mother's dislike for me and was burdened with listening to an accounting of everything I had ever done wrong by her.

Louisa asked me, "Do you want to know the things Mom says about you? Or would you rather not know?"

My curiosity, combined with a desire to defend myself against what I was sure were slanderous stories, urged me to say yes. However, overcoming my desire to be mired in what was sure to be a mudslinging, I chose to decline the offer and to remain apart from the attack on my person. Louisa understood and gallantly continued to bear the burden of playing mediator between the two of us. To make up for her lack of chivalry in defending me against the knife-hiding episode, Louisa arduously set about righting that wrong and spent many hours trying to talk Mother out of her ill feelings towards me.

As Valentine's Day approached and Nora and I met at what had become our table in the sandwich shop, I began with, "Mom sent me a Valentine."

Nora's eyes lit up more than usual and she exclaimed, "How wonderful!"

It had, indeed, given me great pleasure to receive that little dime store piece of paper addressed to me in the unmistakable handwriting of my mother. The last weeks had been almost unbearable jumping at every phone call wishing and hoping that it was from Mother. And then the mail arrived containing the tiny little card with her signature that glowed as brightly as the sun.

"Nora, it was all I could do to keep from jumping up and down. Tom thought I was overreacting, but Mom had reached out to me, and I do not take that lightly."

My eyes glistened with joy and the rest of the evening was filled with happy chatter about Nora's daughter who was taking a cruise, the rain showers that had melted some of the piles of snow that afternoon, and the bonus that my husband had just received. The world was a much happier place and we celebrated by treating each other to sundaes at the ice cream parlor up the block. We laughed as we picked our way across the still partially iced over sidewalks, but somehow the frozen delicacy just seemed the only appropriate way to celebrate.

I rushed home full of strawberries and whipped cream to call my mother, convinced that the phone would be answered on at least the fourth ring, allowing her enough time to get out of her chair in the living room and make her way to the kitchen. The phone rang eleven times and no one answered. Perhaps, she was in the shower. I waited half an hour and tried again, glancing at my watch to satisfy myself that she should be at home at a quarter after nine o'clock in the evening. However, that call, and all others that followed, went unanswered.

"I don't get it, Louisa," I said. "Why would she send me a Valentine and still refuse to talk to me?"

"She sent you a Valentine?" Louisa asked, as surprised as I was. I described the precious little piece of paper with the little lamb asking if "ewe would be my Valentine?"

There was a pause on the line as Louisa hesitantly described the large glittered foldout Hallmark card she had received from Mother. A sudden sadness and envy came over me as I began to wonder if Elena had not been instrumental in providing Mother with one of her grandson's preschool Valentines to send, as if it were an afterthought.

How childish the exchange then seemed – so sophomoric to be playing games with Valentines. Mother's determination to keep me at a distance was actually becoming annoying and ridiculous. How long could she hold on to her resolve to disown me? Chagrined, I wondered if my ability to love my mother was based on that love being returned – a concept which is not part of a Christ-like life, but rather one which is egocentric and self serving. At times I wanted to just wash my hands of her and walk away.

I then posed a question to Nora that had been bothering me for some time, "Can we truly love another, if that love is not returned in kind? Mom is becoming less and less capable of expressing love and it affects my ability to love her in turn."

Nora quickly commented, "You and Louisa and your mother have a strong relationship that is well grounded in a faith-filled home from the time you were both small. God is with you and has given you a support system in each other and in the rest of your family. It is so evident that you love and care for your mother, in spite of what this disease makes her do. That is agape love in the truest sense. You mustn't give up on it, Allison, because dementia doesn't give up. Dementia never stops its forward motion and you must keep looking forward, as well, with those same strong and loving eyes that help you see through the tricks it plays on your mother."

Sometime later that evening, I prayed that Mother's mind would somehow find its way through the murkiness in which the dementia had trapped her and that she would break out into the sunshine again. St. Valentine's Day seemed like an appropriate day to revisit scriptures and rehearse the beloved lines.

Love is patient and kind;
Love is not envious or boastful;
It is not arrogant or rude;
Love is not proud.

Over the next few months and well into the summer, Mother's memories of her stay in the hospital became more and more clouded until she was convinced that I was the perpetrator of a plan to "put her away." She steadfastly maintained that the doctor told her the only thing wrong with her was her eldest daughter.

"Nora, can we just talk over the phone this week?" I inquired, not wanting to bare my soul in a public place, for my heart just wasn't into getting together for dinner. Food held no interest and I had slept very little in the last few days, calling in sick to work more than once.

She was open to the idea, although caregivers were encouraged to meet with their care receivers in person; I suppose in order to make that emotional connection that only a look or a nod can convey. Besides the fact that she was a good friend, Nora was part of a volunteer care ministry in which our church participated and had spent many hours training to support and encourage those going through difficult times. The uncertainty and pain of losing my mother to Alzheimer's prompted me to reach out to this unique ministry, and Nora was the logical choice to walk this path with me. Even if she had not spent many of her weekends and evenings learning how to work with those who were suffering, her caring ways would have naturally lifted my spirits, for Nora had a deeply rooted gift for listening and offering encouragement. Regardless of the pain I may have borne going into a conversation with her, I always emerged feeling hopeful and blessed in some way.

She picked up the phone promptly at eight o'clock that evening and asked her usual leading question, "How are you, and how is your mother?"

There could not be a more open-ended question, and I usually hesitated searching for a place to begin, but that night there was no hesitation. Not really knowing how to begin, I managed to speak in spite of the lump in my throat.

"Mom has written me out of her will. I have been disinherited."

The lump rose until I could no longer talk and tears stung my eyes and cheeks.

"Oh, Allison, I am so sorry."

Her soft voice conveyed genuine concern. A long silence followed, allowing me to become further engulfed in the stillness of our living room where I usually sought refuge.

"Are you alright?" she asked with compassion, and I knew that she had dropped all else to sit down in her own living room to talk with me.

"I don't know how I am supposed to feel, but...it's like walking into a completely dark and silent room," I slowly answered. "There is just...emptiness. It would almost have been easier if she had died... that I would have understood. Death is not a mystery to me."

Choking on the words, I said, "Being divorced by my own mother just... leaves me blank... like a chalkboard that has been erased."

I had suffered the pain of a divorce several years before meeting Tom and knew the emptiness of neglect and abandonment, but this was different. Being divorced by one's own mother was unspeakably difficult and left me completely void, as if the life she had given me had been sucked into a vacuum. I had little energy for the things of daily life which ordinarily would have given me purpose and motivation.

"So, all the lawyers visiting your mother were for the purpose of changing her will," Nora conjectured.

I held the phone closer to my ear, grasping it as though it were the only lifeline in an ocean of darkness.

She gently continued with familiar words that I needed to hear yet again, "This is not your mother. Alzheimer's takes away a person's ability to think clearly and to make sound decisions. Many times they become suspicious of those they love the most."

There was silence on the phone for a moment while I struggled to gain control of my emotions.

"Louisa didn't want to tell me. She cried and cried and apologized that she wasn't able to change Mom's mind. She begged me not to give up on Mom. She said she can't do this alone."

"Dorothy and I were very glad to have each other to lean on," Nora agreed. "When one of us was having a hard time with it, the other one was strong and vice versa. There were many times when I swore I was never going back to see Mommie because she was so mean. Sister and I really had to rely on each other to get through it."

We talked on into the evening, and as dusk became darkness, Tom quietly came into the living room with a fresh box of tissues in his hand. He was a welcome sight and as Nora and I said goodnight, we curled up on the sofa together to let the last of the day close around us. His strong and comforting arms cradled me as I wept and I slowly fell asleep exhausted from emotions finally spent.

One evening shortly thereafter, a box was waiting for me on the front porch when I came home from work and, much to my surprise, it contained a miniature rosebush from my sister. The card simply read, "I love you." Always the considerate and sensitive one, Louisa's gift was the ray of sunshine that I needed just then.

Sitting behind my desk at work that day had been excruciatingly difficult as my very well-intentioned boss had innocently asked how my mother was. Much to his dismay, tears welled up in my eyes and I could only say, "She is continuing on her journey." It was a rather lame, but truthful answer – the short, polite version rather than the long involved answer which I doubt he wanted to hear. He is, none-the-less, a kindhearted family man and later that morning on one of my trips into his office he said how sorry he was to hear that Louisa and I had to bear this burden. The mother of a close friend of his had recently died from Alzheimer's, and he offered the only consoling words he could by saying that the hardest part of this disease is that you lose your parent twice. The truth behind his words stuck with me and somehow made me feel better from the simple knowledge that others knew the same heartache.

Louisa's gift of the rosebush warmed my heart, as well. It suddenly dawned on me that she must be going through a difficult time caught between her mother and her sister, but she had taken the time to reach out to me. In all of our phone calls across the miles we had focused on me - always my thoughts and my feelings. My grief pulled the two of us closer together, and she had been a willing support to me in my anguish. Now, it was her turn. I picked up the phone to thank her and to ask for the first time how she was doing in dealing with all the changes in Mom.

The steadfast duplication of our father, she simply replied, "It's been difficult."

I smiled weakly knowing the depth of that statement and said, "Tom opened a chocolate drop last night and offered it to me. The saying on the inside of the wrapper was, 'If you are going through hell, keep going.' That's you, Louisa. You amaze me with your strength. You just don't give up."

We spent the next hour talking about Louisa's resolve to deal with both the illness of a mother whom she loved, and a sister who, hurt by that same illness, she also loved. I began to hear overtones of acceptance in her voice for the first time. Perhaps, she, too, was beginning to work her way through the sadness of the long goodbye.

"Louisa called last night and was very adamant in telling me that she did not approve of the way in which Mom was treating me," I told Nora.

It was with a small sense of relief that I passed on this news, for here-to-fore, Louisa had not defended me against the barbs Mother hurled my way. I had no idea what prompted Louisa to decide that she and her family would no longer allow Mother to speak ill of Tom and me.

"She was almost angry about it all and said she had lost her patience with Mom," I said, feeling a bit guilty about the fact that this pleased me. "This disease should not be a battleground, but it has become one where even our family relationships are threatened."

Nora understood and nodded, "Family members rarely look at dementia from the same viewpoint without eventually walking separate yet parallel paths. I am glad that your sister now sees how tough this has been for you and is ready to affirm your relationship."

We soon found ourselves deep in discussion while seated on a bench in the midst of a colorful display of blooming bulbs. Springtime had managed to peep out from under the piles of snow, and the sight of purple crocus and bright yellow daffodils always helped to brighten my mood. Nora and I chose to abandon the sandwich shop that week in favor of a stroll through my "secret garden". There was an historic home hidden in the thickly wooded hills not far from our house that, while frequented by deer and squirrels, saw few humans enjoying the estate's English gardens. Tom and I had discovered it quite by accident in one of our Sunday afternoon drives and enjoyed slipping onto the grounds for many hours of respite from the din of the city and nearby highways. We called it our secret garden and had only shared it with our closest friends, among whom I counted Nora.

Her encouraging words and the evidence of new life in the earth gave my spirit hope that someday my mother and I could be reunited in each other's arms. Louisa's timely gesture of solidarity warmed my heart and drew me closer to her when we had been in danger of tearing apart.

Holidays are always a difficult time for families in turmoil, and as Mother's Day approached, ours proved to be no different. So often in the weeks prior, Mother had energetically maintained that I made no effort to reach out to her, in spite of a constant stream of cheerful greeting cards and voicemails. Straying from the traditional choice of white roses for a woman whose own mother was no longer living, I ordered a Mother's Day bouquet carefully selected for its bright colors and fragrant message – roses for love, orchids for beauty, and iris just because I knew she loved them.

The gift went unacknowledged, not that I really expected her to break her silence. I had skipped church services that day, certain that my grief would be too public in the choir loft in front of the congregation. Nora understood, for this was her first Mother's Day without her mother. We shared a simple hug when we met at the garden, the usual greetings silenced in lieu of an unspoken embrace. We did not talk about Mother's Day, choosing to let a private grief cleanse our hearts and prepare us for the next part of the journey.

For the next several weeks, Nora and I met at the garden in search of renewal through the freshness and beauty of the out-of-doors. Temperatures were unseasonably mild, and we took advantage of the natural breezes blowing across the hills to go for walks out under the arching maple and oak trees.

Spring turned into summer and Mother's mid-July birthday presented a challenge for me as I pondered what to give someone who resisted any outpouring of love. Remembering my sister's words, "It would be so easy for you to give up on Mom, but you keep at it anyway," rang in my ears, and I struggled to push aside the anger that kept welling up and to find instead even tiny pieces of forgiveness.

"Fruitcake! I decided to give my mother a fruitcake," I excitedly exclaimed when Nora asked if I had solved the birthday dilemma.

Nora laughed out loud, "You have to be kidding."

"No, I am not. My mother is part of the one percent of the population that actually likes - no, loves fruitcake. So, I ordered one from the best bakery in the South and had it shipped to her. Louisa said that Mom was put off by it until she reminded her of how much she loves fruitcake and that it is the perfect gift anytime, not just for Christmas. I didn't hear from Mom, but Louisa told me she ate it all, in spite of her protestations that it was a 'stupid gift.'"

The mood lightened a bit as Nora and I continued our conversation on a bench overlooking the garden's vintage herbs and vegetables. The soil had warmed enough to give the region's tomatoes a sweetness that was hard to match anywhere else. We didn't dare pick anything in the garden and had brought our own picnic basket full of vine-ripened tomatoes, mozzarella and fresh basil.

"Nora, I truly care for Mom, but I'm really disgusted that she is being so childish. It's as though she is throwing a two-year-old tantrum. In my music classroom I would have put that child in timeout. How do you do that with an adult? How do you talk to and reason with someone who has dementia?" I asked pleadingly, fully expecting the answer to be "you don't."

"Think of Edith," Nora answered quite simply. "How do you talk to Edith?"

She was referring to our mutual friend Edit Solomon. Nora and I take a spiritual and musical retreat once a week by attending church choir rehearsal. I am a second soprano and sit between two other seconds, one with a bubbly personality that just overflows with enthusiasm, and the other is Edith, who is quite the opposite. She has the very quiet demeanor of someone with dementia. We share moments of pure and simple joy by just sitting next to each other talking about the weather and what she had for dinner, which many times she can't remember but does recall that it was satisfying and good. Her favorite color is pink, and I always find something quite beautiful and delicate embroidery on her clothing about which to compliment, and her face beams from the praise. Although she often has no clue what piece of music we are rehearsing or where her hymnal is, she knows many of the tunes and words by heart and sings the melody even if the second soprano part is different. Her voice is very small, like her person, but her spirit is large. She seems to be blissfully unaware that her memory is not what it should be, but she cheerfully accepts guidance and it doesn't seem to bother her a bit.

"We talk about simple things," I replied to Nora's question. "I told my sister that Edith is a gift from God. She sits quietly next to me and we talk and sing... and it is almost like I have a proxy for my mother. I always feel like I have been mothered when I am with her – such a counterpoint to the mechanical voice on my Mom's answering machine."

"Your mother, too, will become sweet at some time along the way. Mommie was very peaceful near the end." Nora paused before saying, "It doesn't sound like your mother is ever going to accept or understand her illness. In fact, dementia patients actually do better if you never mention the word. Do you think it would be helpful for you not to try any longer to make her understand?"

Nora's suggestion was an interesting one. I sat back on the bench, taking in the perfumed air around the wisteria dropping down from the pergola above our heads. It felt peaceful in the garden and it was easy to bare one's soul in such pastoral surroundings.

"Probably," I finally admitted with reluctance.

The teacher in me wanted Mother to understand and to accept her illness; but, the daughter in me had grown to understand that she could not.

"So, how do you talk to someone with dementia?" I repeated my earlier question, although I already knew the answer.

Nora replied with a little smile on her lips, "You talk about the weather, what she had for dinner...and wherever the conversation takes you - which might be someplace very sweet."

Chapter 4

*T*wo weeks went by before our schedules allowed us to sit down at the dinner table again. The weather has turned hot and so Mora and I found refuge in a secluded spot in the sandwich shop, sinking down into the familiar leather cushions of the booth, surrounded by chatter of other patrons and the wonderful smells of baked bread. It felt comfortable there, and I wished that same feeling of security and warmth for my mother.

"Mom has wonderful memories of bits and pieces of her life. Her long-term personal history seems to be somewhat intact, but events of the last five years or so are slipping away," I began. "We worried that Mom would chose to stop using the memory patch, which she still refers to as a pain patch. Elena assures us that on the days that she is with Mom, the first activity of the morning is to reapply a fresh patch."

Louisa had related to me that Mother growls at Elena whenever she goes near her medications. Elena has tried to help her sort out all the pill bottles, but Mother is very protective of them. She isn't using a pill sorter, but has worked out some other system that supposedly helps her remember what she has taken and what she still needs to take.

"Nora, there is a very real possibility that Mom's memory and cognitive issues may be caused by over- or under-medicating herself," I observed. "Without a consistent physician following her case, and with Mom's insistence that she can manage her own medications, we can only wait until some incident allows us to penetrate the defensive wall she has built around herself. It's scary to think that she has to harm herself before we can step in."

"That is so wise of you to realize that your mother has the right to lead her own life. Unfortunately, you see that her ability to take care of herself is faltering, and you naturally want to protect her from what could be a serious mistake," Nora observed. "There is little that you can do except to encourage her to have her caregiver there as much as possible."

"That's part of the difficulty, Nora. She resists accepting help, probably because she grew up in hard times during the Depression and everyone had to be self-sufficient or they didn't survive. That has carried her very well through life – until now, when she needs to let go of that stubborn streak."

Nora laughed and asked me if there was any other news from Elena. We ordered dessert and waited for the decaf coffee latte and iced chai tea to arrive before continuing.

"Elena now tells us that Mom is more and more confused when they are out driving together. She is worried that Mom will become truly lost when she is driving alone and may not be able to find her way home. Elena thinks Mom goes out driving just to be driving, thinking that she can prove to us that she can still safely operate a car."

My mother's knowledge of anything mechanical, much less an automobile, is comical. She grew up in the backwoods where the modern conveniences of a washing machine and indoor plumbing were rare. She never had to learn the intricacies of operating an electric can opener, a remote control, or a garage door opener. It was not until she graduated high school and moved into the "big city" of Nacogdoches to attend secretarial school that she was introduced to a mechanized world of business machines and household gadgets, whose operation never came easy for her. Only after she had been married for a year did Mother venture to learn to drive.

Prone to excitability, Mom's driving lessons must have been a challenge for Dad, who was the exact opposite of Mother in temperament. Ever afterwards, the calm, rarely flustered executive vowed he would never teach another female in his family how to drive. To his credit and Mother's perseverance, she learned to keep the car in the proper lane and obey all the traffic laws, but that is as far as her knowledge of the world of automobiles extended.

"Mom tells a story on herself about the time she had to show a car that Dad had listed for sale in the classifieds. She met the prospective buyer in a department store parking lot, supervised while he drove the car around the lot, and fielded his questions as best she could. His primary concern was the loud noise under the hood, to which my mother quickly replied, 'Oh, that is just the dipstick rattling.'"

Nora and I broke into peals of laughter, bringing smiles from those around us.

"The man bought the car from my father in spite of Mom's very creative selling techniques," I said through the laughter.

Through the many years of their enduring marriage, Dad maintained our little fleet of cars. His meticulous service books on each car showed the last tune-up, how many miles per gallon the car achieved, and the date and mileage of every oil change. Just keeping the car full of gas, the tires and brakes maintained, much less the oil changed, proved beyond Mother's abilities as a widow. The service book fell out of use. Her sons-in-law came to her rescue on their visits every few months and regularly took her car out to pinpoint any problems. Tom pointed out to me on one of these routine inspections that she had been running into things and "touching up the paint" with fingernail polish, which was close to the car's bright maroon color, but not an exact match.

"What would she have done if the car was green?" Nora glibly asked as the waitress refilled her coffee cup.

"She is actually rather creative in her efforts to cover up what she perceives to be her faults," I said. "We never mention to her that we know her ability to control the car is declining due to the number of scrapes and dings it has acquired."

Nora put down the spoon she was using to stir in sugar and cream and said, "Do you think that may actually be doing her a disfavor?"

"Yes, I suppose it is like ignoring the elephant in the room. We are not completely sure that she is having little mishaps, but I suspect that more is happening than we are aware of when she is behind the wheel."

My suspicions were soon confirmed when she and Elena were out on a shopping excursion for new living room draperies and she gunned the accelerator to beat the cross traffic in a parking lot. Ignoring Elena's pleas to stop, Mother ran up over the curb of a median before screeching to a halt with the car precariously perched atop the grassy divider between two parking areas. Her reaction time was too slow and, although the only moving violations she had ever received were for speeding in a school zone and for rolling a few stop signs, she broke numerous laws in those few moments. Mother, shaking from the experience, allowed Elena to drive them slowly homeward with a strange new sound coming from beneath the car.

"She can't cover that up with fingernail polish," Nora said excitedly.

"No, she can't, but it's interesting that the first thing she said to Elena was not to tell Allison, a vow which Elena solemnly made, but knew she would not keep," I said, grateful that Mother's caregiver loved her enough to break that promise.

The difficulties my mother had with cars went back as far as any of us could remember, and lately she admitted that sometimes she forgot "what all the levers and knobs are for." I shivered at that thought and recalled the almost comical, but frightening, conversation that Louisa's husband Matt had with his mother-in-law about the air conditioning controls. Mother was positive that the buttons with little pictures of people on them were to adjust the position of her seat and, even after many demonstrations by Matt, she was not convinced that those buttons actually directed air flow. As funny as the image of Mother repeatedly pressing the air conditioning buttons to move her seat forward or backward, all the while sitting in the same position, the idea that she was behind the controls of two tons of machinery that could harm someone else or herself was very sobering.

When the old car finally breathed its last two years ago, we all encouraged her to purchase an automobile with fewer bells and whistles. After searching the local newspapers she reached out to her friend S.T. for his assistance in evaluating an almost new Impala which she saw advertised in the newspaper. Together they examined the car, and the owner, "a nice lady whose son used to be a policeman," allowed her to take it to a mechanic for an inspection. Satisfied that this was the car for her, Mother jumped at the chance to buy it and immediately wrote out a check for fourteen thousand dollars and gave it to "the nice lady."

"Imogene, did you get the title with the car, and switch the insurance from your old car to the new one?" Tom had asked.

"Oh, she promised to send the title to me. The car belonged to her husband who passed away, and the estate hasn't been settled, yet. I haven't had time to get the insurance for it," was her ready explanation.

As a genealogist, estate settlements were something Mother believed she understood, but it did not occur to her that the car may not have a free title, or that the "nice lady whose son used to be a policeman" may not have actually even owned the car. When Tom pointed out that she had just given away fourteen thousand dollars to a stranger in exchange for a car that very well could have been stolen, she became quite defensive, and for the next few days drove her new car around town without a title or insurance in spite of his warnings. I hurriedly flew to San Angelo and walked Mother through the steps to successfully procure the title from "the nice lady," register the car, obtain and install the new license plates, have the car inspected, and secure the insurance.

"Nora, she doesn't remember any of that now. Not one bit of it! Louisa tried to help her recall the assistance I gave her in hopes that she would think more favorably of Tom and me, but Mom has no memory of how she obtained the car," I said incredulously. "She stubbornly maintains that she and S.T. bought the car and he took care of everything."

Nora, having a way of asking those questions which I did not ever want to hear, redirected my line of thinking onto a more positive course, asked, "Allison, how important is it that she remembers and gives you credit for the assistance with the car?"

Her question hung in the air until I lifted my eyes from my cup of tea, and peering over the rim of my glasses, reluctantly admitted it would only serve the purpose of feeding my own ego. No, it was not important, and I struggled to let the memory of it pass into history, just as my mother had without any effort at all.

"We now have the very difficult situation of convincing Mom to stop driving and to give up the car," I said, moving on to my second cup of tea and the second elephant in the room.

"That could be as much of a loss to her as losing your father," Nora commented. "Her life as she has known it will completely change, and perhaps most significantly, her image of herself."

We both parted that evening contemplating the impact of loss – loss of a family member, loss of independence, loss of abilities, loss of memories. My mother's journey was not unusual, for many had walked the same trodden down path before her and many would follow after her, each of them desiring to grow old on their own terms. Growing old gracefully is something we all aspire to, but those with dementia approach their aging through the eyes of someone who believes their years of experience should allow them to continue living exactly as they have for the majority of their adult lives, not realizing that the ability to remember how to live may have vanished.

Nora helped me to understand that memory-challenged individuals cannot make the decision to stop driving on their own, whereas some of their peers who do not have the same obstacles, can analyze their own decline and make the wise decision to turn over the car keys to sharper eyes and quicker feet. My mother obviously did not fall into the latter category and was not going to stop driving on her own - certainly not when her baby sister, who is in far worse physical shape than she - continues to "tootle about town." Mother simply could not envision herself relying on others for transportation, for that would be a mark against her very character. She never found it easy to ask others for assistance, feeling like it would be an imposition for them and would bring embarrassment upon her. My willful and courageous mother did not possess the ability to age gracefully, and gallantly fought every passing day to retain her rights and her independence, in spite of the fact that her driver's license had expired.

"Nora, my father was a very quiet and gentle man. He did not speak often, but when he did, his words always spoke volumes. When I was struggling to regain my life as a newly-divorced single woman and showing my stubborn side by refusing to reach out to my parents for assistance, he took me aside and quietly said to me, 'Allison, there is a fine line between independence and stupidity.'"

Nora's eyebrow raised and she cocked her head, contemplating the depth of his words.

"I want to say that very same thing to my mother, but I

know she would not understand it. She is fiercely independent and will do anything to remain autonomous, even lie to her children and break the law without any regard for the consequences," I said.

"She doesn't have a license?" Nora asked incredulously, eyes opening wide.

She and I had not met for dinner for several weeks because of summer vacations, and there was much to catch up on. We studied the menu, and placed our orders before I ventured to tell her the latest news.

"Mom's birthday just passed in the middle of July, and her driver's license expired at that time," I explained. "In Texas, there is a law that on your seventy-ninth birthday you are automatically required to go into the department of motor vehicles in person to renew the license on its next expiration date. Coincidentally, hers expired on that birthday. Mom thinks that because she mailed in a check, her license will be renewed automatically like Aunt Minnie's had been. Her license has expired, but she continues to drive, thinking that the new license will come in the mail any day."

"Oh, you have to do something, Allison, before she hurts herself or someone else," Nora urged.

Nodding my head in agreement, I explained that an unsafe driver can be reported and an anonymous request made that the individual be retested. Unbeknownst to Louisa, I made the difficult decision to file a report. I hoped that the state would intervene and force Mother to stop driving because my sister certainly was not going to take any action.

"I feel badly that I am going behind my mother's back and forcing legal action against her. I never dreamed that I would do anything like this. Isn't this the opposite of honoring thy father and thy mother?"

"It takes strength to do the right thing," Nora reminded me. "And you have shown that strength. What she is doing is incredibly dangerous, and you have to take action. This is actually the ultimate in honoring your mother. You are caring for her when she can't care for herself."

Prompted by yet another report from Elena that Mrs. Adams had hit the bank drive-thru booth and was running up over curbs and onto sidewalks, I faxed a letter the next morning to the appropriate official in the state office to anonymously report my mother as driving, not only illegally without a license, but also as an impaired individual with dementia. The letter was not signed, but I did identify myself as the driver's daughter and that the driver, Imogene Adams, lived in San Angelo at Waverly Place. Much to my surprise, Deborah Barnes called my office that afternoon to pass on a message from the local motor vehicles office. The license renewal officer wanted to speak with me about my mother's case and asked that I contact her. I reluctantly decided that this was not a time to be shielded by anonymity – although my efforts were only thinly veiled - and to protect my mother from herself, I made the call.

"The agent was empathetic in listening to my description of Mom's situation, but until Mom goes into the local office to be retested, they can take no action. The problem is how to get her there. She is still not taking my phone calls," I sadly reported.

"How does your sister feel about this? Do you think she is willing to take any action herself?" asked Nora before noting that Louisa may not be in total accord with my actions.

"She might not, Nora."

I was amazed that she had picked up on my sister's reluctance to force the issue with Mom. "Louisa would like for someone other than the family to step in and say that Mom must stop driving and take away the keys. She wants the state, or Waverly Place, or …well, anyone other than us to have to do this to our mother. Tom thinks she is afraid and not willing to stand up to Mom."

"And what do you think, Allison?" Nora asked me with directness.

I paused for a while trying to sort out the words that would most accurately describe the situation.

"Louisa is a strong individual – as strong and stubborn as our mother."

Having said that, I smiled to myself, realizing how similar I am to Mother and Louisa.

"The three Adams women are alike in more ways than we care to admit. I must be careful that in judging their actions I don't bring that same condemnation upon myself."

"Louisa comes by her stubbornness quite honestly. I don't think she wants to make that kind of judgment. She is fine with Mom just driving around the streets inside Waverly Place, but, Nora, she does not understand that a fatal car accident at Mom's hand can happen in her own driveway just as well as it could driving the five miles to a department store."

I had raised my voice to the point of yelling at Nora who understood my vexation and continued to encourage me to present Louisa with the facts in order to protect our mother. Communicating with either one of them had become laborious – actually non-existent with the latter and confrontational with the former. I desperately needed to talk to someone who would not fight my every word. Even Tom was wont to fall into his familiar pattern of "you should do this" and "you should do that," punctuated by "you have to…"

Nora's approach was refreshing. She was a listener, and only when I had exhausted my pent up emotions did she gently push my line of thinking further, helping me find my own solutions and answers.

While the waiters delivered a plate overflowing with mussels and linguine for me and a sumptuous bowl of salmon Caesar for Nora, she pulled out a little book from her handbag. The pages were well worn, and while at first I thought it to be a Bible, the palm-sized literary work was filled with inspirational gems written to encourage, enthuse, and energize the weary. Once again, Nora had seen my need and risen to the occasion. Scripture was sprinkled throughout, but, the quote she chose to read to me was by Marie Curie.

Life is not easy for any of us.
But what of that?
We must have perseverance and above all
confidence in ourselves.
We must believe that we are gifted for
something and that this thing,
at whatever cost, must be attained.
                    ~ Marie Curie

Putting down the book and resting her chin on one hand, Nora continued, "Allison, you have taken many, many steps of faith, and yet you continue to be worried that you can't see the outcome. Your mother's journey with Alzheimer's has been full of twists and turns, even backtracking at times. It is unpredictable and by its very nature, frightening... to your mother and to your sister."

I lost interest in the mussels on my plate and folded my hands over the white cotton napkin in my lap to take in more fully what my friend had to say.

"You are the strong one right now. You have been given the gift of perseverance to be used exactly for this moment in your mother's life," Nora's gaze seemed to be focused on the center of my heart. "Have faith in your God and faith in yourself that answers will soon be evident."

Surely, the depth of her convictions spoke so loudly that those around us would stop their conversations and the sound of utensils on china would cease as they turned to hear her next words, but the din of the restaurant continued to swirl around us. Nora's words were meant only for me and only to my ears and heart did they seem to cut through the cacophony of everyone's lives and come into focus on mine. Instantly, I knew that she spoke the truth. My eyes began to match hers in joyful intensity and the ends of my mouth rose in a smile, the first genuine expression of joy in a very long time. A new surge of energy ran through my body and an indescribable feeling of strength rose in my heart. My mother would find peace and safety and contentment someday, perhaps not in this life, but in another beyond the boundaries of the mental imprisonment of Alzheimer's. There would be an answer to all of our prayers, those spoken out loud, those murmured in our hearts, and those we did not yet know would be needed.

"Thank you for being the answer to my prayers for a guide through all this," I simply and sincerely replied. "Nora, there are so many prayers finding their way to God, and you are the answer to one of my most fervent – for someone who understands what it is like to be faced with the indignities and the uncertainties of this disease. You know what it does to families and to individuals. Thank you for being my answer."

She smiled back at me and before her face began to blush

ever so slightly she said, "...and there will be an answer for your mother."

The answer for the problem at hand came the next morning, as it had many mornings before, in the form of Elena. Angels come in all shapes and sizes, and Mother's personal guardian angel was not quite as tall as she, had jet black hair and a round face that broke easily into a smile. Elena had become our confidant, our partner in crime, if you will. Coaxing Mother to take her medications, to go for a walk, or even to take a shower required all the energy and creativity that this exceptional caregiver could provide. She had inexhaustible ways to make her elderly charge think an activity was her own idea.

Once again, when it seemed that Louisa and I would have to physically take the keys from Mother's hands or take steps to sabotage the car, Elena came to the rescue by reminding her that she needed a government issued photo ID in order to cash checks. We joyfully gave our blessing as the two of them headed off to obtain said ID. Of course, Mother wanted to drive them there, before Elena convinced her that it would not look good to pull up in front of the state trooper's office with an expired license. Mother acquiesced and let the determined caregiver take the car keys from her hand.

All was going well as they waited for their turn at the counter until Mother saw an elderly woman in line ahead of them successfully receive a driver's license. She decided that she, too, deserved a license and, instead of applying for a government ID as agreed upon with Elena, she would "march right up there" and demand her license back – which she did, pounding her walker on the floor with every shuffling step. With halting words and rambling sentences, Mother presented her case to the officer at the desk. Elena was amazed that the officer had any idea what her elderly charge was talking about. The officer nonchalantly checked the computer screen and, without revealing the source of the information, flatly informed Mrs. Adams that her license could not be renewed because the records showed that she had dementia.

Stunned at first, and then quickly becoming enraged, Mother began screaming at the officer that it was all her daughter's doing and that she did not have dementia. Although the officer had spoken with me earlier in the day - a fact which she did not reveal - as a public servant she was obligated to listen to the ranting of the woman standing before her, giving her the benefit of the doubt as was due her by law. In response to Mrs. Adams tirade, the officer kindly suggested that there were two things Mrs. Adams could do to have her license renewed. The first was to obtain a letter from her doctor stating that she did not have dementia, and the second was to retake and pass the written driving test.

Elena giggled a bit as she described to Louisa and me how Mother snatched the exam booklet from the officer's outstretched hand and indignantly shuffled into an adjacent room to prove to all the world that she was more than capable of driving herself to the grocery store and back again. The female officer and Elena silently watched her go in and waited for the door to close behind her before either of them spoke. The two women's eyes met and the officer asked Elena what she knew about Mrs. Adams' situation. The devoted caregiver made a quick decision not to stand on the elderly woman's right to privacy in favor of her right to be safe and boldly spoke up telling the attentive policewoman that "Mrs. Adams takes a medication for dementia," to which the officer replied without hesitation, "Then we will not be able to issue a license to her."

Mother, indeed, failed the written test, but begrudgingly agreed to take a study manual home to practice and to retake the test again in a week's time. Upon leaving, Elena diligently followed her client's heated request to drive them directly to the doctor's office where she would demand a letter stating that she was of sound mind and fit to drive. Elena parked the car in a handicap space in the shade as instructed by her irate charge.

The duo arrived at the doctor's office in the midst of summer cold season because the waiting room was standing room only, adding to Mother's agitation as she impatiently stood in line leaning exhausted on her walker. They finally moved to the front of the line and stepped up to the receptionist who listened quite patiently while Mother awkwardly explained that she needed a letter saying she did not have dementia. The receptionist was very familiar with Mrs. Adams and quickly retreated behind the steel cabinet stuffed with files to whisper the request to the head nurse.

The nurse knew her by sight and gently motioned for her and Elena to come through the door, and standing in the hallway halfway between the noisy waiting room and the handicap restroom, she explained that the doctor could not provide such a letter because her diagnosis was, indeed, dementia.

Mother was completely taken aback and beyond angry, shouting at the nurse that her daughter was behind this and it was a plot to just get her money and put her in the loony bin.   All eyes in the waiting room turned to watch as Elena forcefully took Mother's arm and guided her and the walker between the tight rows of chairs and out the front door. Other times Elena had taken her discreetly out the side door when she forgot her public decorum, but the rows of turned heads and staring eyes told Elena that the fastest retreat route would be best this time.

"Nora, when my sister and Elena told me that evening what had happened, all I could think of was how Mother's world must have felt like it collapsed in on her. She lost so much that day and I really cannot blame her for feeling deeply unhappy with herself and angry towards everyone else," I said, describing the scene. "Louisa told me to stop trying to reach her on the phone. It disturbs her even more to hear it ring and know that I am on the other end. Mom and Elena now spend a lot of time just talking.   Mom is embarrassed and her pride is hurt. She has entirely stopped calling friends and going to church. Her confidence in herself and who she is are badly shaken.   Louisa is worried that Mom has lost her purpose and is slipping into depression."

Feeling partly responsible for her blue mood, I had difficulty rejoicing over the fact that Mother had finally gotten the message that she should consider relinquishing her car. Much to my dismay, however, Elena soon told us that Mrs. Adams had continued to drive inside Waverly Place and was gradually venturing out onto city streets once again. As autumn approached, we decided to enlist the aid of Mother's sisters, whom we had not told about her diagnosis out of deference for her privacy, but at this point self-esteem had to take a backseat to safety, and we moved forward with a plan to call the aunts that same evening. As Louisa was uncertain that she could find the right words, I was elected, perhaps drafted is the more appropriate term, to make the calls.

My Aunt Goldy, to whose side Mother had rushed a few months prior, was not surprised by my call, and calmly told me that she could tell her sister was becoming extremely forgetful and repeating herself quite often. She told me that Cricket would call her and then a few minutes later call again, completely unaware that the previous conversation had ever taken place. The blonde, blue-eyed Aunt Goldy had a great capacity for compassion and understanding, in particular toward those in need of extra care and pampering. She quickly came up with ideas for making her sister's trip down for Christmas as easy and low key as possible, and sweetly promised to try and work in a conversation about Mother giving up her car keys. We laughed openly at such a thought, for we both knew how strong willed she could be. In fact, it was Aunt Goldy who once told Tom that everyone usually just gives in to Imogene because "it's just easier that way."

The second phone call was to Aunt Minnie and was conducted even more delicately. Aunt Minnie had suffered a stroke and was residing in an assisted living community. According to Goldy, my youngest aunt also had difficulty remembering details accurately, was legally blind in one eye, and relied on a motorized wheelchair to get around. I had never found anything lacking with Aunt Minnie's heart, though, for she was as kind and gentle as Goldy herself who had suggested that I not go into as much detail about Mother's strange behaviors. Goldy was not sure that Aunt Minnie would understand, nor be able to keep my confidence, as she and Mother were very close. So, I did not tell her the purpose of my call, nor that Mother believed a giant worm was living in her dishwasher, that she refused to sleep in her bed because "the ants were so thick they turned the bed covers black," that there was a negro man trying to break into her backdoor every night, or that she could no longer read a calendar or operate an answering machine. Rather, we talked quite sweetly of Aunt Minnie's three grown children, memories of my kind and very religious Uncle Earl, and how her eyesight was fading…and only then did we talk about Mother's forgetfulness. Much to my surprise, Aunt Minnie said in her very soft and warm fashion, "That's not unusual for people with Alzheimer's."

"She knew, Nora! She knew that her dear eldest sister had

Alzheimer's. I let her tell me how she knew, and then we comforted each other. I don't remember exactly what she said, but I always feel as if she has given me a big hug when we hang up," I said tearfully.

I shared the conversations with Louisa, who was so relieved to hear that the aunts were sensitive to Mother's changing ability to remember and had already noticed that she was not herself. It should not have surprised us, as they had been sisters for over seventy years and, although separated by hundreds of miles, knew each other's souls intimately. There is no relationship longer lasting than that of a sibling, and none as strong, or as fragile, as that of a sister.

My own sister and I had been friends for a half a century. We love each other dearly and find joy in every phone call and every opportunity to get together. Louisa has always had great focus in her life and knew from her teenage years that she wanted to follow in our father's footsteps and work for a non-profit. After graduating college with a degree in humanities, she became a professional development expert and conducted training seminars for philanthropic executives across the nation. As she crisscrossed the country teaching and training, her destinations would occasionally bring her near to where Tom and I lived, and we enjoyed her company for a few days, treating her like royalty at the Babstock B&B - the name we had affectionately given our quaint two-bedroom apartment at the time. Those were special times as she and I spent precious hours together relaxing in the beautiful countryside of Upstate New York. It was then that we came to love each other as adults well-established in our own careers, happily married, and in love with life. We enjoyed the same pleasures – strolling through secret gardens, picking herbs at a local farm, and making trips into the city for a show or to visit an art museum.

Having caught the wanderlust of our parents, Louisa and I loved to travel together. Packing up Charlotte and Charlie when they were little, we fearlessly started out on treks across country in search of a mountaintop observatory, or a fireworks display, or the perfect swimming hole. As the kids ventured off to college, Louisa, Matt, Tom and I sought faraway places like Paris and the Pacific Northwest, taking in the beauty of man's creations in art and architecture, as well as the wonders of the master Creator.

Louisa and I both excelled in school in our own areas, I in the expressive realm of music and she in the study of humanities. Louisa is a people person and she has a natural charisma about her that endears her to all. She finds the good in everyone and has that unique gift to motivate and encourage, a quality which served her well as a highly sought after expert on volunteer leadership. She and Matt had the opposite arrangement of most career couples in that she was the one that traveled, and he ran a local business and kept the home fires burning. Their marriage was strengthened by an uncommon bond of fidelity and longing for each other brought on by the many days of being apart. In spite of Louisa's long absences, they raised their children in a close and nurturing home, devoting all their time and energy to shaping them into people of integrity and caring.

Louisa's life, however, has not been without its challenges. While Mother's pathway was strewn with fading signposts, Louisa paralleled that journey with an uncertain walk of her own, which had resulted in unmitigated pain, permanent disability, and premature retirement.

"Nora, my sister has lived with pain of an intensity that I can only imagine. About eight years ago she started experiencing facial pain so severe that she would pass out and have unexplained seizures. After a few years of struggling to manage the pain and the seizures, she was forced to take early retirement. It was a huge loss for her. She told me that it was like dying. Who she was – her very identity - no longer existed. Executives from all the philanthropic agencies that she served throughout the country sent her gifts and retirement well wishes. I don't think very many of them knew that it was an illness that stopped her in her tracks. She has had to reshape who she is, and it has been extremely difficult on her family. After years and years of seeing neurologists and pain specialists, she finally has a bit of relief thanks to a neural stimulator implanted in her brain. In spite of the implant, though, her days are sometimes just a blur of pain and narcotics that dull her senses, making it nearly impossible for her to focus on anything. She is asleep more than she is awake, which concerns me when it comes to making decisions on Mom's behalf."

Nora listened intently.

"Is Louisa homebound like your mother? Maybe that's why she seems so reluctant to take action that would affect your mom's independence."

"Yes, a lot like Mom, Louisa has to rely completely on others for transportation," I explained. "Matt is a wonderfully caring husband and he devotes his evenings to getting her out of the house. They run errands together and usually go out for dinner. Their maid is a good friend from their church and once a month she takes Louisa out on a shopping spree. Josephine is a true gift from God. She and Louisa are very close and their monthly excursion is a day for splurging on themselves. Louisa pampers them with manicures and afternoon teas. She comes home exhausted, but happy to be enjoying some of the things she used to do on her own."

Nora and I were reviewing the events of the last few days in the seclusion of the dinner booth. The sky outside had darkened with rain clouds, and hungry patrons were scurrying in with raincoats flapping and umbrellas dripping. We were glad to have arrived before the late summer rain and, ignoring the impending thunderstorm, I continued to relay the week's events, but was interrupted by a group of school girls who had come in out of the rain, giggling about a picture on their cell phones, their heads close together intently studying the images. Tucking the phones into the pockets of very tiny denim skirts, they fussed with their hair and applied lipstick before making their way up to the counter. After discussing which pastry under the glass had the least amount of calories, the girls all settled on non-fat chai tea lattes, while Nora and I returned to enjoying the calories in our croque-monsieurs.

"You still seem troubled over your relationship with your sister," Nora noted.

"There is more to her story, and I'm wondering if we should save it for another time," I began and then decided to plunge in and lay all of my feelings on the table.

"Another physical burden has been placed on Louisa, and I am torn between the responsibility I feel toward my mother and the compassion I feel for my sister. I don't want to push Louisa beyond her physical and emotional strength. She has been the one to step in and deal most directly with Mom's behavior, and we have both agreed that because Mom is so unwilling to respond positively to me right now, Louisa must be the one to work most closely with her in conversations – many, many difficult conversations about what kind of care she needs and now to bring about a change in her financial situation. As someone with dementia, Mom is a very needy individual and Louisa is the one that has been on the front battlefield with her."

"Are you feeling guilty about that?" Nora asked as she cut into the cheesy crust in the pottery bowl and steam escaped filling the air with the hearty aroma of ham and onion and port wine.

I took a deep breath and allowed the smells of comfort food to calm my anxiety before answering, "In some respects, yes, I feel guilty because I am not physically present for Mom even though I know that my role has been equally important. It has carried its own degree of heartache because I see what should be done to assure Mom's safety and happiness - if happiness is at all possible for her – and I just can't seem to make Louisa understand the need or the urgency."

There was a pause in the conversation – a quiet space of time filled with silent thoughts as Nora searched for words to reassure me, to calm my distress over the disagreements with my sister. Walking the tightrope between what is and what should be – at least from my point of view - had proven to be wrought with painful realizations of just how tenuous our family ties had become.

"If we are to weather this storm, we must pull together. The ship will just bob up and down on the waves unless all of us understand and accept our part in this journey. I feel as though the oars are only pulling on one side of the boat and we are going around in circles discussing the same things over and over."

Nora quickly understood the analogy and replied, "Even though we are twins, Dorothy and I also move in different directions at times. You would think that our approach to life would be similar, but it isn't. We had very different understandings of Alzheimer's. Every sibling has a different relationship with their parent and their other family members, and approaches the disease from various perspectives. Dorothy let me take the lead in decision-making, essentially becoming Mommie's guardian," Nora said.

"When Brother died, we were all sad, of course, and Mommie never understood why he did not come to see her anymore. He was never an influence in the decision-making process, though."

She paused to stir sugar into her coffee.

"It was easier for us than it is for you and your family."

I sipped from my tea cup and thought about each of the six people in Mother's immediate family has a distinct role in her life. We walk with her along similar but different paths, and the task which has fallen to me is to research this awful disease and to understand its hold on her. Louisa's role is more hands on - more present with Mother - and I find that I am jealous of that relationship.

"I sense that you and Louisa want to share the burden equally, but at times there is more weight for one or the other of you," Nora quietly observed. "I would think you could expect that and to accept that there will be ever-changing responsibilities depending on where your mother is in the progression of the disease. Every Alzheimer's individual is just that – an individual – and there is no magic formula or solution to the many, many issues that will arise, both with your mother and with your sister."

Nora put her coffee cup down and intently holding my gaze, said, "You have such love and caring for them. It must hurt terribly to see them both suffering."

My words came slowly and haltingly, in part because I was choking back tears, but mostly out a feeling of helplessness.

"Yes…. Mom's eyes are clouded by dementia and Louisa's by pain. I pray nightly for healing for both of them - and understanding and patience for myself," I whispered, not certain that Nora heard me above the juvenile chatter of the girls at the next table.

Initially irritated, I wished the girls had chosen another part of the restaurant to invade, but soon saw Louisa and myself and our own noisy group of friends decades earlier gathered around a similar table after a Girl Scout meeting. Just as these girls were completely unaware of anything outside themselves, we had been protected from the uncertainty of life's natural progression. Back then, I had only known death briefly when my grandfather died when I was four, and my only real understanding of that event was that my mother cried a lot. We never talked about it and I had nightmares about it for years. The only other mishaps in our young lives were my broken collarbone, Louisa's concussion, and the usual childhood bout of mumps, tonsillitis and measles. We knew nothing of cancer, senility, or strokes. How I wished for the blissful naivety of those days.

"Louisa is facing several major surgeries in the next few months. She now has an additional physical burden to bear, and that is scoliosis. Adult onset scoliosis is very rare, and her doctors have suggested that it has actually been caused by the neuro stimulator which is implanted in her head for the control of her facial pain," I said while tracing my finger through the salt that had spilled on the blue and white checkered tablecloth.

"Apparently, the stimulator has been known to cause a weakening of the muscles surrounding the spine. Her spine started collapsing and twisting around a few months after the stimulator was put in, and her body is basically closing in on itself. Her spine now has a seventy-five percent twist in it and she is unable to stand up without a great deal of back pain. One leg has become shorter than the other because her pelvis is crooked. Her organs are slowly being crushed," I said numbly.

Nora's silence and the expression on her face told me she was listening with every beat of her compassionate heart. Her unspoken words comforted me as tears rolled down my face. My body shook with stifled sobs. The thought of losing my sister was unbearable...the thought of adding to her burden with that of our mother was equally unbearable.

"The tilt in her pelvis must be corrected," I eventually managed to continue. "Only then can the surgeon attempt the two surgeries to straighten her spine. He has never seen this combination in an adult – in children, yes. But, an adult's bones have already calcified and he does not know how to do the surgery. .... She will die without it."

A small gasp escaped from Nora's lips and she reached across the table for my hand, squeezing it and urging me to go on.

"The surgeon is looking for a specialist somewhere in the country who might know how and be willing to take on her case. In the meantime... she waits in so much pain. The hours that she is awake and feeling relatively good are very, very few, and I feel terrible taking those precious moments to talk about the problems with Mom. We have agreed that at least every few weeks we will have a Mom-free conversation where neither of us is allowed to talk about her."

"What a refreshing solace that must be," Nora offered brightly, raising her eyebrows conveying the smallest spark of hopefulness.

I smiled at the remembrance of my last phone call to Louisa – it had been declared a Mom-free time – where we chatted about my niece and nephew, caught up on the antics of their new puppy, and compared notes on growing roses. We laughed about our husbands' latest adventures and proudly bragged about their accomplishments. It was a sisterly call – a time to reconnect, just the two of us.

The conversation with Nora had not been filled with such laughter, and I said goodnight to her out on the brightly lit sidewalk wet from the rain. She promised to keep all of us close in her heart and always in her prayers until we could meet again in a few weeks.

"Call me before then, if you need me," Nora always said before we parted.

The summer heat soon set in and the air was humid, making it hard to breathe. Our spirits were not dampened, though, as Tom's birthday the first week in August was always a happy event. This year he celebrated by taking nine friends to a ballgame, enjoying my office's corporate suite. The day was punctuated by phone calls from his parents, other family and friends, including my sister who had also sent him a GPS for our next geocaching excursion along the shorelines near our retirement property in Bliss, Massachusetts. The only mar on the day was that Tom's train buddy Imogene had not called him with her traditional rendition of "Happy Birthday" sung very ceremoniously over the telephone.

A few days later the chirping of my cell phone told me Louisa was calling and it rang several times before I could dig it out of my purse. She laughed at my breathless hello.

"You sound like you had to run to catch the phone," she giggled.

"No, just rummaging around in my purse is always an adventure. How are you?" I merrily asked.

"Just the usual round of doctors. I'm trying a new medication that makes me kind of loopy, so if I sound goofy…" she started and let out another giggle.

I finished for her, "…it will just make the conversation that much more fun."

"How was Tom's birthday? Did the Mets win?" she asked, referring to another dismal season for his favorite baseball franchise.

"He had a great time. Even when they don't win, Tom always manages to have a blast. He missed hearing from Mom, though. I don't know if she is just continuing to ignore us, or if she just simply forgot his birthday," I sighed.

Much to my surprise Louisa suddenly outburst, "Oh, this is ridiculous! Her behavior has just gone far enough. I just don't understand how she can continue to believe that you and Tom don't care for her."

As we knew, there would be not be a resolution to Mother's reticence nor her forgetfulness, so we gratefully agreed that the rest of the conversation would be Mom-free, mainly because we had exhausted anything more to say on the subject, but also desiring to preserve our bond as sisters rather than adult children of a senile mother. We caught up on the progress of the new puppy training at their house and my attempts to start an heirloom dahlia garden from a little patch of stubborn ground behind our townhouse.

Another week went by with summer thunderstorms bringing a welcome cool front that lowered the temperatures down from unbearable to slightly above tolerable. It would be a very sultry summer and I clicked on the weather report as another round of thunder passed through. Out of habit my eyes tracked down the east coast, around Florida, and across the Gulf waters to Texas where most of the temperature readings hovered around ninety-eight degrees. As I was wondering if Mom's air conditioning was working well, the phone rang and I picked it up to hear her voice, "'Allie?"

She called me by my childhood nickname. My heart skipped a beat. My mother's silence had been broken.

Her voice sounded so sweet in the earpiece as I closed my eyes and envisioned her sitting in her favorite chair in the living room with the sun streaming through the windows bathing the room in brightness. I captured the warmth in her voice and held on to it as we gently worked our way through the pleasantries of "hello" and "how are you." Neither of us mentioned the fact that we had not spoken in many months, but just reveled in becoming reacquainted after a long absence. I didn't think my heart could stand to hear her words if perchance she remembered the reason why she had not spoken to me, but I did wonder what unlocked her heart and cleared her mind enough to call me - and then the answer came.

"I feel so badly. I missed Tom's birthday," and there was a plaintiff sound in her voice as she waited for my reply.

"Oh, Mom, please don't feel badly. You have so many relatives' birthdays to remember, and I don't know how you did it all these years. It has always been so sweet of you. Besides, sending him a belated birthday card just makes his celebration last longer. He would love it if you just sent a card," I said cheerfully and quite honestly.

"Do you really think he would like that?" she said, slightly more upbeat.

"Of course, he loves anything you do for him," I reassured her, and the conversation continued in a lighter, happier mood, as if celebrating a reunion of sorts. I let her lead, and we wound our way through several topics before she tentatively offered, "I love you," and hung up.

There were a thousand people I could have called to give them the exciting news that my mother had finally wished to speak with me, but I relished the sweetness of her voice and the plaintiff gentleness of her words and chose to hold them close in the privacy of my own thoughts for just a while longer.

❖

Chapter 5

Summer melted into fall and with it came more news from Elena. Mother's phone calls were not as frequent as they had been in years past, but each was more precious than gold to me, and I savored every word - all the while realizing that the world she was describing to me was far different from that portrayed by Elena. The security guard at the front gate had responded to emergency calls from Mother several times in the previous weeks, each time reporting back to the front office that there had been no threat, just fear and panic on the part of the resident at 421 Emerald Drive. Her paranoia was becoming more deep seated, and the hallucinations more frequent. She was positive that men were roaming the outside of her cottage peering through the windows at her, thus prompting multiple calls on the distress button hanging from a lanyard around her neck.

Louisa and I were thrilled when Mother had moved to Waverly Place, not only because the old house on Humboldt Street had become more than she could manage, but mainly because of the emergency call system. Help would never be far from her as long as she wore the lanyard or could reach a call button in the kitchen or bathroom. Mother utilized this system a bit too frequently, however, with only two real situations where she needed anything more than reassurance. The true emergency events involved falls in her bedroom, but fortunately, Mother comes from hardy stock and suffered only bruises. As a matter of fact, Elena passed on pointed concerns from the EMTs and the security guards that Mrs. Adams was wasting their time with unnecessary calls and wild stories of gangs of teenagers robbing the residents.

"Nora, I called the head of security at Waverly Place to check out Mom's story about the teenagers raiding residents' garages, and to see if there had in fact been any strangers walking through the gated neighborhoods. He said there had not been any robberies, and furthermore, with all the Waverly Place staff on the streets throughout the day and the security carts patrolling at night, my mother was quite safe. Without coming out and saying so, he hinted that she was having psychological problems," I sighed, not really sure of how to respond to his implication. "She seems to be easily worked up these days by imaginary people,"

"Fear is all too much a part of Alzheimer's," Nora gently pressed upon me. "Paranoia and suspicion can be overwhelming and very difficult for caregivers to deal with.   Has her doctor prescribed anything for it?"

"Are you kidding? She's in a stage where she is even suspicious of doctors and keeps making appointments with this doctor and that doctor and then cancelling them. If she had a true emergency, there would be no primary care physician with her complete history to treat her," I said in a disgusted tone.

Mother's poor decision-making regarding her medical care was so frustrating to me, and I had already pushed her buttons too many times by urging her to see a doctor.   I suspected that her darting from doctor to doctor was her way of running away from the issues she secretly knew she should be addressing. However, now that she was receiving my calls, I had no intention of alienating her from me again - which meant I had to let many sensitive issues slide by.

Louisa, on the other hand, could freely discuss almost any topic with her, and Mother listened to her for as long as her memory and attention span would allow. Any progress Louisa thought she may have made with Mother, though, would be completely forgotten by the next day, forcing Louisa to patiently revisit the same issues over and over. At times we were certain that she knew something was terribly wrong with her memory, while at other times she pushed any signs of disease into a dark and rarely visited corner of her mind.

With every passing week, Mother's mind fought with itself, frequently calling up visions and hallucinations of intruders, both human and animal. Repeated assurances by Elena and the security guard failed to assuage her fears of ants crawling all over her bed, "so thick that they covered the spread and turned it black." From then on she chose to sleep on the sofa rather than encounter the insects in her bedroom. Similarly, she pressed her security alarm for a worm that she was certain had taken up residence in her dishwasher. The security guard rushed over to find her hysterical over a long strand of onion caught in the bottom of the dishwasher. He removed the "worm" and went back to his security post at the gate shaking his head at the crazy woman at 421.

"Elena has such a beautiful way of reassuring and working with Mom. We are so blessed that Mom has her because we can't physically be there for her. I wish Mom would agree to hire her for more than six hours a week. Mom gets so irritated because she has to pay Elena. We think she is pushing her security button rather than phoning Elena for several different reasons – loneliness, fear, and also because she doesn't want to hire Elena for the additional hours."

"She is in such denial of her condition, isn't she?" Nora commented more than inquired. "She will probably never accept that Elena can be a huge help to her in so many ways. Interestingly, a part of her belligerence may be the fact that dementia often brings out an inability to accept guidance from someone younger than oneself. It is seen as an affront to them as the older and wiser adult parent image they have of themselves. She is not ready to give that up and become the child."

"But, Nora, She has so many irrational thoughts and images. It's so difficult to talk to her without wanting to laugh or get angry. I feel like we had a breakthrough last night, though, when she and I talked for a long time. Her phone calls these days are usually very abbreviated, as if she loses interest or forgets what she is talking about. Sometimes I am certain she has forgotten even who she called, but last night she stayed on for a long time and wanted to talk. So, I let her lead the conversation and it was such a soul-baring moment. Mom may not have realized that she was talking to me rather than to Louisa, who she usually speaks with quite freely."

My eyes sparkled and there was excitement in my voice as I told Nora, "For a rare few minutes Mom talked about her feelings. Most of the time with me she covers up any emotion that she thinks might be construed as weakness, but this time she talked about her worries and things that frighten her."

I remember the conversation so well. It wasn't one particularly filled with sweet morsels of praise generally shared between mother and daughter, but it was a conversation none-the-less – one for which I was grateful. One tiny little ember of my mother's former self still glowed under the spent tangles of her mind. Her mind was full of dread for so many things and was a trap for long-held prejudices and horrifying tales of things and persons she was seeing in her dreams… and in her living room…and at the foot of her bed. My response to her attempt to reach out would be a crucial step toward her letting go of at least some of her fear – the fear of judgment and criticism from her eldest daughter.

"Mom," I began. "That must be so terrible to think that someone is lurking outside your house. I know that worries you a great deal."

"How do you know that? You aren't here," she suddenly countered, as if jolted out of her sharing mood and back into one of suspicion.

Determined not to be put off by her accusatory tone, I slowly and softly replied, "I know because I am your daughter, and I am exactly like you. I look just like you. I have the same actions and mannerisms as you. I think like you… and I am afraid just like you are."

I paused to listen to the silence on the other end.

"Together, we can get through this because we know what worries us and what makes us feel better."

Nora's eyes were moist as she listened to my retelling of the phone call, "Beautiful words, Allison. I hope that she responded positively to you."

"It was very hard to tell. She changed the subject and then ended the call," I replied.

The abruptness of my mother's response was not unexpected, and I could only hope she had heard the warmth and sincerity in my voice.

"Nora, even if she doesn't remember the exact words I said, perhaps she will remember the sentiment," I said hopefully.

"I'm told that is true. Even in the last stages, which we pray is far in the future for your mother, they can sense emotions when all other forms of communication are gone. It's as though the heart feels what the mind cannot comprehend, and that feeling lives on in the individual."

Her words took me back to a scene at Waverly Place that Louisa and I had witnessed when taking a tour of the Alzheimer's unit. Mother was so determined to prove to us that she did not have dementia that, when we arrived at her house shortly after that fateful Christmas diagnosis, she arranged for us to take a tour of the community's two memory assistance units. Her long time friend and Sunday school teacher, Howard Spears, picked us up at her cottage and gave us a personal tour of the two facilities, one being the assisted living unit for those who needed memory assistance and the other the Alzheimer's unit.

Howard was well-versed in the dementia unit as his sister-in-law was a resident there. He easily gained access to the locked down facility on the pretense of visiting her and showed us every aspect of the daily care of the individuals entrusted to a team of professional caregivers and doctors. Howard was quick to point out that the residents of the dementia unit seemed only present in body and that their minds seemed to wander off somewhere that only they were permitted to see. Howard demonstrated how many of them simply shuffled along with their heads down, concentrating on the floor as if it would disappear beneath their feet.

I knew then that Mother had impressed upon him the purpose of the personal tour, and I wanted so badly to tell him about the events that had brought us to her side. However, out of deference for her dignity, I remained silent. He would learn soon enough of the difficulties she faced and would subsequently see that his friend also shuffled her feet while studying the strokes of the vacuum cleaner in the carpet.

"At what point do we tell her friends, Nora? Do we even say anything at all? Louisa is not in favor of talking to anyone, but I somehow want to let them know that she may need a little extra care and understanding. Is that too much to ask of friends who, although they have known each other for forty years, may have aging issues of their own?"

My questions came in rapid succession, quizzing Nora on

her own history with her mother.

"We had the advantage of living in the same town as Mommie. We knew her friends and were there when they came to visit. It was easy for them to see what was happening because they were witnesses to our interactions with her," she said as she cocked her head and looked away, as if seeing the gallery of her mother's friendships. The number of portraits in her mother's personal gallery would have been large, but none outlived her, as Nora's mother was one-hundred-two when she passed.

Mother's collection of close friends was small, about a dozen who still lived nearby. We were not certain at first if any of them sensed the things we did, but as the months passed it became obvious that her friends were either completely oblivious to the changes in her or were irritated by her strange behaviors and just thought she had "gone off the deep end." Thinking back to those few relationships of my own that had gone sour – or at least the ones that could not be attributed to my own missteps or lack of attention – those friendships that had been the most difficult to maintain were with people who had emotional issues that simply could not be overcome by any amount of love or caring. I feared that Mother had fallen into this latter category and her mind did not remember how to be a friend. Those that were still left in their tight-knit little community did not know how to love the forgetful, the unkempt, and the unlovable person that my mother had become.

Nevertheless, Louisa and I elected to stay out of Mother's personal relationships with her friends and neighbors – for the moment. As an adult, she deserved the right to conduct herself in a manner of her own choosing, and we could not protect her from any missteps or misunderstandings, much like an adolescent forging new relationships – she had to do this on her own. She and her friends had to find their own way through the maze of aging minds and bodies and to determine what shape their new relationships would take.

Howard continued our tour of Waverly Place with a final stop at the Alzheimer's unit where he wanted to visit a longtime friend of his. We were given access through a double set of locked and alarmed doors. He stopped to be certain the first door had closed behind us before going on through to the second. The three living areas were noisy and full of activity. Some residents were seated in chairs around a common living area, engaged in nonsensical chatter not really directed at anyone in particular, while other residents gathered at the lunch table with attendants close by to assist with a spoon or a fork. Another resident was led across the room, clutching a doll while screaming out that nobody loved her.

We walked as unobtrusively as possible through the large communal living area, stopping to examine a resident's room that was empty at the time. Along the outer perimeter of the room were a family conference room, a glassed-in aviary, a well-stocked library, and an inviting patio completely empty of anything but sunshine. It was next to the patio that Howard found his friend and his family. After whispered introductions, Louisa and I pulled away to explore other areas of the Alzheimer's unit, giving him a few private moments with his friend, for it was obvious that it would be the last time they met. The man was seated in a reclining transfer chair, draped in blankets, head lolling back. His eyes were closed and his mouth slightly parted. We could hear the soft rattle of what would soon be his last breaths. His wife and daughter sat near with hands lovingly placed on his arms, occasionally reaching up to stroke his face. In spite of the noise and activity in the room he looked peaceful...at rest...waiting.

This was a place of beauty and of solace and of rest, more so perhaps for the families who could no longer care for their relative than for the relatives who did not know nor seem to be concerned about where they were. I hoped on the one hand that Mother would never need to come here, but felt blessed that she did have that option if the time came when we could not care for her. We returned to the cottage and she seemed satisfied that Howard's tour had squelched any thinking on our part that she was demented, for how could we possibly compare her to any of the residents of the Big House.

Not too long after Mother and I talked so intimately about her fears and worries, my sister excitedly telephoned me.

"You will never guess what I got in the mail today," she exclaimed. "Mom has put you back in her will."

I was dumbfounded, and then elated, and then speechless.

"When… how did that happen? How do you know?" I asked, barely breathing.

"She mailed a handwritten note to me that said 'My daughter Allison is to receive her fair share,'" Louisa said. "I have no idea what prompted her to change her mind. This came out of the blue."

Louisa's voice was overflowing with excitement, and as she told me again and again how unexpected and miraculous this was, I smiled, knowing that Mother and I had finally reconnected by way of that one phone call where she had dared to bare her soul to me and I had taken on the burden of knowing her secret anguish. She could not deny that I was her flesh and blood, her heart and mind, sharing joys in days past and now holding her tight as if to chase away her fears. I was welcome once again in my mother's arms.

"Thank you for telling me, Louisa. That means so much," I said, wanting to reach out over the miles and hug her. I wanted to tell her about my conversation with Mom, but felt that the sanctity of those precious moments should not be diminished by sharing it with others and so I let Louisa exclaim over and over, "This is so exciting."

But, being the more practical of the two of us, I deigned to interrupt her.

"You know that the note isn't admissible in court as part of her will, Louisa."

"Why not? It's in her handwriting and it's obviously her intention," Louisa sounded worried.

"Wills have to be witnessed and more importantly, the testator has to be of sound mind. Anything Mom does at this point is highly questionable," I argued.

Louisa followed up with a conviction that I had not heard in a long time, "Well, my family and I have talked about it, and we decided that Mom striking you from her will was not fair, especially since she did it out of unjustified anger. We decided that when Charlie executes the will, he will divide it evenly between you and me - the way Mom and Dad always intended."

My heart was immediately crowded with warmth. For the first time in many months, I felt surrounded by the care and support of my sister and her family. The determination and force in her voice gave me that vote of confidence I so desperately sought. I closed my eyes and relaxed into the joyfulness of that feeling.

And then the impact of Louisa's words hit me.

"When *Charlie* executes her will? But, but... I am Mom's executor," I stuttered, hoping that I had misheard.

There was a silence and then a sigh on the other end of the phone line.

"When Mom wrote you out of her will, she also changed the executor from you to Charlie," Louisa said very slowly, as if implying that the slower delivery lessened the sting. "She didn't want me because she thinks I am too sick, so she chose Charlie..." Louisa's voice began to break, but she managed to say, "... and I think it is a marvelous idea."

There was an odd mixture of contempt and, yet, at the same time approval in the tone of her words. It was the first time that I could remember my sister openly admitting that she was not in control of her life and that her disability had forever taken away so much of whom she was. Louisa and I had never spoken of her struggles on such a personal level. Like the true Adams that we were, one's challenges were rarely discussed. Disappointments, fear, loneliness, depression were all borne privately. The simple utterance that Mother perceived her as too ill to take care of her family and professional responsibilities was an admission that she, too, was suffering from Mother's harsh and judgmental attitude. I realized that Mother's illness and subsequent lack of sensitivity had touched a raw place in Louisa's heart.

My mind raced. In spite of her attempt to bring a positive light to bear on Mother's actions by lamely adding that she approved of the choice of executor, the raw truth was there. Our mother had shunned both of her daughters, and in a state of mind blurred by dementia, she selected a teenager to execute her estate. The warmth I had felt only moments before suddenly turned to ice and crawled throughout my whole being until I was numb and could feel nothing at all. The phone became heavy in my hand and I desperately wished for a few minutes of solitude as a myriad of thoughts swirled around in my mind like a vortex.

Sensing pain by my silence, Louisa continued to press on, "At least the executor is another member of the family. She could have chosen an outsider."

Regaining my composure and fighting back that all too familiar ball of anger rising in my throat, I breathed a deep cleansing breath and said, "I am going to do the right thing and accept Mom's attempt to reunite us. If she believes that a simple handwritten note is a legal and binding statement, then I will not tell her any differently. I really appreciate you and your family wishing to keep to the intentions that Mom and Dad built together. Thank you," I added very sincerely in spite of the robotic way in which I had delivered my decision.

"No, thank you for not giving up on Mom and our family," Louisa was quick to say before dissolving into tears. "This disease has been so awful. I just hate what it has done to us and to Mom."

Nora had listened very intently to my story when I too began to cry, and she simply reached out her hand across the table to touch mine. There were no words to comfort me at that moment, and in her wisdom, Nora let me weep. The little scrap of paper should have been a reason for great rejoicing, but rather served to drive home the fact that my mother was struggling with many demons. We could only imagine the pain she must have felt radiating throughout the depth of her being, believing that her family had either turned against her or that they were too sick to function. Not that I wished my father would have had to witness this terrible thing happening to her, but I did yearn for his presence and wisdom in helping us face this terrible thing that had taken over my mother. Nora understood all too well and silently offered her support as only a dear friend can.

When I could finally speak some time later, my first words to her were not about Mother's will, nor about her choice of executor, nor Louisa's pain. Rather, I wished to change the subject in a feeble attempt to put it behind me and move on.

"Well…, Mom finally went to see a doctor. She went to a new guy, a cardiologist," I said with as much positive energy as I could muster. "She went in complaining about a pain in her abdomen."

The mood in our corner of the restaurant brightened considerably as Nora's ready smile appeared and her blue eyes twinkled.

"She went to a cardiologist for a pain in her abdomen?" she almost giggled as the question came out.

"Yes! Louisa tried to explain to her that he was not the right type of specialist, but she wouldn't listen. Consequently, he is sending her to a gastroenterologist," I said, smiling back at my friend.

"After the visit Mom told me that she really resented the fact that the doctor had a copy of her files. So, at least we know that he is aware that she was diagnosed with dementia, although at this point it is probably fairly obvious to any medically trained person," I quipped.

"She seems excited to tell me now about all her doctor visits, and I have to be very careful not to interject too many comments or suggestions. Mom gets defensive if I sound in the least way like I know anything at all about her condition. She wants to be in control and I suppose that makes sense. None of us want to be shepherded around like a little child. Elena tells us in our weekly calls that Mom keeps missing appointments or shows up for them too early or on the wrong day entirely. I don't think she actually knows what is happening. She tries to see the wrong doctor for the wrong symptom on the wrong day."

We found our sense of humor again over dessert when Nora reminded me that chocolate is actually an antidepressant and we, subsequently, ordered several pieces of chocolate cake and pie between us before I continued.

"Elena - bless her, she is such a patient dear one to Mom – said that last week Mom was confused about the time and place of an appointment, but Elena drove them to the office as directed by Mom. Nora, they sat in the doctor's waiting room for close to three hours before she would let Elena approach the receptionist and inquire about the supposed appointment."

"Three hours. You have got to be kidding," Nora exclaimed before attending to the last slice of chocolate pie.

"Yes, the receptionist explained that Mrs. Adams did not have an appointment and was not a patient of theirs and suggested that she try the doctor next door," I couldn't help but laugh at the thought of Mother stamping her feet and yelling at the poor girl behind the glass.

"They went next door and the equally young receptionist there said she had missed her appointment two days ago and they would have to reschedule. Elena said she wanted to tell Mom, 'I told you so,' but decided there was no virtue in pointing out the faults of others. She took her back home after making another appointment, and in front of Mom wrote it on the calendar."

"Can your mother still read a calendar?"

"It's very odd. She can still write checks, but she can't read a calendar very well. I have been finding out in the research literature that graphs and the relationships of numbers are a problem for dementia patients," I said. "And recipes are impossible. Completing sequential steps and measuring out ingredients seem to be the issues. You should have seen the congealed dessert she tried to make for us when we were there."

We were both glad at that point not to be eating fruit cocktail encased in gelatin and polished off the last of our dessert before I continued.

"Mom asked me why it never turned out right for her anymore - which just her asking me for my advice was miraculous. We have never been able to cook together in the kitchen, but that is a long, long story which I will save for another time. I suggested that she be really careful when measuring out the water, and I showed her the instructions on the side of the box. She took the box from me, but shook her head and put it back down again."

Looking furtively into Nora's kindly face, I sighed, "We don't think she can read and follow a recipe anymore."

Nora's knowledge of dementia had been gained over decades of time watching both of her parents die from the disease. Most of us would have shut those memories into a deep corner of our minds and refused to revisit them, but Nora chose to share those moments with me and sincerely hoped that the coping skills she had learned during her parents' journeys would be helpful to me. There was a comforting solidarity between us, and I welcomed every piece of wisdom that she could share.

"At a certain point numbers and graphs become meaningless. The ability to read the symbols and to comprehend them is lost. Your mother may have reached that stage," Nora gently said.

As we talked about the many things in our daily lives that required an understanding of numbers and graphs, letters and words, symbols and concepts, I nodded a reluctant acceptance of the fact that my mother now needed constant assistance with most aspects of daily living. We parted with a hug and I drove home slowly, noticing as if for the first time, the hundreds of messages conveyed through symbols and words on the dashboard, street corners, and on storefronts. I wondered how much of it my mother could understand.

"How does one survive in a world full of coded messages that no longer make sense?"

As the weeks passed and reports of doctor visits became more and more garbled, Elena eventually created a system to keep track of appointments, and after a few thwarted attempts to go into the examining room with her, Mother finally acquiesced and began to request Elena's presence at every appointment.

"Elena is a miracle worker," I routinely told Nora. "Neither Louisa nor I can get a peep out of Mom regarding her doctors' names or even why she is going to see them. Either she genuinely doesn't remember why or she is being stubborn again and shutting us out of helping with medical decisions. She is seventy-nine and should not be making such decisions on her own."

My sister had slightly better success in discussing medical issues with her, and one afternoon Mother called to tell her that he – Louisa eventually surmised that "he" was the gastroenterologist - was scheduling her for surgery and announced that she was having a colostomy. Louisa said the call was an interesting combination of *"look at me, I'm having surgery"* offset by genuine despair at the thought of wearing the contents of her colon on the outside of her body. I am not certain which of our relatives actually had a colostomy bag, but do recall that Mother was repelled by the inconveniences that the procedure forced upon one and avoided associating with anyone who could not "control their bodily functions."

Mother has always had very interesting prejudices toward this person or that person for reasons varying from the color of their skin to how they greeted her. Most of her prejudices I suspect were driven by a fear of the unknown, of the "what if." The origin of this extreme wariness of most people and things around her remained a mystery, but it was becoming evident that paranoia was to be a permanent and gripping part of her newly emerging personality.

Louisa listened to her talk at length about how painful and inconvenient it would be to have a portion of her intestines cut away, but that it would take care of the problem she was having. Exactly what that problem was remained a mystery, for she could not describe nor explain it to my sister. As Mother struggled to recall exactly what the doctor had said and to decipher what was written on the doctor's orders, Louisa suddenly asked her to spell the name of the procedure.

"Oh, Mom, you aren't having a colostomy! You are having a colonoscopy," Louisa cried out, laughing with relief. "That's just a test to see what's going on in your colon. There is no cutting involved."

This did little to assuage Mother's fear and was not retained in her memory any longer than it took to hang up the phone. In every subsequent conversation with either of her daughter's over the next month, Mother still referred to the procedure as surgery and called the church office to put her name on the prayer list for her upcoming colostomy. She called her medical buddy Sylvia to take her for the surgery and started packing her suitcase for a long hospital stay.

"I think the clothes were getting dusty sitting in the open suitcase on the guest bed. If it weren't for the sad fact that Mom is so completely confused and simply cannot grasp what procedure is going to be performed, it would be comical, Nora. I have explained to her numerous times that she won't be spending the night, that it's just a test, no surgery involved," I explained to Nora over the phone.

We had agreed that for the next few months we would suspend our dinner engagements and visit on the phone instead. I actually found our phone conversations to be more helpful than trying to keep our voices down in public. Free from the distractions of other diners, I enjoyed curling up on the comfy green upholstered loveseat in the living room to talk with Nora. The loveseat was within earshot of Tom's favorite recliner in the family room, and I think he felt more in tune with what was running through my head and heart. We both knew that his skill, like most men perhaps, was as a fixer. This disease cannot be fixed and we found ourselves at cross purposes many times as I tried to find a trail through the endless maze that is Alzheimer's. Talking on the phone with Nora, therefore, met two needs – my needs to have a caregiver who was a listener rather than a fixer, and his need to know what I was feeling.

And so the conversation began, "Mom has already tried to start drinking the colon prep, and the procedure is still a month away. Elena caught her just before she was attempting to measure out how much to drink. She took everything away from her and hid the preparation supplies - which made Mom very mad."

"Oh, the poor dear. I can't believe that the doctor is making an elderly woman with dementia go through this," Nora said, shaking her head.

I shook my head in agreement as if Nora could see me in the front room of our townhouse. Dusk was beginning to fall and children's voices could be heard from the sidewalk just beyond the open windows. I watched them happily drawing chalk faces and making up stories for their imaginary friends, not unlike my mother.

"Mom also swears that the doctor put her on a liquids only diet and she hasn't had anything solid to eat in over a week," I said, rising to close the windows. "Elena called me yesterday and said Mom is not doing very well. She is getting sick from taking medications on an empty stomach. Mom is having trouble keeping even liquids down, and she feels so weak she can't stand at times. As much as Elena has tried to get her to eat and prepares and leaves meals for her, Elena finds them in the trash the next day."

"Why doesn't Elena stay and see that she eats?" Nora queried.

"Mom sends her away. She is indignantly refusing to have Elena more than two hours three days a week, and that is just not enough time to cover doctor's appointments and mealtimes. Elena has no choice, she has to leave," I bemoaned.

I paused, not knowing what else to say. Mother's confused state was leading her to make unhealthy decisions, and much like the four-year-old who refuses to eat, she was completely unmovable and stuck firmly to her resolve. I hurt for her and longed to be with her, if only to sit next to her while she dutifully drank a cup of broth.

Dusk had begun to fall quietly in what had become my sanctuary in the living room. The children playing outside the windows had been called indoors for dinner, and the sunlight was low and dappled as the day disappeared. The rhythm of life began to slow in preparation for sleep and rest. My thoughts turned even more inward as I silently prayed for guidance.

"She needs help, Allison," Nora's soft voice whispered in my ear.

A moment or two passed before I responded, "Louisa and I have tried talking to Mom about having Elena for longer hours each day. That would be so helpful in getting her back on a proper diet and to regain her strength."

"She is going to need it for the colonoscopy prep. That is the one procedure that I just dread every year," Nora said with laughter in her voice.

Mother had insisted so vigorously that the prescribed solution be brought out of hiding and put back on the kitchen counter where she could see it, that Elena had to comply.

"Every time Mom gets up from her rocking chair in the living room and starts back toward the kitchen counter, Elena heads her off and distracts her until she forgets why she was going for the jug of limeade flavored mix."

Nora and I laughed at the image of the kindly caregiver blocking the way of her elderly charge and gently, but firmly turning her around like a sheep dog would with a member of its flock.

In spite of the ingenuity of Elena's actions, it bothered me that such steps were necessary. This was my mother.

Why was it necessary to take away her self-will and independence? Why had she become like a little child in an adult's body?

I was suddenly grateful for the comfort of the sofa and its overstuffed pillows, and cocooned myself, wrapped up in a blanket that somehow protected me from the uncertainty of the future.

"She has no idea what the colonoscopy prep is going to do to her. Even if Mom could follow the directions correctly, she moves very slowly because of arthritis and might even forget where she is headed and wind up in the garage. This is just going to be a disaster for her," I predicted.

Nora quickly agreed and again expressed consternation at any doctor who would impose this procedure on a dementia patient. She urged me to find out who the doctor was and to contact his office to discuss it. We both knew that the privacy laws would most likely prevent me from being successful, but I promised her that I would try, and we said goodnight.

I sank even further into the pillows and tried to clear my mind. Hearing that the phone call had ended, Tom came in to the living room and held me close until I found enough peace to fall asleep in his arms.

Two weeks passed as Mother became weaker and weaker, and I decided that I had to enlist the help of the doctor's office. Elena secretively told me the name of the doctor, found the number for me, and I made the call. As Nora and I suspected, Mother had not indicated anyone's name on the release forms and the receptionist made it clear that the doctor would not speak with me, but she reluctantly called the nurse to the phone. The nurse listened for a few minutes – only listened in keeping with privacy regulations – as I explained the situation. Once I said that my mother had dementia, the nurse's lips were unsealed and she immediately understood the problem. She agreed to call Mother with an additional "doctor's order" that she must have someone with her for the preparation, as well as for the day of the procedure.

Mother called me that night to complain about the pain in her stomach and that she hoped the surgery would take care of it. To my surprise she also told me that the doctor's nurse had called to inform her that someone must be with her for the surgery. I knew that she had not completely understood the message and that she still did not accept the need to have Elena help her the afternoon and night before. Risking that my mother would shut me out again, I perilously ventured forward to describe what the preparation entailed and what it would do to her system, and to her clothes, and to the floor. The sound of Mother's jaw setting could almost be heard through the phone lines. For the next few days both Elena and I pleaded and cajoled until, in a final move of desperation, I told Elena to just show up at the house mid-afternoon the day before and more or less bully Mother into letting her help with the measuring, the pouring, the drinking, the waiting, and the inevitable cleanup to follow.

Elena did just that. She faithfully guided her very surprised and bewildered client through every stage of the preparation, until exhausted, Mother fell asleep and Elena went home in the wee hours of the morning, pledging to be at her side the next day. Mother had insisted that her medical buddy Sylvia would take her and stay with her for the week that she was sure would be needed. However, true to her word, Elena joined Sylvia in the waiting room for the "colostomy" to be completed.

A group of faithful friends and church members had also gathered at the hospital to support her, but upon finding out that this was only a routine colonoscopy, left the waiting room in disgust to return home. Word would quickly spread that their dear friend Imogene was having a touch of senility and the request for prayer was delicately reworded. Only Sylvia remained to wait with Elena. A few hours later, she helped Elena put her dear friend of thirty-five years into the car and thanked Elena for driving Mrs. Adams home and settling her back into her own bed for the remainder of what they hoped would be a quiet day.

In later conversations with Mother, she repeatedly told me every detail of Elena's assistance, right down to her sliding around on the bathroom floor in an attempt to clean up the results of the prep.

"It was everywhere, Allison. I just couldn't get my pants down fast enough," she exclaimed.

"Now, aren't you glad that I suggested you have Elena there with you?"

"Oh, yes. She really worked so hard. I could not have done it without her," Mother said gratefully.

Elena's attentiveness and caring solidified the bond between the two of them, and Mother began to rely on the kind woman for more everyday things, no longer taking the reins, but relaxing in the trust she now had in Elena. The two of them began to walk down to the mailbox together and Elena guided her charge back home again. The caregiver was there to wash out Mother's hair and restyle it when she mistakenly sprayed it with bug spray instead of hair spray. On grocery shopping day they compiled a grocery list and went shopping together with Mother haphazardly loading up the grocery cart and Elena coming along behind and re-shelving the items. Perhaps most importantly from my perspective, Mother gradually began to allow Elena to sort her many pill bottles, reorder prescriptions, and administer her medications.

Louisa and I rejoiced at this small triumph and were very thankful for the inconveniences of Mom's "colostomy." She never complained of stomach pain again after the colonoscopy and spread the good news to all her friends and to the pastor that the "surgery had cured her." For a few precious weeks following, life for us all seemed to slow down into a predictable pattern of mornings and evenings, days and nights, weeks and weekends.

"So how are you and how is your mother?" came the almost routine, but very welcome, inquiry from Nora as we finally sat down together some months later in the empty restaurant down the street from the sandwich shop. Our dinners had followed the same pattern for months, and feeling the need for freshness in the venue, we decided to try the restaurant in the new hotel near Nora's workplace as an administrator for a women's fertility clinic, something that suited her well. Her life was constantly influenced by her desire to be in ministry, whether with friends, family, or at work. Helping women achieve the joy of conception and childbirth was the perfect outlet for her energies. In spite of coming straight to dinner from a long day at work, I never found her without a smile or words of cheer. She was a remarkable person with the glass always half full rather than half empty.

"I noticed a difference in Mom almost overnight after the colonoscopy in that she seems calmer and happier. Part of the daily burden of managing her life is being shared by someone, who is not her overly-pushy daughter, but a gentle person who knows how to help her at just the right moments," I enthusiastically told Nora. "She is actually sedate, and that has freed her mind somehow."

"That's wonderful," Nora exclaimed.

We ordered from the menu and then set about catching up with each other's lives.

"Thank you for my birthday card, Nora. That was so nice,

and I was surprised that you knew the date."

"The birthdays of all the choir members are listed on the rehearsal calendar. I took at peek at it and wrote down your birth date," Nora confessed.

"Well, it was very sneaky, but thoughtful, of you," I said and rejoiced to tell her that my mother had remembered my birthday, as well.

Perhaps Louisa or Elena had made sure that Mother knew, but a card and package arrived a few days before my birthday. Never knowing whether to open the card or the gift first, I chose this time to read the card and found the words, "I love you" to be especially sweet. The card went on the mantle above the fireplace in the family room as was our custom. The flowered and glittered sentiment was a nice balance to my husband's card with a picture of a bowl of peanuts on it and a greeting that read, "I'm nuts about you."

Picking up Mother's package, I tore off the brown grocery bag wrapping to reveal a smaller box swathed in toilet paper. Her gift-giving practices were always entertaining, and it seemed that this birthday gift would be no different. I carefully unwound the toilet paper and found a little plastic box that had been partially crushed despite the copious amounts of cushioning. The box was vaguely familiar, and I opened it to discover an ivory lace butterfly lying on another padding of toilet paper. The butterfly evoked pleasant memories of a trip that my high school choir had taken to Europe some thirty-six years earlier. While on that trip, I carefully selected the perfectly starched lace butterfly pin from a Viennese street vendor and gave it to my mother upon our return home. The threads holding the little pin and clasp on the butterfly were now unraveling and hanging off the back, but otherwise it was in pristine condition, just as it had been when I gave it to her.

A range of emotions swept over me, the first being a warm sensation at the thought that my mother had saved this little gem all these years, like a child's crayon drawing on the refrigerator. The warmth gradually gave way to a question mark, however, "*Why was she giving the butterfly back to me now?*"

I got out needle and thread to repair the damaged clasp and then called my mother to thank her for the birthday present.

"Oh, I'm so glad you like it, dear. I picked it up at the Hallmark store and thought of you," she chirped happily when I called to thank her.

"That was very sweet of you," I managed to say as my mind returned to the question mark.

I later asked Nora, "Why did Mom go into her own jewelry box and claim it was something she picked out especially for me? Did your mother shop for presents in her house and then pass them off as hand-selected treasures?"

Nora did not know whether to laugh or to sigh. "Mommie did that, too. I won many Academy Awards unwrapping and thanking her for presents that I knew had come out of her closet. Regifting is epidemic among the elderly. I suppose it's because of a fear and inability to get out of the house and actually go shopping, in addition to their worry about the cost of a gift when there is a perfectly suitable gift sitting right there."

"I shouldn't be surprised. Mom has done this for several years now. I've received everything from her old exercise bike all wrapped up in Christmas paper complete with a huge bow to a silk scarf that Louisa had given her a few years before. I don't want to say anything because it will make her feel badly, but it's just such a letdown," I said.

"She is not trying to snub you, I am sure. She thinks she is honoring you by giving you something precious of hers."

I took those words home with me and let them sink in, hoping that they would push out the more hurtful thoughts and feelings of disgust for my mother's lack of understanding and initiative. Over the next few weeks I began to research online why dementia individuals are so inclined to re-gift their possessions and soon discovered that those with memory impairments also display a declining ability to grasp and follow society's rules of etiquette and begin to lose the manners taught to them during their upbringing. Once again, what I perceived to be Mother's insensitivity was, in fact, my *own* insensitivity to her diminishing skills in following often nebulous and somewhat esoteric rules of behavior.

I doubted that she had the opportunity to learn or practice the finer points of etiquette and good manners while a child, as my grandfather and grandmother were focused on their jobs at the state prison and at the local cannery, respectively. The purpose of a salad fork and how to make introductions did not come up as topics in family discussions, I am sure. Somewhere along the way, however, Mother did learn the finer points of etiquette, perhaps in secretarial school or from the many ladies journals that she loved to read. She was a very gracious hostess and loved to entertain, although we did so infrequently in our home. Her models for the social graces were her mother-in-law and Jacqueline Kennedy, who captured the hearts of every young homemaker in the early 1950's. It may be interesting to note that Mother followed Mrs. Kennedy's lead with enthusiasm and Mrs. Adams' example with a sense of dread and duty. Nevertheless, Mother did become a lady, far removed from her wood chopping and milking days. My father loved her dearly for all of her skills, those that were finely polished and those that were still rough around the edges.

My birthday in early November was followed by a Thanksgiving that was truly unlike any our family had ever had.

"Louisa, I am concerned about Mom flying to you at Thanksgiving. I can see her hopping in her car and driving herself to the airport. Elena says she is still driving even without a license and has started going on short errands to the pharmacy and the grocery store. She's becoming more and more brazen because she hasn't been caught by the police. She isn't open to having Elena drive her because she doesn't want to pay Elena to do that. I tried to explain that the cost of parking the car there would equal more than Elena's fee, but she just doesn't get it. Do you have any ideas?" I asked my sister.

"That's a good point. I didn't even think about that, I have been so busy trying to get everything done. It's been really crazy here with Mom arriving the day before Thanksgiving, Charlie's Eagle ceremony the day after Thanksgiving... and then we are celebrating Christmas with Mom the next day because she will be in Nacogdoches this year for Christmas, and that is the only time we will have to exchange gifts with her," Louisa spoke breathlessly. "And, I am really not feeling very good right now. The weather has made my face hurt even more."

"Sister, no matter what you are able to get done, everyone

always loves going to your house. You are such a wonderful hostess. Mom will just enjoy seeing you. She won't care if things aren't exactly the way you want them to be."

"Thank you, Allie. I'm trying…" and her voice trailed off.

She had been close to tears in so many of our conversations lately. The chronic and debilitating pain that she experienced every waking hour required so much of her strength to overcome, and with the pressures of holiday preparations, Louisa needed a respite from the added burdens of caring long distance for our mother. That respite would not come, however, for many months.

I could hear her gathering her strength again, and breathing through the pain, she said decisively, "I will call S.T. to see if he is available to take her and pick her up from the airport. She will probably get mad at me for going around her, but we can't run the risk of her getting in the car and driving herself."

"Good plan. Let me know if you need my help with any of that," I offered.

We would not be going to Louisa's for Thanksgiving this year. It was our turn to be with Tom's family who were gathering at his sister's house in Raleigh. In one sense, I was glad to have a reprieve from always being on my toes with Mother, for I was still not used to the delicate way in which I had to talk to her. Not one to hide my feelings and reactions easily, I am told that my face and body language speak very loudly when in her presence. Mother could pick up on any little prickle that I felt when she repeated the same story for the third time in five minutes. Shielded behind the telephone, I could practice reacting positively to her new personality quirks without worrying about the message my body was delivering.

"Nora, how was your Thanksgiving?" I asked as we settled into the familiar old leather booth on one side of the sandwich shop a few days after the holiday had come and gone.

The hotel restaurant had not been anything to write home about, so we had elected to return to our comfortable booth where we knew the food was good.

"Wonderful! We had such a good time with my daughter and her family. Ate too much, but that is what it's all about – family and feasting," she shared merrily, her blue eyes sparkling. "How was yours?"

"Tom's family is a riot. There was plenty of fun and visiting – never a boring moment. Everyone is doing well," I answered, holding a spoonful of tomato basil soup over the bowl to cool.

"And your family..." Nora began, and for the next half hour, I updated her on my mother's visit to Louisa's.

Just as promised, my sister had arranged for S.T. to take Mother to the airport the day before Thanksgiving, getting her there at four p.m. for a six o'clock flight that evening. Louisa was frustrated that Mother could not remember the day or the time and kept giving S.T. conflicting information, finally telling him to arrive at her house a day too early at four in the morning. S.T. had the presence of mind to call Louisa and reconfirm the day, time and flight number, and managed to dodge his eccentric friend's anger by showing up at the correct time on the correct day. He commandeered a wheelchair and shepherded her through security and on up to the gate before seeing her off as she was happily rolled down the causeway by a flight attendant. She always looked forward to trips to see Louisa and Matt, and had packed her suitcase days in advance.

Louisa and Matt built their house sixteen years ago in The Woodlands north of Houston. It is a beautiful slate blue ranch house sprawled across two acres of rolling hills. Matt is a master craftsman in wrought iron with a thriving business in custom decorative pieces primarily for homes in the affluent Post Oaks area of Houston. Finishing out their own home in a rich mahogany mission style, many of the rooms showcased his skills with wrought iron.

"Nora, Mom has been visiting them in that house since it was in the sheetrock stages, but when she walked in this time it did not look the least bit familiar to her," I explained. "Louisa was stunned when Mom asked her for a tour, but politely showed her around just as if she had never been there before and reminded Mom where her bed would be nestled into the front room which doubled as a study. After asking for the second time where the bathroom was, Mom settled in for the weekend. My sister called me that night and was concerned that there had been such a huge change in her memory since she last saw her. Mom didn't even remember that they had a dog."

The Butler family consists of Louisa and Matt and their children; Charlotte, now a junior in college, and Charlie, a freshman in college; plus the family dog. Roger, the Labrador, exuberantly greets every person who enters their house, and unashamedly demands one's attention. Mother has never been a pet-friendly person, and the closest we ever came to owning a pet while growing up was a goldfish in a glass on the kitchen windowsill. Because of Roger's size and playfulness, she usually turns her back to him with her arms raised high to protect herself from his happy lunges. After the initial inspection of each visitor, Roger waits for them to be seated on the sofa before presenting his backside for a good scratching just above the tail, which Mother generally declines to deliver.

"Roger knows something is different about Mom. He didn't jump up like he always does with her. This time he just walked up to her and put his body next to hers and just quietly stayed by her side the whole weekend," Louisa told me several days after the holiday had died down and everyone was back in their respective homes. "It was the strangest thing. He senses that she needs something, and she actually started petting him and talking to him. They have become good friends."

"Well, I know that the dementia unit at Waverly Place has dog therapy for its residents," I noted. "Roger would be a good candidate. I wonder what it is that he senses."

"I don't have a clue, but Mom has started calling Roger her Granddog," Louisa said with amusement. "Mom did really well once we got her oriented again. She enjoyed seeing Matt's parents, and they had a nice conversation. She didn't say anything weird and didn't repeat herself with them too much. She ate everything at the table, not just onion dip," which we both agreed was a good sign.

"It was sweet how Mom doted all over Charlie when he got his Eagle. I put Char in charge of her grandmother because a lot of the time my head and face really hurt and I had to go to bed. She made sure that Grandmother was ready on time for everything we did and that she didn't get lost in the house or when we were out somewhere."

I wondered how Charlotte liked that assignment. She is always the grandchild that winds up looking after her grandmother, but she always rises to the occasion and treats Grandmother with great respect and care. Their relationship has reversed from the time when Charlotte was the child who climbed into her grandmother's lap for a story, innocently calling her Grandfather. Now, it was her grandmother that was confused and needed the loving care. Ironically, Charlotte is the member of the family who most genuinely emulates her grandmother's gift for caring. Her heart is soft and warm, and she puts her hands and feet into action to reach out to others, not always willingly, for as a young adult she has not yet found the maturity to reach beyond her own needs and to serve others without a great deal of complaining along the way.

"A lot of caregivers have that same difficulty," Nora said when I paused in the story. "Balancing the needs of someone who requires constant supervision and attention like your mother with taking time to meet the needs of yourself is very tricky. Caregivers can just simply give away too much and have little left with which to nurture themselves."

"As Christians, though, that is what is required of us - to give completely without prejudice even for ourselves. So, how do we find that mid-point where both persons are fulfilled and neither is totally spent?"

"I don't think we are asked to completely pour ourselves out until there is nothing left to pour. God only asked that of one person – his Son. The rest of us mere mortals can take time to breathe in fresh air, to rest our bodies, and to restore our minds. There should be no guilt in doing that," Nora suggested.

I stored those thoughts away for future reflection and continued to describe the family's celebration of Charlie's Eagle Scout award. Coming from a Scouting family there is no higher achievement, and Charlie had worked diligently to earn it. He proudly pinned the mother's emblem on Louisa's lapel, who in turn pinned the Eagle on his uniform. Grandmother could not have been happier. She and my father had encouraged him up through the ranks, and now she stood proudly by, with Charlotte at her elbow, while her only grandson received this honor.

The moment of triumph passed all too quickly, though, as Grandmother pointed to Charlotte and blurted out, "Now if this one would just graduate and get a job...."

"Oh, my," Nora gasped. "Has your mother always been so judgmental, or is this part of her latest personality change? Unfortunately, Allison, you can expect more outbursts like that as she progresses through the stages of the disease."

I looked at Nora with a troubled face, wishing that I could protect my niece from further abuse at my mother's hand, all the while knowing it would probably not be preventable.

"Louisa told me that she jumped in between them at that point and announced that it was time for pictures. Cameras came out all around and happy chatter picked up again as family members posed beside Charlie in his uniform. Charlotte said that even Roger found a spot in the portrait as the mascot for the whole affair." I said. "But then, more drama with Mom..."

"Mom, where is your camera, the one we gave you for Christmas last year? We need to get some shots with your camera," Louisa said.

"Oh, I used it up and threw it away after the pictures were developed," Mother answered.

In the silence that descended Charlie spoke up, "Grandmother, that wasn't a disposable camera. It was digital. They should have printed off the pictures and given you back the camera."

"They did and I threw it out when I got home because it was all used up," she insisted.

Charlie and Louisa glanced at each other and, realizing that Grandmother's technical knowledge was limited to the operation of a manual can opener, silently agreed to buy her nothing but disposable cameras from that point on. For several years Charlie had served as the official restorer of all things electronic at Grandmother's house. He had magically retrieved over two dozen voicemail messages from her answering machine, "fixed" her garage door opener by replacing the batteries, and patiently explained to her the difference between her cell phone and her cordless home phone. When she accidentally turned off the cable selection on the remote control and could only receive four network channels, Charlie again worked his magic and reprogrammed the television and the remote so that she could browse through more than fifty channels, provided she remembered to aim the remote at the television rather than at the ceiling.

While Charlie was the fixer, like his father and grandfather before him, Charlotte was the helper, pitching in with a hand to hang draperies in Grandmother's living room, to reach for a pitcher on a high shelf, or to plant flowers in her patio garden. She was also the designated chauffeur since both her mother and grandmother could not drive, all the while keeping up a constant dialogue of happy chatter. Charlotte was also the one who helped rinse out Grandmother's mouth when she brushed her teeth with liquid hand soap rather than toothpaste.

"She did what?!" Nora's eyes grew big.

"The soap dispenser looked like a tube of toothpaste, I suppose. She came out of the powder room with soap bubbles coming out of her nose, complaining that the toothpaste tasted funny," I said, trying to hold back the laughter and not succeeding. "Charlotte said it was hilarious to see Grandmother standing there in her flannel robe and silk nightcap blowing bubbles every time she spoke. It probably tasted awful and Charlotte took her by the hand, led her back into the powder room, and began giving her glasses of water to gargle with. "

Her ill-timed comment about Charlotte's hope to graduate from college had stung, but Charlotte shrugged it off and willingly went to her grandmother's aid.

"Char and I are kindred spirits when it comes to Mom's stinging words. We have both borne the brunt of her callous comments, which have taken us both off guard. Her dismissal of me was so hurtful, and my niece is equally puzzled at the treatment she has received. She asked for the opportunity to meet Grandmother's plane at the airport. She wanted a private time to visit, just the two of them. None of us knows what transpired in that conversation, but after Charlotte arrived back home with her grandmother she exclaimed to Louisa, 'You are right, Mom. Grandmother is crazy.'"

"This disease impacts everyone in the family, Allison, as you have said before," Nora acknowledged. "There must have been some precursor to Charlotte's comment for her to agree with your sister. It sounds like a consensus had not been reached until then, and that is really tough on a family when members are at cross purposes."

"Well, Charlotte did not share with any of us what they talked about on their hour long ride from the airport, but it seemed to have changed her from a grandchild into an adult, partnering with the rest of us to look after Grandmother," I noted with a certain sense of pride in the once gangly teenager with braces.

Thanks in part to my weekly discussions with Nora, I now knew with my whole being that dementia teaches humility and selflessness. It is an illness carried by the whole family, and Charlotte and I hoped to carry that burden with patience and understanding in spite of the heaviness of the load. Her grandmother's comments showed a lack of understanding and support for her evolution from an unsure teenager into an adult with a clear focus for her life. Charlotte wisely chose to let her grandmother's comment go unanswered, saving the family from another unpleasant holiday scene.

In the three days that Grandmother was at the Butlers, Louisa orchestrated the family celebration to move from Thanksgiving dinner, to the Eagle ceremony, and finally to Christmas morning. The day Mother was to fly home, the five of them, plus the two dogs, gathered around the Christmas tree, which had been erected and decorated right after the Thanksgiving leftovers had been put away. As the tree went up, Grandmother's suitcase was opened to reveal a treasure chest of items which she carefully removed one at a time and painstakingly delivered to the tree - walker in one hand, present in the other. None of the gifts were wrapped, and when Charlotte offered to wrap them for her, Grandmother replied that she didn't want them wrapped because she wanted to explain each gift. Her granddaughter argued that she could still do that after the present was unwrapped, but Grandmother insisted, "Let me do it my way." Charlotte backed away and left her to continue the task of taking one gift at a time to the tree until the space beneath the boughs was filled with an assortment of items that would rival any garage sale.

The family gathered around the tree at the appointed time,

and as was our tradition, each member in turn unwrapped a present, or in the case of Mother's gifts, feigned surprise at the presentation of a pair of pants hangers or a turkey baster and then politely listened to the explanation of the gift. Charlotte won the acting trophy for her portrayal of the delighted granddaughter when Grandmother gave her back the scarf that Char had knit for Grandmother the previous year.

"Nora, it just didn't make any sense. Previously, Mom always wrapped her Christmas presents, and rather creatively, I might add. Why she chose to forgo wrapping this year is a mystery...and Char was so bewildered by Mom's regifting of the scarf," I said, shaking my head.

Our dinner had lasted longer than usual and the restaurant was nearly empty, but we had not yet reached the conclusion of the conversation.

"Social conventions are set aside and new, seemingly illogical, ones take their place. It all makes sense to her," Nora reminded me. "Which is more important – to make sure she follows tradition and society's views of acceptable behavior or for her to be happy in her own recreation of a world she can understand?"

"That is a rhetorical question, right?" I inquired, squirming in my seat. "It is very difficult for me to see the world as she now does, and to accept it without wanting to correct the course of her life and to bring it back into line with reality. I desperately want her to wrap the Christmas presents."

Nora waited before taking the last sip of coffee to gently say, "You have already adapted to her needs just by realizing that dementia has changed her and that she will never see the world as it really is. Who does it hurt if she leaves the presents unwrapped?"

I felt myself slipping back into a state of grief at the loss of my mother, but at the same time found a greater resolve to assure her happiness no matter where this journey took us. We parted with Nora's question hanging unanswered in the crisp night air.

Shortly after thanksgiving, a teller at Mother's bank notified Elena that Mrs. Adams had run her car into a pole their parking lot, scraping some of the paint off the pole and putting a long scratch in the side of the driver's door. Mrs. Adams was sitting in the bank lobby crying hysterically and begging them not to tell her daughter Allison. Of course, I was the first person that Elena called after she and another of the aides safely ferried the car and Mrs. Adams back to the cottage.

"Louisa, what are we going to do about Mom's driving? She doesn't seem to care that she is having accidents and is driving illegally, and is not making any moves towards relinquishing her keys."

I was more insistent than usual in voicing my concern.

"Oh, I know. She kept telling Matt at Thanksgiving that things are easier now that she isn't driving. She didn't have to worry about filling the car up with gas or paying for the insurance. We wanted to laugh because we know she is still driving, and whether she drives or not, insurance still has to be paid for as long as she owns the car."

Whether out of avoidance or lack of a plan to separate Mother from her car, Louisa had not answered my question. Every second Mother spent behind the wheel of a car she put herself in peril, as well as the lives and property of those around her. Elena had become a master at convincing Mrs. Adams to let her drive them wherever they needed to go, but she was certain that Mother was sneaking out on her own between the caregiver's visits. Groceries suddenly appeared in the refrigerator where the day before there had been none, or prescriptions miraculously refilled themselves. But, the evidence against her came down hard when she could not operate the garage door opener properly and lowered it on top of the trunk, trapping the car beneath the garage door. Somehow she managed to get out of the car and called Elena in a panic. Mother said nothing to either Louisa or I about the extra cost of having Elena come over and release the car from the clutches of the garage door.

Louisa, however, was as immobile as the garage door in her reluctance to force the issue with Mother. Her hope was that Mother would voluntarily come to her own conclusion that it was no longer safe for her to be behind the wheel. No amount of persuasive arguments caused Louisa to give up the notion that Mother was still capable of rational thought and would eventually come to the decision on her own.

"She could go to jail if the police stop her. The fines are in the hundreds of dollars and she could be sued if she causes property damage or injury to someone...and, how can we live with the thought that she might actually kill someone or herself," my voice raised in pitch and volume.

It had been many, many years since I had raised my voice at my sister. Not since we were children had I yelled at her, but Louisa's own thought processes were dulled by the massive quantities of narcotics she had to take to even begin to live with the pain of intractable trigeminal nerve neuralgia. Our phone calls always had to be timed for that small window in the day when she was awake and free of most of her pain. I was in awe of her fortitude, but frustrated when her disability clouded her mind. I would never tell her that, but like my mother, she was acutely aware of when I was displeased with her and none more so than now.

"Please don't be angry with me," she cried. "I'm doing the best I can."

I lowered my voice and apologized for pushing her.

"*Dear God,*" I prayed. "*Of the four women in this family, why was I the one to receive the least amount of patience?*"

Louisa regained her composure and proposed that we leave things in the hands of our aunts who Mother would be seeing in a few weeks. It sounded odd just to say that. For the first time in our lifetimes, she would not be spending Christmas with one or both of us. I knew her decision was more a product of running away from me than of a desire to go to Nacogdoches for the holidays. Mother told me that it was because she had not seen her sisters in two years, which I countered with a reminder that she had just been there for Aunt Goldy's hip replacement.

That resulted in the very defiant comment, "But I never got to see her."

"Then how could you describe the flowers in her room, if you weren't there?" I retorted, and so the argument continued until she hung up the phone in the middle of one of my irritated comebacks.

After a final very hollow click followed by deep silence, I knew that I had most likely caused another retreat of Mother's presence in my life. I was deeply ashamed that I had instigated yet another heated exchange with my beloved parent.

"How can I continue to be so insensitive, Nora?" I bemoaned with my head in my hands, gripping the locks of hair between my fingers – the hair that was thick and brown and wavy just like my mother's. I wanted Nora to excuse my behavior, but knew that a reprimand was more in order.

"You have a strong desire to be right," Nora stated very simply. "It supersedes everything else, which in one sense is a testament to a strong orientation to the truth. However, truth is not always appropriate. Sometimes, loving kindness must override truth."

"Loving kindness must override truth" echoed in my head, which was empty of anything but remorse at that moment. I had not turned on the light in the now darkening living room, and gentle shades of purple, gray, and green swept over me, washing away all thoughts but those of the sage that God had provided.

Judging from my lack of response that she should continue, Nora said, "Your mother only wants to be loved. Truth - in this case the reality of her situation - scares her and she is running to those that she believes will support her."

Louisa believed that the impending Christmas trip would be the key to moving her to make the right decision about driving. I was not so certain that our aunts would readily agree to be the catalyst for Mother to turn over her car keys. Aunt Goldy was still driving and Aunt Minnie had only recently given up driving because she simply could not see the road any longer. Louisa was recalcitrant, and against my better judgment, I agreed that we would leave things in the hands of Mother's sisters. I added one condition to this agreement – Elena would do everything in her power to assure that Mother rely on her for transportation from that time until Christmas. I had no difficulty asking this of Elena, who was only too happy to prevent Mother from getting out on the streets. Elena set about calling her employer several times during the day to see if she needed anything, to keep her occupied and distracted from anything having to do with the car. All went well until the week before Christmas when Elena approached Mother about driving her to the airport.

"No, no, Sylvia is taking me," she insisted.

Not satisfied that she had indeed made these arrangements, Louisa called Mother's friend to confirm the day and time of her flight bound for Nacogdoches. Sylvia knew nothing about it, but volunteered to take her anyway, and on Christmas Eve arrived at Mother's doorstep only to find S.T. helping her into his car for the ride to the airport. The longsuffering Sylvia graciously turned around and went back home to call Louisa.

"Nora, it seems that Mom knew she had contacted someone about taking her to the airport, but couldn't remember who," I said with a sigh. "It's a wonder she has any friends left at all."

As Mother was arriving at her sisters in Nacogdoches, Tom and I arrived at Louisa and Matt's in The Woodlands, and our two families fell into the joyful and familiar routine of going to the movies, playing games, taking in a concert, cooking our favorite recipes together, and just generally enjoying each other's company. Christmas was celebrated the next morning with the traditional exchange of gifts, every one of them carefully selected and brightly wrapped. Louisa and I set aside time after Christmas dinner had been devoured to call Aunt Goldy's house, hoping to catch the trio of sisters there. And they were – complaining of having eaten too much and laughing over the antics of the newest great nephew. It was good to hear Mother's laughter and we savored it.

"Have you had a good Christmas?" she asked us. "Where did Tom go for Christmas?"

Louisa and I looked at each other. I answered, "We are all here at Louisa's together, Mom. You are the only one that isn't here and we miss you. Did you get the presents we sent to Aunt Goldy's house for you?"

"No, there were no presents from you here."

"Mom, I made a photo album for you and shipped it with two books for Aunt Minnie and Aunt Goldy," and I described the photo album in detail.

"Oh, that. Yes, it came," she said, moving on quickly to, "How is the weather there?"

"What was that all about?" Louisa asked when we hung up. "Why did she change the subject so quickly, and why on earth does she think Tom was not with you?"

"She is so easily confused these days and very focused on herself. Haven't you have noticed that her attention span is only as long as she can remember a train of thought?"

I explained what I had read in the Alzheimer's Association literature about the different stages of memory loss. "Did you have a chance to view the video I sent to you, Louisa?"

She had not, but I was not surprised, due to the her own short attention span because of the cocktail of narcotics she took to kill the pain in her face, which unfortunately also took away most of her ability to stay awake. I gave her a hug and let it go. I was learning that forcing things on my family was counter-productive, particularly with a subject as difficult as Alzheimer's. Tom told me in private one evening as we prepared for bed that Matt had said, "Just let the woman grow old in peace."

He was still in denial and not ready to see the truth about Mother's illness. There it is again, the word "truth." In this context, however, it was important that the truth be known, and I wondered how to bring my family into a sense of understanding and acceptance of Mother's condition, for only then could we assure her wellbeing. Mother's daily living skills were comparable to an elementary aged child. Dementia was reversing her memories and abilities, causing her to forget the very foundations of a happy life.

Occasionally, I would hear glimmers of understanding in Louisa's words, such as when she told Char that things would never be the same again – that we would never go to Grandmother's house as a whole family again. Her head knew the truth, but Louisa's heart had not completely accepted it. That realization could not be forced upon her – she had to grow into it.

I asked Louisa, "Did you notice that there were no Christmas presents from Mom to Tom and me?"

Louisa gasped, "No, I didn't. Are you sure?"

"Yes, little sister, I'm sure. Mom either had no intention of giving us presents or she just forgot, bless her," I answered, and turned away with a heavy lump right above my heart.

❖

Chapter 6

"*H*appy New Year, Aunt Goldy," I cheerfully greeted my aunt when she answered the phone. "I just wanted to call and thank you for the marvelous time you showed Mom at Christmas. She was so happy to be with you and Aunt Minnie. I think it was the break she needed. How did things go?"

"We loved having her. It's been too long since the three of us were able to spend a lot of time together. We just sat here at home and let everyone come to us, except for when we went over to Jess' for Christmas dinner. Cricket knew everyone's name and I think they really enjoyed seeing her," Aunt Goldy said. "Cricket was a little confused about where the bathroom was and whose house we were in, but seemed to be doing pretty good otherwise."

"Cricket" is a funny little term of endearment in the Hickson family, one of three, in fact. Aunt Goldy's name is actually Fanny, but she had been nicknamed Goldy because, as a baby, her hair was reddish-blonde and shone like gold. Aunt Minnie is named after her mother, Oleta Minerva, and like myself uses her middle name as her given name. I wonder if she looks at her photo ID with surprise upon seeing the name Oleta, just as I go through an identity crisis every time I see my first name, Amanda, on my passport.

Cricket is my mother's nickname, and there are two stories of how she acquired this name. The first is told by Mother who claims that an uncle, upon the first time seeing her, declared she was as cute as a Cricket. With a full head of dark brown hair and very plump cheeks, she was, no doubt, a darling baby. The second story is told by Aunt Goldy and is just as likely to be true. According to Goldy, the three sisters, relatively close in age, were placed on a quilt in the shade of a fruit tree. The grass was inhabited by various creatures, including all manner of things that jumped onto the quilt. Goldy still laughs to recall how, at the sight of crickets hopping toward them, Imogene jumped up and began running around the outside of the quilt screaming, "Crickets, Crickets." The nickname stuck. Whether decreed by her uncle or by her sisters, we will never really know how Mother acquired the name Cricket, but it was always used to show affection for the most extraverted of the sisters.

Aunt Goldy continued to tell me about Mother's visit, and chuckling at the remembrance of something, said, "You know that Edgar's father-in-law is a pastor, and so he is really friendly. Cricket was positive that he was trying to pick her up, even though his wife was standing right next to them. She was sure he was putting the moves on her when all he was doing was striking up a conversation. Cricket didn't like it one bit, but it was funny!"

I was happy to hear that Aunt Goldy enjoyed Mother's visit, and I then placed a call to my Aunt Minnie.

"She was a joy to be with. We had a lot of laughs," her youngest sister said cheerfully.

Of the three, Minnie is the most jovial and in spite of her own physical hardships, always left me with the loving feeling of our strong family ties. I hated to ask her if the subject of her sister's driving had come up, but needed to know how Mother may have received the gentle prodding from her baby sister.

"She told me about the DMV taking away her license," Aunt Minnie began. "I think she can still drive around Waverly Place, though, without a license and not have any problem."

"I appreciate you talking with her about it, Aunt Minnie," I said, carefully choosing my words. "Mom has told me that she has trouble remembering what all the knobs and buttons are for in the car, and we are concerned that it might not be safe for her to continue to drive, even inside Waverly Place."

"You don't need to do anything about her driving right now," she said in her slow and reassuring way. "Oh, she had difficulty remembering things when she was with us. We had to help her a little bit with dominos, but otherwise she did real fine."

Her words were anything but reassuring. Playing dominos and driving a car are not comparable activities, and it was clear that

Mother's sisters were as reluctant as my own sister and certainly not willing to provide the support I had hoped for. We were no further along in Louisa's resolve to coax Mother to come to her own decision about driving than we were six months earlier when she had been declared unfit to drive by the State of Texas.

"Louisa, do we have a plan B?" I asked her that night on the phone. "I think you have to go there and just *take* the car."

Louisa was quite disappointed to hear that her hope to enlist the aid of our aunts had not panned out, and after enduring a very pointed monologue from me on the dangers of an individual with dementia behind the wheel, she finally came to the conclusion that we would have to force Mother to give up the car. We both knew, however, that simply showing up on her doorstep one day and demanding the car keys would not accomplish the objective. Our very resourceful mother would simply have new keys made. No, the car had to disappear, hopefully taking her desire to drive along with it.

We also knew that it had to be Louisa, accompanied by Charlie and Charlotte. Louisa's thought was that they would drive up before the kids had to go back to college. Charlie would tell Grandmother that his personal car had been recalled, and he could not drive it until the part came in, which was not to be for several months. He needed a car to go back to college and wondered if he could buy her car since she no longer drove. Charlie would drive the car back to The Woodlands with Charlotte and Louisa trailing behind in their family car. That was the plan - neat, quick, and clean – like ripping a bandage off.

It had taken several months to convince Louisa that our elderly mother should stop driving. Taking away her independence would be painful on many levels and my sister placed more value on Mother's feelings than, perhaps, she did on her life. It wasn't really, forgive the expression, driven home in her mind until quite coincidentally a few days after Christmas that an elderly driver forgot which pedal was the accelerator and which was the brake and killed over a dozen shoppers at a flea market. Louisa had not heard of the accident, not able to stay awake long enough to view the news or read a newspaper. I found the most detailed account of the incident that I could and emailed it to her, hoping that something would spark her into action – and it did.

Mother was surprised that her daughter and grandchildren wanted to come so soon after just having seen her. She forgot whether that had been Christmas or Thanksgiving and in whose house they had gathered, but she told them to "come on" in her beautiful slow drawl. They timed their arrival for well after dinnertime the day after New Year's, and spread out into the guest bedroom, the living room sofa, and an air mattress on the living room floor. They all chatted about nothing in particular for a few minutes and then headed for bed. Grandmother saw that her grandson had claimed the sofa, her usual sleeping spot now that ants had invaded her bedroom. She wandered around the small kitchen and dining room adjacent to the living area for some time before going into her own bedroom for the night.

Conversation had been light when they first arrived as everyone was tired, and there was no hint from any of the three of what was to transpire the next day. The night was quiet until close to midnight when Grandmother suddenly appeared in the living room wildly waving a flashlight about the room.

"Are you okay, Char?" she asked, truly concerned for her granddaughter's safety. "I heard a gunshot and thought you were hurt."

Char groggily lifted her head from the air mattress and said, "No, Grandmother, I am fine."

Charlie sat up on the sofa at the sound of his grandmother and reassured her that everything was fine and that she should go back to bed. As Grandmother shuffled away leaning heavily on her walker, Char glanced at her brother and said, "Thanks for checking on me." There was no reply from the hunched over figure retreating down the hall.

The lights were turned back out and calm reigned until the next morning when Elena arrived for the usual routine of changing her client's memory patch, making sure she ate breakfast before taking her morning meds, sorting pill bottles for the lunchtime allotment, walking her down to the mailbox, and taking out the trash. With all the chores out of the way, the five of them sat down around the table for a mid-morning cup of tea. Louisa, and Mother, too, learned all about Elena's family and her history. Mother seemed surprised that most of what she had told us about her caregiver was, in fact, not true.

Then Louisa took a big breath and launched into a speech that she had practiced in her mind many times during the three-hour drive the day before.

"Mom, there is something that we hope you can help our family with," she began. "Charlie's car has been recalled."

"WOO!" exclaimed Mother.

None of us had any idea what that word meant, but she had used it for as long as I could remember to convey alarm and surprise, invariably accompanied by a shaking of her hands to emphasize the point, whatever that might be.

"The part for the car is back-ordered and won't be in for a long time, so he can't drive the car. He really needs a car to go back to school. We wondered…if you would sell him *your* car since you are not driving any more. It would really help us out," Louisa beseeched, stretching out her hands to touch Mother's arm.

"No, I need the car," was the very quick reply as she removed her arms from the table to clamp them tightly together in her lap. "My two caregivers use it."

This surprised Elena who gently reminded her that she had her own car and was only too happy to drive her client anywhere she needed to go.

Puzzled, Louisa asked, "Mom, who is your second caregiver?"

"Amelia – she runs errands for me," was the curt response.

"Amelia is your housekeeper, and housekeepers aren't allowed to drive residents' cars," Elena gently contradicted her.

Louisa was grateful that Elena was there because Mother had come to trust her caregiver and relied on her for guidance. For the next half hour, the conversation went back and forth across the table, with every objection that Mother made countered by one of the other four. Charlotte brought up the fact that she would not have to buy car insurance or worry about maintaining the car. Charlie reiterated how much he needed a car and offered to buy it from her for $1,000. Elena pointed out that Waverly Place knew her license had not been renewed and would become suspicious if a household without a driver had a car. Louisa listed all the transportation options that were at her disposal between Elena and Waverly Place, as well as help from her friends. One by one, her strenuous objections were quieted until she was backed into a corner and begrudgingly gave in to her grandson's request to buy the car.

"Nora, that afternoon they all piled into the car and went down to the county registrar's office to change the title on the car, over to the bank to deposit Charlie's check, and then to the insurance agent to cancel the insurance policy. All that before dinner! Louisa said she did not want a night to go by with Mom thinking about getting rid of the car. She just wanted to get it done. Mom's spirits softened slightly at the local diner, where Louisa treated everyone to dinner."

I smiled to myself, imagining the quick pace at which Louisa and my niece and nephew must have moved. They were all focused on the mission at hand and did not let a second go by that was not filled with activity or chatter, leaving no room for Grandmother to change her mind.

The next day was Thursday - beauty shop day. A caravan of cars – Charlie, in what had been his grandmother's car; Charlotte and Louisa in their family car; and Elena, with Mrs. Adams safely buckled into the passenger seat, all drove over to the administrative building for her weekly beauty appointment. They went in to be introduced to her hairdresser because Grandmother liked to show off her grandchildren - and while she was being shampooed, Louisa and the kids said their goodbyes, walked out into the parking lot, and drove away in the direction of The Woodlands.

Louisa called me as soon as they reached the edge of town and the cruise control was set on seventy miles-per-hour. We had been out of contact while she and the kids were with Mother. I purposely remained apart from the intervention at Louisa's fortuitous insistence. She feared that my involvement might send Mother into a deeper resolve to keep the car, and there was a very real possibility any suggestion of my support would alienate her from me even further, if that were possible. Louisa was now my protector...as much, I suspect, as Mother's.

"We have the car," were Louisa's first weary words. "She was dead set against it initially. The first time I mentioned it she crossed her arms and just refused to give it up. Charlie, Char, and Elena were great. They helped so much at just the right time. Mom really had no choice with the four of us sitting there."

"That is fabulous news, Louisa. I am *so* relieved," and I congratulated her on a job well done. "How are you doing? You sound tired."

"I am. My head and my back hurt. There must be a storm coming in. That always makes it worse. Plus, I'm not used to getting in and out of a car so often and cannot lie down when I need to," she said wearily. "It was a really difficult time both physically and emotionally. We had to be on our toes every minute to avoid making Mom defensive or mad. I think we accomplished that, and she has some sense of having done something good with the car, instead of just having it taken away, even if we had to lie to her to get it done."

"Thank you for taking on the burden of doing this. It was so absolutely necessary," I said with genuine gratefulness. "I hope you can get some rest now while Char drives you home."

It was hard to wait a few days to call my mother, but it was necessary to continue the illusion that I had been removed from the activities of those few days. I never knew when I call if Mother will receive my voice with joy or with consternation. Some days were better than others, and at times I simply told her I would call again when she was in a better mood. "Hey, Mom, how are you?" was the usual beginning of our conversation. Her answer determined the course from there, whether it would be light and happy or dark and negative.

"They ganged up on me. My family ganged up on me," was her somber and immediate reply, cueing me to take the encouraging and sympathetic track.

"What happened, Mom?" knowing full well what she was referring to, but playing my out-of-the-loop card.

"I sold the car to Charles. I had no choice. They ganged up on me," she repeated.

"Oh, Mom, I am sorry. You must be feeling a great loss without your car."

"Well… I am," she said with a note of surprise that I would understand. She continued to open up and pour out her emotions,

"It's hard to go into the garage. It's so empty. I cried and cried... How will I ever get along without it?"

My mind flashed back to a moment when she had asked almost the identical question, except that then she was wondering how she would get along without my father who had just passed away. We were sitting elbow-to-elbow under a funeral tent next to my father's gravesite. Mother had held up well under the stress of the previous four days and was a figure of strength for us all until that moment when the reality of his death hit her. Tom had just lowered the urn into the ground and each of us dropped a single red rose onto it. As the first shovelful of dirt was unceremoniously shoved into the hole by a very disrespectful groundskeeper in a dirty gray uniform, Mother let all her emotions out in a loud shriek.

Unlike many of her outbursts, this one was real, and she began to sob, "How will I ever get along without him?"

Louisa and I wrapped our arms tightly around her, as much to console her as to comfort ourselves. The three of us dealt with his passing in different ways, but, Mother, who had the greater share of grief, and true to her indomitable nature, nobly rose to the challenges of widowhood - until now, when her diminished mind would no longer allow her to remember how strong she really was. My thoughts turned back to the present and to my mother who had another difficult loss and transition to overcome. I tried to be as encouraging and supportive as possible; although I must admit, my heart was doing a happy dance of its own.

"You have Elena. She can take you places - and doesn't Waverly Place offer rides to doctor's appointments and grocery shopping?" I said, knowing that the answer was yes.

"I don't want to use the shuttles. The drivers are grumpy."

I was glad that the conversation was steering away from the family and more into the logistics of how she could get around without a car. She was no longer interested in talking about what the family had done to her, which told me that she had no ill will towards them. Perhaps she felt relief that the decision had been made for her and had moved on to a new stage in her life where relying on others for her needs was the new norm, an uncomfortable, yet necessary norm.

"How do you know the drivers are grumpy, if you have

never used the shuttle?" I quizzed, knowing as soon as I said it, that challenging her was a mistake. It really wasn't important that she believed the drivers were grumpy or not, as it was clear that she had no intention of utilizing their services.

"I heard them one time when they drove up to the house where my mailbox is," she retorted, making up the lie only milliseconds before it exited her mouth.

Changing the subject, I brought the focus back to Elena and the services that she had to offer. I urged Mother to hire her on a more frequent basis to help with shopping, errands, and doctor's appointments. She realized how fortunate she was to have Elena and fervently sang her praises for the next few minutes. Thankfully, we were able to end the phone call on that positive tone.

Louisa was relieved to hear that Mother had not vilified her for asking that she sell the car to Charlie, and over the next weeks we all praised Mother profusely for helping out by making a car possible for her grandson, reinforcing the positive impact of her generosity.

"She must feel thrilled to have done something so wonderful," Nora exclaimed. "You gave her a dignified way to relinquish the car. Bravo."

"It did seem to work out well," I replied. "Mom has been telling her friends that her grandson was in a bad way and that she came to his rescue and offered her car to him. It is such a sweet feeling to finally have made a positive step or two in the right direction. We all needed this break in the storm, and Louisa and the kids did a marvelous job. It was hardest on my sister, not just because it is heart wrenching to play the part of the parent to one's own parent, but traveling always takes a lot out of her."

When I described the conversation about Waverly Place's shuttle service, Nora observed, "It's amazing how good she is at covering up. She is so adept at creating stories, and most of the time they make such good sense that you don't know what is grounded in truth and what is not."

We spent the rest of our hour on the phone comparing notes on the tales our mothers wove. Her mother often believed that hurricanes were pounding down the doors of the nursing home, while my mother swore hordes of people were rushing her house. Although there were no real solutions to helping either understand the difference between fact and fantasy, I found some comfort in knowing that adopting one's own picture of reality was quite normal for a person with Alzheimer's.

My sister, however, was still a long way from confronting the reality of Mother's condition. She could not bear to think that our mother could be so severely stricken and staunchly stuck to her own delusional belief that Mother would snap out of if she just regulated her medications or started eating more healthily. Phone calls to Louisa always left me in a state of disappointment, impatient for my sister to come to the realization that Mother was seriously ill.

"By the way, we got a package from Mom today, which I assume is a belated Christmas present," I told her when next we talked on the phone right before Valentine's Day. "The box is nicely wrapped in Santa Claus paper. Tom and I will open it together when he gets home tonight."

"That's wonderful, Allie," Louise cried out. "That was really nice of Mom to send you a Christmas package. I truly think that because you weren't going to see her at Christmas, she thought presents for you weren't necessary. It's so funny how quirky her logic has become."

I once told Nora that my sister could take any negative situation and put a positive spin on it, but Tom and I firmly believed that Mother never had any intention of including us at Christmastime as part of her punishment to us for whatever wrong she thought we had done.

"We called her to thank her for the presents. She was pleased we called and apologized that they were so late. Sometimes, I don't think she remembers why she is mad at us," I said - to which Nora mildly laughed, for although there is a certain sense of comedy in the games Mother plays, we know they are brought on by great insecurity and loss of memories.

However, in all truthfulness, the box of presents had been a great source of amusement when we opened it and saw the array of items that had been carefully assembled from her own closets and drawers. For Tom she selected the charger for the digital camera which she had thrown away, and for me she chose the devotion book which Aunt Minnie had lovingly inscribed, "To Cricket, with love, Minnie." The rest of the box contained the usual toothpaste and toothbrushes, sticky notes, potholders, and gloves to "keep us warm in the cold winters in Massachusetts." Mother explained every gift and its purpose in detail, with the exception of the camera charger.

"I don't know what that is, but I am sure Tom can use it," she said. Changing the subject, she asked, "How is the house building coming along?"

"Uh....it's great," Tom improvised. "The house plans are perfect for what we have in mind. We hope you will come see us when we have retired there in another eight years."

Elena had forewarned us that Mother's sense of time had become quite skewed. She knew we planned to retire in Massachusetts, but was telling everyone that we had already packed up, moved north, and were busily building a fourteen-room house. Mother's hairdresser had argued with her that I was not old enough to retire and surely she was confused, which pushed Mother to the edge and she became quite hostile in the beauty shop. Elena intervened, and after calming her client down again in the chair so that the other half of her head could be cut, she pulled Carolyn aside to advise her to just go with whatever stories Mrs. Adams comes up with.

Carolyn, however, felt the obligation to let Deborah Barnes know about the decline and hostility of one of the residents and went to the independent living office to voice her concerns.

"Can Deborah do anything to encourage your mother to have a caregiver with her more often than six hours a week?" Nora asked.

I frowned and shook my head.

"Deborah has a responsibility as a social worker to look out for the welfare of residents in independent living, in addition to protecting the property of the corporation and well-being of other residents. Contractually, independent residents may live without supervision unless they pose a threat to themselves, others, or to any physical property that belongs to Waverly Place. Only then can Deborah impose any type of restrictions or conditions on a resident.

In Deborah's history with Waverly Place, there have only been three cases where residents were asked to seek other living arrangements. Mother, fortunately - or unfortunately, depending on how one sees it - does not fit any of those scenarios, unless we are completely unaware that she has been streaking through the neighborhood, missing her monthly payments, or having hallucinations which took her screaming into the street."

"You will get a kick out this, though," I said with a chuckle. "Elena said Mom has enlisted her help in getting another car. She wants to go car shopping."

"Oh, my," Nora said, staring at me with disbelief.

"We aren't surprised. Mom is such a stubborn individual and has not quite let go of the fact that she really had to stop driving. She never believed it would happen to her, and it is a blow to her image of herself. I think she secretly knows it was necessary, but is putting up a show for the sake of her pride," I said. "The good news is that Mom is relying on Elena more and more, and hopefully Elena will be able to redirect her attention elsewhere. I really think it's a passing fixation."

"Do you realize how calmly and easily you said that, Allison?" Nora asked with warmth in her voice. "You are beginning to find an acceptance of your mother's new normal."

"Thanks, Nora. That means so much to me," I said, appreciating the praise. "Just one more thing before we say goodnight. Mom has asked Elena to park her car in the garage and has started referring to the car as hers."

"Oh, my! She has such delusions. That must be difficult for you to hear things like that," my friend replied. "But, as you know, it really doesn't matter if she wants to pretend..."

"As long as she doesn't steal Elena's keys and take the car for a spin...," I said, and we ended another phone call with a parting prayer on our lips for greater understanding and patience.

Louisa and I did not hear anything from Elena for the next few weeks, and took it to mean that "no news is good news." My phone calls to Mother were uneventful, and a comfortable routine settled in, affording us all a much needed respite from the drama of the last few years.

Nora and I settled into a rhythm, as well, and talked about

the peace and calmness that was beginning to come over my mother, bringing a period of relaxation for Louisa and me. Nora shared with me what to expect during this time and applauded me for the transformation in how I saw my mother. While I continued to stumble and react badly to Mother's new personality, and she in turn countered with her own ferocity. Love continued to prevail in spite of the rockiness of our paths.

I was reminded of the church marquee I had seen some years ago which read, "The brook would cease to sing if the rocks were removed." That brief little sentence had a positive impact on my life in so many ways, but none as profound as when applied to the relationship between my mother and me. Water tumbling over boulders and logs strewn across its span makes a musical sound that is sweet to the ear. The larger the quantity and size of the obstacles, the mightier the sounds. Mother and I kept our stream perpetually littered with old grudges, hurtful words, and haunting actions – all the more to make the stream churn and gurgle along its way – and when it reaches a smooth spot, the shade trees overhead make the water a sweet refuge. It is my hope that we will continue to churn and bump our way along until we finally fall exhausted into each other's arms, glad to find a calm sort of respite in one another. She and I do love each other, in spite of the rocks along the way.

One afternoon in late February, I called Nora at work.

"Can you talk?" I asked.

She had always encouraged me to call her anytime I needed to talk, but I had not felt comfortable contacting her at work. None of our conversations had ever been of an emergency nature, but that day, I felt an unusual yearning to talk to someone who knew what it was to have a parent fade away. I took a break from my desk to reach out to Nora from the refuge in an empty conference room.

"Certainly," came the ready reply. "Are you alright?"

"Not really. Elena called with news that Mom is very disoriented today and even has trouble remembering her own name," I barely whispered for fear I would choke on the words.

"It is a shock to hear that, I know," Nora quietly replied, perhaps recalling the same moment with her mother when the loss of self added another sad dimension to their journey together.

I held my head in one hand, while clutching the phone in the other.

"Elena said that Mom walked down to the mailbox, which is just four houses away on the same side of the street. Mom told Elena that she crossed the street and went down a few houses before she realized she was on the wrong street and didn't know where she was. We aren't sure if she saw a neighbor in the yard, or went up and knocked on a door, but apparently someone two blocks away walked her home. She has lived there for eight years. How do you forget something that you have done every day for eight years?" I questioned.

"It is not unusual for someone to become lost in familiar surroundings. Places no longer ring a bell," Nora explained.

"According to Elena, the same thing happened in the grocery store. They went to their old standby grocer where she has shopped for over two decades, but Mom swore she had never been there before. Elena took her to each department and showed her the produce and the paper goods and the pharmacy. None of it looked familiar," I said. "She must have been frantic, knowing that this was someplace she was supposed to know and didn't."

I was thankful for the seclusion of the darkened conference room for the image of my mother wandering around in search of something she recognized was all I could take in at that moment.

"You are so fortunate that Elena was with her," said Nora, interjecting a more positive outlook on the sad news of my mother's abject confusion. "How much time is she spending with your mother?"

"That is part of my anxiety. Mom is only allowing Elena to be there a few hours on three or four days a week, if that much. Louisa is not willing to push her to hire Elena for any an extended length of time. I am so frustrated with her for that," I said, not even trying to hide my exasperation. "Mother does not respond well to my prodding, and in fact, she is probably more likely to do the opposite in an effort to prove to me that she can live independently."

"You said your mother can't remember her name?" Nora prodded.

"Yes, in the grocery store. She remembered how to run her

credit card through at the checkout but when the clerk asked her to sign her name, Mom told the clerk that she didn't know her name. She asked Elena to sign it for her, which Elena did," I explained as calmly as I could. "Mom, of course, has not told Louisa and me about this. We are only hearing of it through Elena."

"Most likely she will not tell you, if she even remembers it happening at all," Nora assured me. "One of the blessings of Alzheimer's, although it sounds odd to call anything a blessing, is that the individual will soon forget that these things ever happened. Her distress over it will disappear along with any memory of it. Your mother is in that in-between stage, which is so full of uncertainty. She knows something is wrong, yet cannot do anything about it."

"Nora, I want to go to her and help her, but that won't really solve anything. I can help her find her way home from the mailbox today, but tomorrow when I am gone, it will happen all over again," I said with increasing speed and intensity.

Nora's reply was slow and measured.

"You're right. You and she can only live in the moment, one moment at a time."

As someone who is constantly planning, coordinating, and organizing something, the idea of living only in the moment was totally foreign to me, and ordinarily would have seemed equally odd to my mother. But, life had become out of the ordinary and the rules had changed for both of us.

"I have noticed in my phone conversations with Mom that sometimes she remembers what she had for lunch and sometimes she can't recall having lunch at all. It is difficult to go into a conversation with the expectation of a pleasant visit, knowing that it will end in frustration because she can't remember what we are talking about. The other day, Mom had absolutely no memory of the many years that she and Dad faithfully went to water aerobics at the YMCA. Even after Dad died, she continued to go on her own and really enjoyed it because the warm water and the exercise helped her arthritis so much. She doesn't remember any of that, Nora. She asked quite surprised, 'I used to do water aerobics?' I guess it never occurred to her why she has so many bathing suits in her dresser," I said, envisioning Mom pulling suit after suit out of her dresser drawer and puzzling over them.

"Allison, how can you help her with this? You can't rely on past memories to make her smile and she no longer has a concept of planning for the future, so every moment is precious just for that fleeting spot it occupies in time. How do you plan on reacting to this new and different way of viewing the world?" Nora challenged.

The challenge was laid before me, and sitting in the quietness, I slowly began to change the way I related to my mother. I could no longer be certain that she would find pleasure in the memories of our family when we were growing up. Even events of last week or this morning were only present in her mind for as long as they took to occur. The future was clouded, as well, for she could not distinguish between tomorrow and next week. The magic time machine that most of us could utilize to go backward into a huge warehouse of happy memories, or forward into visions of future trips and events, did not function for Mother. The only time she knew was right then. Every moment on the phone with her was an opportunity to make her laugh, to revel in a kind word... to feel loved... before that moment passed into history.

Making each small droplet of time beautiful and free of rough edges would be a challenge for me. Nora knew that I was a planner and a perfectionist, an impatient one at that. Conversations with my mother, heretofore, had always been laced with an undercurrent of conflict. I resolved to soften my natural tendency to correct any outlandish statements she made and instead to build up and affirm her new sense of self. I had to become a caregiver.

Interesting word – caregiver - the one who provides care. This is a much different objective than that of a teacher – one who guides and corrects. Granted, guiding and correcting can be done in a caring manner, but their primary purpose is to teach, to increase someone's knowledge and skills for use in the future. Caring lasts only for the moment, leaving in its wake the feeling of having been loved.

As an impatient perfectionist who loves to plan for the future, the idea of lavishing attention only for the sake of a small piece of time, would be next to impossible except that I could feel my mother's hunger for it. I sensed that she wanted to be affirmed for who she was at any given moment because she had no realization of her past or her future. I ended my call to Nora with a new resolve to be more caring, more loving, more attentive to my mother, without tarnishing the few moments we had remaining. I left the conference room with a plan

The relaxed feel of Sunday afternoon came and with it a desire to talk to my mother.

"Hi, Mom. How are you this beautiful Sunday?" I began after her familiar voice finally sounded in the earpiece.

"Well, not very good," came back the forlorn answer.

Undaunted, I asked with genuine concern, "Do you want to tell me about it?"

"Well, I went to the emergency room in Sterling City with an *acute* urinary tract infection," she said with great emphasis. "I'm on antibiotics which make me feel sick."

Completing skipping over the first question in my mind, *"Why a hospital twenty miles away rather than the one in your own neighborhood?"* I thought better of it and said instead, "That must have been very uncomfortable."

"It was. I didn't go to church. I called Elena and she took me to the emergency room," Mom explained in a slow halting voice.

In my constant search for more information about dementia, my readings had uncovered that individuals become incontinent for several reasons, with the number one reason being poor hygiene. In recent years we had all noticed that Mother was not one to relish taking a shower. It was often a struggle to convince her that it was necessary. Whenever she had been a guest in our home, Tom and I could hear the water running into the tub, but never heard it transition to the muted sounds of spray falling from the showerhead. Having traveled with Mom on many occasions and come to her rescue when the operation of the plumbing was confusing to her, it seemed that she might be forgetting how to take a shower.

My sister always insisted that Mom had taken a shower whenever she was at their house, but I doubted that Louisa really observed that the shower never actually came on, or that the towels were still mysteriously dry. Elena had noticed this, too, but said she never suspected anything from Mrs. Adam's appearance. Mother was a fan of "wash-offs," no doubt a throwback to her childhood days where indoor plumbing consisted of water carried in from a well and poured into a basin. Having been subjected to wash-offs when we were on family camping trips, I was all too familiar with the process and decided that, if she believed she was performing the ritual of daily cleansing, we could not object without creating an embarrassing and unseemly scene. I cautioned Elena to please keep an eye out for signs of further infections or incontinence, as that was sure to be an unsettling change for Mother.

"That is great that you called Elena. I am sure she took good care of you," I said, glad to hear that Mother had the presence of mind to call her caregiver rather than the security guard. "If you eat something before you take the antibiotics, does that help with the nausea?"

Perhaps she would take the gentle hint, but I doubted that she was able to remember that some medications should be taken with food. I made a mental note to talk to Elena about telephoning Mother on a regular basis to urge her to eat.

"I'm very glad you got that taken care of, Mom. Are you feeling any better?"

The conversation seemed to be lifting her out of a dour mood and into a more cheerful one filled with little sparks of laughter over the inconveniences of managing a bladder infection. I should have stopped there and ended the phone call with Mother laughing and feeling better about her situation, but the urge to question her choice of emergency rooms was too strong.

"Can you tell me why you went to Sterling City rather than to the hospital near your house?" I asked in as gentle and unassuming voice as I could muster.

"Well...," she started and then became flustered.

"The emergency room here is just not well thought of," she finally blurted out.

"But, that is where you have always gone and they have always treated you well," I said with a slight edge in my voice.

"Well, we didn't go there," she answered defiantly, making it clear that it was the end of the discussion.

I retreated and circled back to a more favorable topic, "That is great that you got it taken care of, and I know you will be feeling better very soon. How are your little tomato plants?"

She followed the new direction of the conversation and happily launched into a description of the number of little green tomatoes on her patio - and then proceeded to tell me about her trip to the emergency room for the second time - and our conversation started all over again. This time, however, I did not ask her why she went to a hospital so far away, and the conversation had a much happier ending.

I called Elena after hanging up to thank her for taking part of her Sunday to be with Mother in the emergency room.

"I'm curious about something, though. Why did Mom want to go all the way over to the Sterling City emergency room rather than to the one a mile from her house?"

"Is that what she told you? No, she is confused. We did go to the emergency room right over here near the house. I guess she didn't recognize it. Some days are better than others. She has a lot of trouble getting back from the mailbox, and sometimes she recognizes the stores and sometimes she doesn't. You know, when they took her for x-rays, the doctor asked me if she has dementia."

An enduring image in my mind, left over from my trip to see her a year ago, is of her standing between the kitchen and the dining room, half turned in either direction with a glass in her hand, searching for the right way to go. She was not able to remember if she was setting the table or cleaning it up and wandered back and forth between the two rooms several times. Finally, in a complete quandary, she put the glass on the kitchen counter, shuffled into the living room, and sat down and cried. How horrible is this disease that literally makes one lose their mind. At times the image becomes so poignant that I can almost reach out and touch her.

Elena and I noted that with more and more frequency Mother was searching for words, and not finding them, substituted words that were similar, but not exactly right - spoon became fork, and fall became spring. The teacher in me shivered at every misspoken word or phrase, but I refrained from pointing out her errors, as Nora impressed upon me that it was more important that my mother wants to talk to me than it is for her to speak English perfectly. I often found myself completing sentences for her - a bad habit that is not limited to conversations with my relatives. Anxious to get to the end of a sentence, particularly when I know how the sentence will end, I am adept at jumping in to speed up the inevitable conclusion. After moving away from the South where the art of a slow drawl is highly refined, Tom and I relocated to the Northeast where the rate of speech is considerably faster and more amenable to my personality. I forget to slow down to drawl speed when calling my relatives back in Texas, but fortunately, Mother is more forgiving of my assistance with word recollection than she is of my efforts to correct statements such as, "I lost thirty-two pounds this week."

"You are learning to choose your battles, Allison," Nora commented. "Some things are not worth pushing. Did she follow up with her doctor after going to the emergency room the other day?"

"No, she said she was feeling better and didn't see a need to go," I sighed. "We just can't get her in to see a primary care physician. She's only too happy to go to an emergency room and loves the attention, but will not step foot in a doctor's office. Maybe she thinks she will have another colonoscopy, which she now refers to as surgery on her 'female parts.'"

I stayed in constant touch with Mother, checking in on her twice a week, learning her moods, listening to her stories, and yearning to see her. She provided me with many opportunities to reach beyond myself, to put her needs above my own, and to thoughtfully consider my words before speaking to her. I hoped that I provided her with the encouragement and edification for which she hungered.

There has never even been a momentary thought to my mother coming to live with one of us. Louisa struggles with her own physical disabilities and cannot take on the fulltime task of caring for a parent with memory impairment. Meeting Mother's growing needs is a constant calling, a calling which my sister does not have the physical stamina to answer.

I have never felt the call to invite my mother to live with Tom and me. Tom would have loved the idea, as his family traditionally cared for elderly parents in homes of their children, shuttling them back and forth between houses. He grew up with the constant presence of one grandparent or another. Of anyone in my immediate family, Tom is the one who understands and knows how to accommodate caring for an octogenarian. Finding Imogene truly entertaining, he would welcome his mother-in-law into our home with open arms. My arms would be open and welcoming for about three days. As harsh as that may sound, it is a matter of preserving the peace.

Mother and I are too much alike, and in some ways, exact opposites. I inherited my mother's ample physique, her guarded smile, and her sloping shoulders. I am also blessed with her impatience, which on the one hand means we get things done in a timely manner, and on the other hand makes us easily irritated and quick to anger. My anger comes roaring out in the most unpredictable string of words, while Mother withdraws, tightly gathering her hurt feelings and mistrust in around her.

Perhaps the trait that causes the most angst in our relationship as mother-daughter is a penchant toward inflexibility. Imagine two women who are positive they each know how to get something done in the most efficient and correct way possible. Now imagine those two women cooking a meal together. One loves filet mignon - medium rare, and the other loves whatever was on sale - well done. One likes their rice sticky, the other fluffy. One prefers to artfully plate the food on crisp white dishes, and the other serves family style at the table. Throughout my life, most disagreements between the two of us, other than whom I was dating, began in the kitchen and expanded outwardly from there.

No, I never considered for a moment asking Mother to come live with us, and I am sure the thought was not long held in her mind either. However, the time was coming when a change in living arrangements would be necessitated. I approached my sister with the desire to form a plan in advance, feeling certain that any change would happen very quickly. The discussion started with an analysis of Mother's ability to afford in-home care versus going into assisted living with memory support. Louisa was shocked to learn that a home healthcare aide would cost four times as much as moving into the dementia unit, and she slowly began to question whether we would be able to keep our promise to Mother for her to continue living indefinitely in the cottage. Louisa began to add "for as long as possible" to any discussion with Mother about her living arrangements. I was proud of Louisa for taking a more realistic stance and accepting the reality that Mother was quickly coming to the point where it was no longer in her best interest for her to live alone. That is as far as the planning went, however. Louisa was content to leave it at that and did not respond to my prodding for a plan that would take our mother from her cottage into the dementia unit.

The few weeks leading up to Easter were blessedly quiet. Elena called in her weekly report, and Mother seemed to be holding her own without any major incidents. It bothered me that she was alone most of the day, but she did not seem to mind and actually preferred solitude, except for the company of Elena. I loved talking with her on those days when she and Elena had been together, for the caregiver always left her in a state of euphoria. For a short while in the midst of spring, we found a peaceful place in our relationship, perhaps because she had found a new sense of comfort and security.

Mother traditionally anticipated Easter as a time for rebirth. Celebrations of new life erupted from the darkness of Holy Week, families joined together in Easter egg hunts and picnics, and excitement was high as friends gathered to worship. I was expected to come home from college every Easter Sunday, and would leave my dorm as soon as classes let out to drive two hours away to pick up my sister at her dorm before driving many more hours into the night to reach home. Gradually, Louisa and I moved on and had families of our own with Easter traditions much like those we had as children.

This Easter, Mother's little family of friends were gathered around Sylvia Walker's table for an elegant Easter lunch. S.T. picked her up, along with one other Waverly Place resident, and took them to Sylvia's home where they all sat down to enjoy a joyous celebration together.

"Nora, it was glorious for her to be included in this invitation, and she really loved telling me about it, but the sad part is that she barely mentioned the luncheon or her friends. She had no clue what Sylvia served and was vague about who was there. Mom was most excited to tell me about how she got stuck on the toilet and had to scream for help before being lifted off. I know her legs are not very strong and the one knee gives out on her quite frequently. Mom just did not have the strength to rise on her own," I explained.

"Your mother must have been mortified," Nora noted as we resumed our weekly dinners after breaking for Holy Week.

"No, not actually. She seemed quite jovial while telling me the story - several times. Having seen her in embarrassing situations before, I would guess that she went back into the dining room loudly exclaiming about her adventure. It's odd that is how she deals with awkward situations. Mom brings more attention to herself by playing it up, making sure that everyone knows about it. She loves the attention. I've seen her do that many times in the last few years. I imagine that the hostess was the one that was mortified. She had a very beautiful and sophisticated luncheon planned, as only Sylvia could do, and here is Mom yelling about being stuck on the toilet with her drawers down," I bemoaned.

"Sadly, the ability to function in a social setting is compromised for persons with dementia. Social mores no longer have meaning," Nora reminded me.

I blotted my mouth with a napkin and looking off somewhere into the past, recalled, "When we were growing up, Mom was a wonderful hostess. She was the picture of decorum and very ladylike. She took great pride in polishing the silver, ironing the linens, perfectly setting a table with fresh flowers and seeing that none of the guests wanted for anything. That didn't mean her cooking was great, but it was presented very graciously. It's sad to see this change come over her."

"You have noticed this for several years?"

"Well, yes. The older she grows, the sillier and more demonstrative she becomes. Yesterday I was reading about the seven stages of Alzheimer's, and I think she is now somewhere between the fifth and sixth stages."

"Then she has had this disease for a number of years and it is just now becoming noticeable," Nora said. "That is not that unusual. The first few stages are not easily detected and the individual functions with only minor adjustments in their daily living. The fourth and fifth stages are when deficiencies become obvious and they begin to need assistance. She is fortunate to have you looking out for her."

Nora's words are always soothing. She just naturally knows how to lift me up when my spirits were sagging, to calm me down when I become overly excited, and to redirect me when I stray off course. I pondered whether that is the definition of a caregiver, and wondered if I could provide the same comfort to others, specifically to the two women who occupied so much of my mind and heart.

"What do my mother and sister need that I could provide, and just as importantly will they let me?"

One of the hallmark characteristics of my family is that we are so driven to succeed on our own merits without assistance from anyone else that we often don't make willing care receivers. Accepting help is not an easy thing for a strong personality. We view the need for assistance as a sign of weakness, a fallacy that ironically leaves us depleted and exhausted.

Mother's strong desire to live her own life without interference was lessened only slightly by her constant need for attention. She was conflicted between accepting help versus being lonely, and continually wrestled with the notion that others thought she required a caregiver. While at times pleased and proud to tell others that she had a caregiver, she generally sent Elena home early or cancelled her days entirely. In the weeks that followed Easter, I spent much of the time on the phone with Mother building up the idea of a constant companion, but discovered that it was for naught as Elena's hours dwindled down to only a few hours a week. Consequently, the number of hallucinations and other strange events increased, the latest being that her "right shoulder blade had fallen by at least two inches" and that there was a "young girl running along in the alley" behind her house. The short respite that we had all enjoyed was apparently over.

❖

Chapter 7

$\mathcal{D}$eborah Barnes called me at work one afternoon to let me know that the Waverly Place hairdresser had been in to see her. Carolyn was concerned about one of the residents and reported that Mrs. Adams was having some difficulties and had been crying a lot in the beauty shop. She was also having a hard time communicating. Deborah suggested that Mother might be depressed and wanted my thoughts before approaching her.

I appreciated her concern for my mother, and wondered if she might, indeed, be right. Of late, my brother-in-law had come to call Mother's constantly dour expression as Ms. Persimmon Face, and that was not far from the truth. More often than not when at a family gathering, she sat unmoving in a chair and observed activities from behind a frown and furrowed brow, such a contrast to the days when we were children. Family movies document that she was the center of activity at our house, busy directing birthday parties, camping trips, and family holidays. Her side of the family relied on her to gather the troops for volleyball, cookouts, and swim parties. To see her now so sullen and sidelined was disturbing, and those outside of the family were beginning to notice it, as well.

"She goes through phases, Deborah. I had hoped that the sweet mood before Easter would prevail, but now it's like she is having an emotional implosion," I said, hoping Deborah would understand what I feebly tried to communicate.

Deborah decided to visit further with Mother the next time she came over to the administrative building. Louisa and I hoped that if we had not been successful in coaxing her to see a doctor, that a neutral third party such as Deborah might be able to persuade her to seek medical help. For Mother, however, depression fell into the same category as dementia, and proper people such as herself simply did not have mental diseases.

"Depression can be a major factor in a dementia patient's health. The individual's world becomes very somber, and they can't reach outside of themselves," Deborah explained.

"Mom is crying in public, something that she would never have dreamed of doing. As much as she loves attention, this is not the way she would want it," I noted. "She hasn't been very talkative on the phone lately. You know, she has mentioned being tired and going to bed a lot."

The next dinner conversation with Nora focused on symptoms of depression. My friend was well-versed in detecting signs of depression, and I giggle to myself each time she asked me how I was feeling, imagining that she had a mental scorecard on which she marked "Allison is a 7 today," comparing it to my emotional health from previous conversations. The giggle quickly died down, however, because I trusted her ability to recognize declining mental health. Nora was one of two people I would turn to without hesitation if my own mental health score ever took a nosedive; my beloved Tom being the other. Nora would approach it from the viewpoint of someone trained in dealing with emotional turmoil, whereas Tom would look me straight in the eyes and tell me to get a grip. I'm not certain which approach would be most effective, but I suppose it would depend on the source of my sadness or the lack of motivation. Of one thing I am most sure – both would be delivered with the utmost of love and care.

"Your mother could very well be depressed," Nora agreed. "What individual would not be when they realize that their life has taken an unexpected turn for the worse? Most elderly people will tell you that they are more afraid of Alzheimer's than they are of cancer."

Her comments brought Mother's fears into greater focus. Nora is ten years my senior, and although I certainly would not define her as elderly, thoughts of Alzheimer's must be in the forefront of her mind, as both of her parents had this terrible mind-altering disease. We have discussed whether or not we wanted to know if we, too, had inherited the gene which predisposed us to walk this path as both a care giver and, eventually, a care receiver. Nora manages to be more jovial about it than I and laughingly hopes that she will be easier to live with than her mother had been. I cannot ever imagine her as a difficult person, but have no trouble seeing myself as a very belligerent dementia patient.

Mother's genealogy research had uncovered the fact that many of her ancestors were considered to be mentally challenged, and she had written the word "insane" beside the names of those that she thought to be affected by some form of dementia. In an attempt to bravely face our own mortality, I told my sister that Tom and I were preparing for a future with the possibility of dementia in mind; a luxury - if one can call it that – which we had not had with Mother. To know the disease before it knows us could be of benefit.

My family's next generation finds the disease troubling, as well. Charlotte has wondered if her mother or if she, too, might be faced with the same diagnosis someday. It is good to give such things thought, but premature depression over the prospect of mental decline robs us of a joy-filled life in the present because of anxiety about the future. Knowledge can either be demoralizing or can give us the valuable opportunity to prepare and live life with the greatest fulfillment possible.

In response to Mother's apparent depression while fully in the midst of the disease, Nora and Deborah had both asked the same question, "Has her doctor ever mentioned prescribing an anti-depressant for her?"

The answer was a frustrated "No" as Mother had fired yet another doctor.

"She is now on the fourth doctor in a year-and-a-half and has not been with the latest one long enough for him to develop any kind of history with her. Of course, Elena now drives her to all appointments, but like a little child she has wised up and will not let Elena see when the next appointment is scheduled. She uses white out to cover over the appointment in the calendar. The new doctor's office will not let Elena make appointments for her, so we are completely at Mom's whim," I explained. "As long distance caregivers, Louisa and I have to rely completely on Elena for mother's day-to-day care, rationed out over a meager four to six hours a week."

Nora looked up, startled, "That's really not very much at all for someone in your mother's situation."

"Louisa still feels that this arrangement is adequate," I bemoaned. "As long as Elena checks on her every day, either in person or by telephone, Louisa is satisfied that Mom is being cared for. My protests have gone unheeded, Nora, but there is little I can do as Mom does not see the need for more oversight, and Louisa is not willing to press her on it. I am not comfortable with the notion of waiting until something catastrophic happens to force her into accepting more assistance. The thought of Mom wandering outside at night to check on some noise she thinks she heard, is difficult for me, particularly when I know it can be prevented. Until Mom relinquishes her very tight hold on the reins, though, she is in charge of her own life, and long distance caregivers truly have little influence."

I leaned forward across the table to press the point, but need not have, as I was preaching to the choir. The conversation fell silent momentarily as we hungrily eyed the salads and sandwiches displayed on the menu. It was amazing at how distracted we both became with the prospect of food in our sights after a long day at our desks. The restaurant's bakery had conjured up a new bread recipe for ginger lemon pound cake, which caught the attention of both of us, and we decided to split a plate of pound cake before we made a decision on our sandwiches. With the food on its way, we turned our attention back to the topic at hand.

"Louisa and I have discussed having Mom declared incompetent," I was oddly happy to say. "Her ability to carry out daily living skills is declining and, if she is indeed between stages five and six of the disease, she is functioning on the level of an elementary age child. Louisa does not want to own those facts, yet."

"How can we leave an eight-year-old unattended, Louisa?" I had asked her one day.

Louisa countered with, "She will lose so much if declared incompetent."

"But, she could lose her life if she is not," I pointed out, to which Louisa did not immediately reply.

"Mom always tells me that only a doctor can make her move out of her cottage," Louisa remarked.

"She actually understands that?" I asked with amazement.

"Yes, she knows that only a doctor can declare her incompetent and make her move into the dementia unit. What she cannot be convinced of, though, is that we would like to hire someone to be with her for longer periods of time so that she can stay in her cottage," Louisa said. "I just wish it weren't so terribly expensive."

"Do we need to draw the line in the sand for her? Do we need to tell her that having Elena for twenty, even thirty hours a week is a requirement for her staying in her house?"

"I don't think we can get away with that kind of claim because of her nosy next door neighbor. Imelda is such a thorn in our sides," she said with contempt. "She is pretty savvy for an old lady and she knows, and has told Mom, that only a doctor can force them to do anything."

"So, Imelda has stripped you and Louisa of any leverage," Nora summarized.

"It seems so. We need to talk to Mom's doctor, but we can't even persuade her to go see him on a regular basis, much less let us talk to him," I said, feeling my temper rise.

"Nora, this same conversation has continued for months. Someone must be the proactive one. Does that make me a "dictatorial daughter," to quote my mother?" I began to laugh.

She grinned and almost choked on her coffee, "No, I am the protagonist in my family. I completely understand your vexation."

When we had both regained our composure and resumed the attack on our sandwiches, Nora continued in a much more serious vein, "Unfortunately, you are at the point where you really do have to just wait for an indicator that will legally and ethically allow you to act on your mother's behalf. She is still an adult with all the legal rights of a person of sound mind, even though you would question that soundness. Laws protect her, and her next door neighbor - is it Imelda - seems to keep her informed on her legal rights."

My face must have conveyed my distress, for Nora was quick to say, "I'm so sorry that you have to go through this."

"Thank you, Nora," I said, thankful that she was willing to share this burden with me.

"It's interesting that you mentioned her legal rights because

Louisa and I had just been talking about how Mom has not given permission to her newest doctor, a gynecologist, to talk to us, so we can only send him our observations and hope that he reads them. We think he is on board with the diagnosis because he renewed her memory patch prescription, but she has yet to receive a full physical and a definitive answer regarding the extent her memory loss. I am making the assumption that Mom has Alzheimer's because she fits every description I have researched. Without a doctor's input, though, we have to rely on our own research and respond to Mother as we think is most appropriate, but there is so much that we just don't know," I explained.

Nora could say little more than, "This is a time that will try your patience, Allison. Call me anytime you need to."

I thanked her again for her constant support, and as our coffee and tea cups were empty, we said goodnight.

The next Tuesday afternoon my cell phone rang unexpectedly at my desk, the ringtone sounding loudly throughout the office. While I was startled, my co-workers had become accustomed to the sound and knew it was a call of distress from Texas. I had prayed for calmer times, knowing all the while that it could be months, or perhaps years, before smoother waters would be found. The call was from Elena, who excitedly told me that Mother had fallen two days ago, and had been taken by ambulance to the emergency room – this time to the downtown hospital – but was now safely back at home.

"What? Two days ago?" I exclaimed, stepping into an empty office across from my desk.

It was difficult to tell if Elena was more concerned with the fact that her charge had fallen or that she had not been notified until two days later. I shared her concern in that we expected Waverly Place to notify at least one of us when she required emergency treatment.

It seems that early Sunday morning, Mother had pressed her emergency button, sending the security guard and the EMTs skeptically rushing to her door. However, this was not a false alarm as had been the worm in the dishwasher and the figure of a man standing in her living room. They found her flat on her back on the bedroom floor. By her own account, she got out of bed that morning, tripped on the carpet, twisted around and fell to the floor on one hip. Neither she nor the EMTs thought anything was broken, but when asked if she wanted to go to the emergency room for x-rays, she readily agreed.

I thanked Elena again for calling me.

"She didn't want me to tell you," Elena said hesitantly as we hung up, as if to apologize for my mother's reluctance to have me involved in decisions about her care.

Hurriedly flipping through my contacts, I located Deborah Barnes's number. She was most often not at her desk when I called, and I was relieved to catch her in the office this time.

"Deborah," I began, quickly dispensing with the obligatory greetings. "Elena was kind enough to call and tell me that you had contacted her about Mom falling over this past weekend. Thank you for telling her. What can you tell me about the fall?"

The file was still on her desk and I could hear her turning the pages.

"Well, the security report says that she pressed her button at five minutes past eight in the morning, they responded within four minutes, and found that she had fallen in the bedroom. The EMTs did not think she broke anything and asked her if she wanted to go to the ER. She elected to go by ambulance. The ER took x-rays and released her with pain medication."

"Does it say to whom she was released? Elena wasn't called, so we don't know how she got home. Does the weekend security guard call those listed on the emergency contact sheet? I'm a little perplexed that none of us knew she had fallen."

"I was surprised, too, when I read the security log this morning. I will have to check into that," Deborah said. "Imogene doesn't want you to know when she has an emergency, so please do what you can to maintain that confidentiality. In your mother's case, though, if I know about it, I will contact you even if she asks that you not be notified."

I thanked Deborah for her understanding, and we talked briefly about Mother's continuing struggles and how difficult it was to care for her long distance without the support of a doctor.

Then Deborah surprised me by saying, "I don't think a doctor would declare her incompetent at this point, Allison. She has to get much worse. We aren't seeing her setting off the smoke detectors, and she hasn't missed any of her monthly payments; so, other than the usual fears and uncertainties that many of our residents have, there isn't anything that would make Waverly Place ask her to move out. I still maintain that she may be depressed and very lonely, in spite of Elena's attention."

We talked for a few minutes longer about my desire for Mother to have a fulltime caregiver. I promised to keep in touch, and Deborah did the same.

"Louisa, has Elena called you?" I asked when she picked up on her cell phone a few minutes after my conversation with Deborah. "Mom is fine now, but she went to the ER on Sunday. Apparently she fell in her bedroom and pressed the emergency button hanging around her neck."

"Why weren't we called on Sunday?" Louisa jumped at the news.

"Deborah is not sure why the weekend crew did not contact us, but Mom does not want us to know. She could have told the security guard not to call us. Elena wasn't even contacted until today," I exclaimed. "She thinks that Mom called Sylvia to take her back home, but isn't positive about that. Mother seemed evasive about how she got home."

"That's great. Sylvia has been a good medical buddy to her," Louisa commented. "Mom usually tells me things eventually. I will call her and she will probably let it slip and tell me the whole story."

A few hours later, Louisa's number rang back on my cell. I rushed to answer it before my co-workers could be disturbed.

"Allie, Mom told me about it, and she is so upset. When she got to the hospital she called Sylvia, who came down and announced that she couldn't be Mom's medical buddy anymore, and then left her there in the emergency room. She is crushed," Louisa quickly said with anger in her voice. "After Mom was with Sylvia during her foot surgery last year, for Sylvia to treat her that way… it's terrible!"

I, on the other hand, was not surprised that Sylvia would make such a decision, for Mother had been rather needy of late and had not been an easy person to befriend. What did surprise me, however, was the timing of Sylvia's announcement. The very kind and professional person that I knew her to be had more class than that, and it puzzled me as to why she would wait until her friend was clearly in need of friendship and help. To choose that moment to desert Mother was perplexing. That was not consistent with Sylvia, whereas making up that kind of story was totally consistent with Mother. I suspected that Mother was covering up something or trying in her childlike way to pull together a thin web of facts that made sense to her.

"Louisa, I think Mom must have misunderstood what was actually said. I am sure Sylvia had a responsibility as a church elder that morning, and since Mom was not in any kind of medical distress, asked if Mom could find another way home. I truly do not think she told Mom she could not be her medical buddy. I think it is simply a misunderstanding on Mom's part," I said, laying out my case.

"No, Mom is really upset by this," Louisa persisted.

"Mom has been really insistent about a lot of things that turned out to be either the inner workings of her imagination or simply miscommunications," I said, knowing that I should not pursue the argument any further.

My sister was not ready to hear that her mother may have made a mistake – a mistake brought on by illness. For her, Mother was still just an elderly woman with all the natural quirkiness that comes with advanced age.

"*Louisa, she needs help. Why can't you see that?*" I wanted to yell out.

I had not been with the two friends in the emergency room that Sunday morning, and had no real frame of reference upon which to draw my conclusion, but the experiences of the last year had taught me that fear, loneliness, disorientation, depression, and a gift for the dramatic with a dab of factual truth here and there all made fertile ground for storytelling. Once Mother had a thought in her head, nothing will shake it loose. She will forever be haunted with the idea that ants have invaded her bed, that she had been abandoned in the emergency room, and that a stalker roams the yard outside her cottage. Stories or not, Mother believes them to be true. This is her new reality, and her thirty-year friendship with

Sylvia was over as far as she was concerned.

"Nora, I suppose we will never know what Sylvia actually told Mom, but it is another sign of changing relationships. I feel sort of like a parent must feel when their little eight-year-old comes running inside crying about the friend who doesn't want to play with her anymore, except, that for the eight-year-old, it is a moment of teaching. There is no new learning for Mom – only the loss of how to be a good friend. That is so sad," I told my own dear friend, who had listened intently to the narrative of events surrounding Mother's fall.

A few days after Mother was sufficiently recovered from the events of the weekend, she and Elena went over to the independent living office to change her emergency contact information. Mother asked Deborah to remove Sylvia's name and put in Elena's instead, a move which everyone applauded. We hoped that this decision meant she would now accept Elena's assistance more readily, and settle into a quiet routine at home. However, much to my dismay, Elena reported that she was spending even less time at the cottage as Mother often sent her away after they ran their usual errands about town. I could well imagine the exchange between the two of them – Elena insisting that she didn't mind staying to help her with lunch or medications, and Mother insisting that she could do it on her own. Louisa had tried explaining to her that when she canceled Elena's hours, it meant her caregiver's income for the week was reduced. Although Mother is quite charitable toward whatever non-profit requests reach her mailbox, that charity did not extend to her employee, and she steadfastly refused to bow to the perceived indignity of requiring the assistance of a fulltime home healthcare aide.

"I understand her drive to live on her own, but she gets in her own way sometimes. If there were a book written about her, the title would be *The Strong-Willed Dementia Patient*," I said with a smile.

"Your mother is a very interesting person. I would love to meet her someday," Nora eagerly responded. "When you think about it, though, every woman she knows is either married, living completely on their own, or is in a dementia or nursing care unit. She knows she does not want to be in the latter category, so she holds to the ideal image of a strong woman living on her own. She believes that you are threatening to change that dynamic."

"It's a funny mixture of pride and fear," I said as the light bulb went on in my mind. "None of the women who live alone do so with anything other than a maid. On the one hand, she is proud that she has something no one else has – a home healthcare aide. On the other hand, it is also a sign that she is not really able to live completely on her own."

Nora and I had taken advantage of a cool spring day to spread a picnic out on a blanket in the park across the street from the church. I had one of those rare days off and Nora had taken a vacation day to run a few errands and to have lunch with me. We found a fairly flat spot under a thick oak tree and settled down to enjoy avocado and shrimp salad on croissants and fresh orange slices. We laughed at the antics of the squirrels chasing each other around the trees and the funny little sideways hop of the robins. Between courses and laughter, I told Nora about the latest calls from Elena, which had become quite frequent.

"Allison, I wanted to call and tell you about your mother. She pressed the emergency button yesterday afternoon," Elena explained. "You know that low rocking chair next to her bed... well, she sat down in it and couldn't get back up. So, she pressed the emergency button and the security guard came over with the EMTs."

She continued emphatically, "I told her she should have called me. There is a phone sitting right there on the bedside table next to the chair, but she said she didn't want to have to pay me to come over and help her get out of the chair."

"Oh, Elena, I am so sorry. She loves you. I think she is just too hung up on the idea of being frugal."

"Thanks... I love her too. We talk about a lot of things and she is so sweet when she is not upset about something. Anyway, they lifted her out of the chair and put her in bed. The security guard said it was not an emergency and told her that she should not be living alone," Elena said.

I let out a gasp, "Wow - that may be the first time someone other than us has said that outright to her."

"She really didn't like the way the guard talked to her and is worried that they are keeping a list of how many times she has called for help."

It's easy to hear genuine concern in Elena's voice. She would love nothing more than to devote herself entirely to Mother, and calls to check in with her every evening and on her days off.

"I hope she isn't charging me for phone calls," Mom complained once, but her voice gave away the fact that she was pleased with the attention.

They are cute together. Elena is shorter than her charge by several inches, and Mother is not as tall as she used to be. At one time an inch or so taller than I am, she now only comes up to my forehead. The two of them are so comfortable with each other, although Mother is sensitive to any encroachment on her rule over the house. Elena has a way of finessing suggestions by putting an idea in her mind, letting Mother believe it was their idea all along. Mother thrives on that type of attention and allows herself to be led by the caregiver's gentle persuasions, as long as they do not involve finances. I doubt that Mother will ever give up her hold on the checkbook.

Elena contacted me late one night, only because she had forgotten to call earlier in the evening, and although it was not an emergency, she wanted to let me know that Mother was in possession of a large amount of cash. Her concern was that she knew they had not been to the bank in some time. The attentive woman noticed that Mother's wallet was bulging with so much cash that it would not close. When Elena questioned her about it, she could not tell her where it had come from.

"Elena suggested that she not carry so much in her wallet for safety reasons," I explained to Nora before smiling. "She asked Mom if there was some safe place to put the money so that she could at least close her wallet. Mom showed Elena a dresser drawer in her bedroom where she could keep the money, but it was already stuffed with cash."

"Where did she get that much money?" Nora asked before reminding me that dementia individuals often hoard things. "Is she thinking this is a means of protecting her money or saving it up?"

"We aren't sure, Nora. We can't approach her about it because that would break the confidences we keep with Elena.

Mom probably has no idea how much cash she has, but just sticks to the routine she has had for many, many years when my father would give her a monthly household allowance. She kept up that routine and withdrew money for groceries and prescriptions every few weeks, but now she buys those items with a check or credit card. She really has very little use for cash now," I explained. "Lately she has been worried about being able to 'get to her money' when making investment decisions."

"I suppose it could be a type of security blanket for her, to always have access to cash. My mother hoarded food from her food trays. The nursing home thought she was a good eater because everything disappeared from her plate. She would grab a roll and stuff it under her pillow until she could transfer it into the bottom of her closet," Nora smiled sadly at the memory. "They discovered it when her room began to smell…"

"Mom sort of does the same thing with canned goods. When we helped her move from the big three-bedroom house into the little cottage, the guys were hauling box after box of some really heavy items. My brother-in-law asked her what was in the boxes and she wouldn't tell him, so Matt ripped them open and discovered dozens of cans of fruit. She threw a fit and insisted that she needed all of it, so Matt and Charlie dutifully delivered them to her new kitchen," I said. "There was so much of it that there was no way it was going to fit into the cottage's little pantry. They convinced her to let them take most of the boxes to a food pantry. Over the next few years, though, the No. 10 size cans of peaches and pears started appearing again and nearly filled all the storage space in her garage. Only recently did Elena get her to take a box or two over to the church for the food bank."

Nora and I were startled to realize that at that very moment we were enjoying a bowl of peach cobbler for dessert. How sad that the sight of a peach triggered a far different emotion in my mother. We take for granted the plentiful supply of food in a relatively prosperous time, something Mother had not always been able to enjoy. I am certain that she now feels comfort and security in knowing that her pantry is well stocked with food, regardless of the fact that many items were well beyond their expiration dates.

Nora's comments about security resounded strongly with

me as I recalled something Mother had told me many years ago about having lunch at my grandmother's house. Knowing how she felt about my grandmother, I could not imagine why she would be at Nana's house without my father, but nevertheless, she was preparing to leave when she realized that she did not have enough coins in her purse for the bus ride back to work. She was terribly embarrassed to have to ask my grandmother for the money, which resulted in a lecture. Mother told me she vowed that day that she would never be without money in her wallet.

"Elena said there must have been several hundred dollars in Mom's dresser drawer," I told Nora. "She thinks that Mom's next door neighbor is a part of this and worries that Imelda might be taking advantage of her. Mom claims that Imelda drives her to the bank and shopping at the mall. I can't imagine them going shopping at the mall, though. She can barely walk, even with a walker, and gets tired going to the mailbox."

"Maybe this is a story that your mother has made up to cover where she acquired the money," Nora suggested.

"We may never know from where she got the money. Interestingly, she said that Imelda got lost while they were out driving and had to call Waverly Place to come pick them up," I said.

Imelda was becoming a problem. Mother apparently relied on her for guidance and considered her a peer, who, caught up in the same struggle to remain independent, readily commiserated with her neighbor on the many injustices imposed upon them simply because they had reached their senior years. Listening in on the few conversations they had while Louisa and I visited Mother was almost comical as they gossiped about the maids, the postman, and the hairdresser, before moving on to complaining about Waverly Place's monthly fees, the telephone service, and the weather. We doubted that anything they said to one another was completely accurate, but they eagerly entered into a very spirited exchange of gossip sprinkled liberally with numerous profanities, something we had not heard emerge from our mother's mouth before. Mother even confessed that she had imbibed when Imelda offered wine to the maids one day after their quitting time.

"Apparently, Imelda's house is the location for the neighborhood happy hour, and I suppose that because it was not a seedy dark bar, Mother felt that it was alright to join in the festivities, in spite of the fact that she claims to be a teetotaler. Imelda has not been a particularly positive influence," I continued to explain. "If she can so easily persuade Mom to withdraw cash from her account, it is definitely time for Louisa and me to help her simplify her financial management system and remove her neighbor from that equation."

Nora nodded her head in wholehearted agreement.

"By Mom's own admission she has difficulty remembering whether or not she has paid a bill. Now that I am able to view her checking account transactions online, I have also noticed double payments. We know that balancing a checkbook is something she simply cannot do, and we worry when she closes out CDs and money market accounts for no apparent reason well before their due dates."

I enjoyed the last of the orange slices, wiped my hand on the napkin, and turned again to Nora.

"How did you accomplish the transition from your mother handling her own affairs to the three of you doing it?"

"There is no dignified way to do it. I just took the checkbook and files when we moved her into the nursing home and never returned them to her," Nora recalled. "She was so angry with me, but it was not all that difficult. Your situation is different."

The sun had moved further west across the sky and shone directly on my patch of the blanket. I stood up, shook out my napkin and settled down again in a shady spot before continuing.

"My mother just does not see how it would be helpful to her for someone else to handle her finances, and she is totally unable to trust anyone, especially me for some unknown reason. This horrible disease makes her so paranoid and delusional," I sighed.

"You have a financial power of attorney, don't you?"

"Well, yes, but it is contingent upon a doctor declaring her incompetent, and you know how she feels about doctors. The Alzheimer's mind is very perplexing," I said, giving my head a little shake, but determined to find a way to make Mother's life less confusing without taking away her dignity.

❖

Chapter 8

The plan was a two-pronged approach to remove part of the burden of financial management from Mother's shoulders, while giving her the control and continued responsibility of running her daily activities with a small household budget. All of her checking accounts, which we had yet to fully identify, would be consolidated into two accounts: one that would remain the account from which she would write checks and withdraw funds for household items and food; and the other account from which Louisa would pay all of Mother's expenses, including Elena's weekly wages.

Carefully designed to minimize Mother's stress and perhaps to give her the relief she may have subconsciously been seeking, the plan also included a transfer of the home healthcare aide's employment from Mother to Louisa. In this way, Louisa hoped to thwart any efforts to decrease Elena's hours and to keep the amount expended for home healthcare hidden from Mother. As investments matured, she and Louisa would decide together whether to cash or reinvest, with an emphasis on keeping Mother's principal secure from the random management decisions she had been making of late. Insurance premiums and major medical bills would be paid by Louisa out of the primary account, and she would also handle all medical claims. Mother's inability to understand the statements of benefits had already given Louisa heartburn, as Dad had handled everything prior to his passing, and Mother was woefully unprepared to understand the intricacies of health insurance.

"The plan was brilliant, Nora. It still gave Mom the autonomy she craved, yet relieved her of the many of the financial pressures. I drew up a very simple chart showing the components of the plan, and Louisa used it to present the idea to Mom the first time they were alone during Mom's next trip to Louisa's."

My soup was growing cold, as I had neglected it in my long-winded description of our plan. I paused to linger over the comforting aromas of clam chowder before Nora grabbed my arm and insisted that I continue with the story.

"Well, did she go for it?" Nora asked with anticipation upon hearing that Mother had been to see my sister.

"Yes and no. Louisa said Mom crossed her arms and insisted that she was not giving up control of her finances to anyone. I am sure that Louisa tried every motivational trick she knew to persuade Mom to let go of the reins, but she would not budge, claiming that she was perfectly capable of handling everything on her own. Louisa said she made her cry by pointing out the problems with her checkbook balance. That really surprised me, because for years Louisa has stuck by Mom and defended her negligible financial abilities."

"Delusional thinking is prevalent among people with Alzheimer's," Nora reminded me. "From what you have told me, your mother, no doubt, hates to be told that she can't do something."

"Nevertheless, whether she likes it or not, Mom is continuing to mess up on her finances, but won't even consider the possibility that she is making mistakes," I said defensively.

My strong reaction to Nora's words was only a fraction of what my mother must have felt in response to Louisa's presentation of a new way to handle her finances. Knowing that Mother would most likely fly home the next day and immediately move all of her funds out of the joint accounts which she held with my sister and me into some secretive place accessible only by her, Louisa wisely cancelled Mom's flight and insisted on Charlie driving them all back to San Angelo.

"Nora, I was proud of my sister. Not only did she embrace the idea, but she ran full speed with it and would not let Mom off the hook."

"What prompted her to be so forceful this time, when other times she has been reluctant to act?" Nora queried.

"Maybe it was the analysis that Tom did on the cost of living at home with an aide versus the cost of moving into the dementia unit. It is difficult to ignore figures that scream 'Danger,

danger, your mother will run out of funds in twenty-one months.' Louisa and I have both agreed that neither of our families is prepared to bear the financial burden of caring for Mom. Any housing and healthcare that she receives must be funded by Dad's principal investments, his pension and Social Security payments. She cannot afford to make poor investments on her own or to lose money because of a lack of accounting skills. I think that scared Louisa into facing up to the reality of Mom's waning financial management skills. She knows we must make a move to relieve her of those burdens, but our hands are somewhat tied because she has not been declared incompetent. It's a very, very scary situation."

Nora and I batted several scenarios back and forth as the sandwich shop began to close for the evening, and Nora promised to keep us all in her prayers as my sister and I continued to find a way to rescue someone who did not realize that she needed rescuing.

Louisa reported that the six-hour drive to San Angelo seemed longer than usual, in part because her back was in agony, and secondly, Mother had covered herself in a blanket of silence and gave every indication of disowning Louisa just as she had me some months prior. My sister was very brave in realizing that her conversation with Mother over finances could very well be the death knoll of their relationship, but she knew that it had to be accomplished and had placed a phone call in secret before beginning to pack her suitcase.

Upon reaching the cottage, Mother quickly disappeared into her bedroom and shut the door, something she had not done during previous visits from her children. Louisa could hear file cabinet drawers squeaking open and the sound of papers being shuffled. She smiled as she imagined Mother's office area in one corner of the beige and brown bedroom being pulled apart and boxed up in a feverish attempt to hide the years of Dad's meticulous filing of every receipt, every tax return, and every medical claim. When the door opened again and Louisa had a chance to glance in as she passed on her way to the garage where the cold sodas were kept, the usual stacks of papers and file folders on the desk were gone. Louisa's heart skipped a few beats as she realized a paper shredder was nestled underneath the desk, but soon resumed its normal beating as she did not recall hearing the shredder running while Mother had sequestered herself in the bedroom. Dinner was eaten in an unusually one-sided conversation between Louisa and Charlie; the lights went out; and all three headed off to bed, this time with Mother willingly going to her own bed rather than the sofa which her grandson had claimed.

The next day Elena arrived just as breakfast was being cleared.

Surprised to see her caregiver, Mother asked, "Why are you here?"

"You missed your hair appointment last week, so we rescheduled for this morning," answered Elena nonchalantly, knowingly glancing over at Louisa.

"I did not reschedule. Louisa and Charlie are here," Mom said with indignation, as if the trip had been planned for some time rather than spontaneously undertaken only yesterday afternoon.

"Carolyn is waiting for you," Elena matter-of-factly told her, not stopping to argue the point, but with the full expectation that Mother would comply. "You need to have your hair done."

Mother stared at her blankly, trying to process all the information, before dutifully shuffling over to the kitchen counter to get her purse. She put on her head scarf and clip-on sunglasses and followed Elena out the door, grumbling the whole time. Elena glanced back at Louisa and winked one eye. Mother was in good hands.

With the two of them out of the house, Louisa instantly took advantage of the rare opportunity to look through Mother's files and uncover hidden or lost bank accounts and investment statements. She found the straight back chair at Dad's battered old desk to be somewhat comfortable and asked Charlie to hand her files from the institutional gray filing cabinets salvaged from the Scout office remodeling. When they had exhausted the few folders in the file drawers, she instructed him to search under the bed, in the closet and anywhere that he could think of for the remainder of the financial files. He found them in the linen closet in Grandmother's bathroom with a towel draped over them. They opened the files and quickly made a list of account information and contact numbers before returning the files to the closet in the same disarray in which they had found them.

"'Allie," Louisa began her report on Mom's recordkeeping. "She really does a surprisingly good job of keeping up with the filing. I was amazed that we found everything so easily, despite the fact that she had hidden the files in the linen closet."

We laughed out loud at the creative efforts Mother used to keep things from Louisa and me. However, in the eyes of the law, Mother was an adult with legal rights to the sanctity of her home - all the more reason to maintain the illusion that her affairs were safe from her "meddling family." My sister very methodically explained every step they took, and in so doing, I anticipated the obstacle that she would soon lay down before me.

"By the time she and Elena came back from the beauty shop, Mom had forgotten why we had brought her home. Charlie, Elena and I sat with her at the dining room table and we used your chart to explain the plan one more time...," and then Louisa paused.

"I'm sorry, I really tired, but she is absolutely not going to let anyone handle her affairs or make decisions about her money," Louisa said apologetically.

"It is not surprising, sister. It is alright – I know you tried. Did she acknowledge in any way that she is having problems with balancing a checkbook, or any of the other things we have noticed?"

"She started crying again when I showed her my checkbook and tried to explain how to balance it. She kept referring to her list of checks and just doesn't get the concept at all. But, there seems to be a glint of understanding that she isn't doing something right – although, she can't comprehend what that might be or why it is happening. There is good news, though," Louisa said. "Maybe it was a mistake to discuss the checkbook in front of Elena, but it really helped to have her there when I told Mom that in order for her to continue to live alone in her cottage, she had to increase Elena's hours to five days a week for a minimum of two hours on each of those days. I had a contract that I had written up and she begrudgingly agreed to sign it."

My disappointment must have been evident in my halfhearted response, as Louisa went on to say, "I know you wanted it to be eight hours a day, but she insisted she did not need anyone and was barely willing to even add a few hours to the current schedule. The real coupe is that I am now writing the checks for Elena's hours, just as you suggested. We convinced her that worrying with Elena's timesheets was a big hassle, and that I could transfer the funds electronically. She didn't understand that, but seemed more worried over what would happen when I have my back surgery and who would sign the checks. The only way I could get her to agree to this was to add Charlie to the checking account."

I caught my breath and it stopped short in my throat, and I thought I would pass out before breathing again. Mother and Louisa had done it again – given responsibility to a teenager who barely had experience with his own checking account, much less a large account like Mother's. Through no fault of his own, Charlie was caught up in his grandmother's battle to keep me out of her finances and to anoint her grandson as the one who would secure her future. I doubt that she was actually empowering him so much out of her desire for him to one day take over her financial and medical affairs, but more that she was running away from me. I tried to hide my feelings from my sister, as I was certain that she had tried every persuasive tactic she knew, and this was the only solution by which Mother would allow Louisa to take over Elena's employment and service.

"And how did that go when you got to the bank?" I asked, hoping there was not more to the story.

Louisa explained with a lot of stops and starts searching for words.

"The clerk reviewed the account with us and listened while Mom explained that she wanted to add Charlie to the account. A new signature card had to be signed by all four account holders at the same time, but I explained the impossibility of that happening because you were living in the Northeast and could not be there at that time. She didn't want to, but I convinced the clerk to mail the card to you for your signature."

"What was Mom's reasoning for adding Charlie to the account?" I quizzed, hoping that Louisa would read between the lines and sense that I was uncomfortable with the arrangement.

"She wants to be sure that Elena can be paid when I have my back surgery and can't transfer the funds. She wants him to do it."

The silence on my end of the line reverberated with disapproval. Louisa heard it in spite of the silence and forged ahead, describing Mother's reactions in detail, hoping that some of the silence could be replaced with approval.

"Mom threw a fit when she heard that your name was still on the bank account. I'm so sorry. She is just in this habit of being negative about you, although I don't think she remembers why. I am so sorry, Allie. Thankfully there was no way around the requirement that all of us had to be there to take you off the account," Louisa said. "I wouldn't let her do that, big sister."

My heart rose a little upon hearing those words.

"Thank you, sister. Thank you," I said halfheartedly.

Adding Charlie to the account was such a thinly veiled action, but Mother did not have the ability to think beyond that moment and did not realize that he was heading to Scout summer camp as soon as they arrived back home in The Woodlands. He would then be home for a week or two before heading back to university where he was percussion section leader in the band, much to his family's delight. Once he returned to college, his days were highly structured with very little room, if any, for stepping into his mother's shoes to manage his grandmother's affairs. Louisa assured me that Charlie would not take any steps without consulting me should anything happen to her, a thought that I pushed back into the corner of my mind, not daring to acknowledge the possibility that Louisa would not survive the ordeal she was about to face.

The search for a surgeon to perform Louisa's very complicated surgeries had not gone well. The implanted neural stimulator, her chronic pain, and severely deformed body had catapulted her into a high risk category that few surgeons were willing to approach. As the summer passed, the search became more desperate, and she became more and more crippled. From sheer will power and a determination instilled in her by our parents, she rose every morning to meet whatever challenges faced her that day. Our phone calls were primarily centered on Mom; but those that were not, were filled with intimate thoughts and wishes for peace and health for each other and our families.

In one of those phone calls, Louisa said, "I am so glad that you are okay with where Mom is now. It makes it easier on... on us."

Her words made me pause, for there were many layers to think through. I was, in fact, not okay with where my mother was in her journey and, desiring Nora's insight, pulled her into the church library after choir rehearsal the following Thursday evening. The room was quiet at that hour and there was a certain solace just by being in this place full of the wisdom of ancient writers and theologians. Somewhere in the rows and stacks of books were the answers to my many questions, but I would rely this night on someone that I could touch. I was too impatient to stop and read a book or to kneel and listen in prayer.

"Nora, this is not okay. I am far from accepting of Mom's condition. What does Louisa see that makes her think I have accepted anything at all?" I demanded, stopping off at the coffeemaker to start a new pot brewing.

Chuckling, Nora offered, "You have changed so much in the year we have been meeting, Allison. Your anger at what dementia has done to your mother - and will continue to do - has subsided. You are able to step back and look at the disease and its symptoms in a more clinical way, and the emotional sting is hurting less. Louisa probably senses an acceptance of what the disease has done and is moving on," Nora paused before continuing with great conviction. "Your mother is quickly moving along this path... and you have to go with her."

Her words rang true. The initial steps in realizing and therefore acknowledging the presence of the disease in her life, and consequently in ours, had been taken. I knew without a doubt that she was now firmly planted on this path and hoped that my sister would be coming along behind us shortly.

"I do feel a certain resignation and acceptance that this is now her life and it will never regain its vibrancy. In addition to finding ways to secure her future, the focus is also on making her future happy and joyful," I thought out loud. "It is not enough to know that we are beginning to make baby steps in helping her into safer living arrangements, but I want her to be fulfilled - to feel a purpose again - and that fulfillment may take the form of connecting with someone for lunch, or picking green beans in the community garden, or paying her monthly church pledge. Triumphs take on smaller shapes and forms now. It is gratifying to see Louisa take a more active role in this, although I know it completely wears her out."

"You are also giving up the desire to have control," Nora looked over the rim of her coffee cup to check my reaction.

We paused in our conversation as other choir members who had followed their noses to the source of freshly brewed coffee found their way into the library. The coffee maker was soon emptied and we found ourselves alone again.

I laughed out loud, "Ha, ha – I will always be a control freak, Nora, but I now know better than to try and control someone with dementia. It's like trying to herd cats. It can't be done. The only solution is to build a safe environment for them and let them play within the confines of that sanctuary."

I leaned forward to emphasize my point, as it had suddenly materialized in my mind, *"That is where I am not okay with this. Mom does not have a safe sanctuary."* We finished our coffee and giving each other a quick hug, headed toward our cars and home to our husbands who waited patiently every Thursday night for their songbirds to arrive.

During the half-hour drive home, I realized that Mother's situation was becoming more and more complicated and less and less secure for her. When the big mustard-colored house on Humboldt Street - the home I knew as a teenager - became a maintenance nightmare, I urged her to sell and move into Waverly Place. It took two years of encouragement before the bottom of the water heater rusted out and became the final mark against the aging house. Out of the blue, she called me one week after Christmas when she had just returned home to a flooded garage, kitchen and dining room to tell me that she had been to Waverly Place and signed a contract on a two-bedroom cottage. Everyone in the family applauded her courage and decision to simplify her life and to buy into a more secure environment.

Sadly, she was now aging faster than her cottage and it was no longer that secure environment we desired for her. The greatest difficulty lay in the fact that she was in denial, just as she had been before deciding to sell the Humboldt Street house. She did not see the need to leave her cottage, or probably more accurately, she did not relish the thought of moving into the dementia or the Alzheimer's unit. However, her ability to operate the stove, oven, icemaker, door locks, and the garage door opener were waning. By her own admission, she told me that security had knocked on her door one night and told her that she needed to put her garage door down at night.

One morning, after discovering that she had been vulnerable to the "man who wandered the streets" after her garage door had mysteriously opened by itself sometime during the night, Mother called security. Tired of the false alarms and having to answer to an old woman who was as crotchety as an old hen, the guard repeatedly told her that she really shouldn't be living alone. He laughed off her request to check for anything missing in the garage and suggested that she call the maintenance department to check out the garage door. She called Elena instead.

A few weeks passed before Nora and I found ourselves seated in a quaint soda fountain enjoying ice cream treats. We picked up where we had left off with where the previous conversation had ended – with Mother's garage door.

Nora smiled, "Does she really believe that the garage door magically opens by itself during the night?"

"Oh, yes, she is emphatic that the door opens by itself. Elena has seen her try to use the garage door opener and she just can't figure it out. I am certain that the operation of a safe household is now slipping out of Mom's grasp like so many other things," I paused, partly because the ice cream had frozen my tongue, and partly because I hated to say the next words out loud. "The guard is right – she should not be living alone."

Nora nodded in quick agreement, "That's interesting that she still sees the man walking around outside. That seems to be a recurring hallucination of hers, doesn't it? I know that an Alzheimer's individual can't make sense of their surroundings sometimes. It is as if the sensory parts of their bodies are receiving signals, but the brain cannot interpret it correctly. As a result, they sense things that aren't really there – people, smells, objects. Trying to convince them otherwise is usually unsuccessful and only makes them defensive. Dorothy and I found that it calmed Mommie to just validate her feelings and redirect her toward something more pleasant."

Shaking my head because my mouth was still too cold to speak, I took a sip of warm water and replied when my tongue had thawed a bit, "To answer your earlier question about whether she still sees people who aren't there – yes, Elena says that she does. Last week Mom asked Elena if she saw the two girls running through the living room and out the front door. I'm not sure what Elena said, but it was, no doubt, something reassuring and it calmed her down. She hasn't mentioned ants on the bed in a while, and I think she may have started sleeping in her bed again rather than the sofa."

Nora and I were sitting on a bench in the sun trying to warm ourselves after indulging in ice cream for dinner. The long days of summer had arrived. Usually the blazing heat of the sun drove me indoors, but today was milder than usual and we enjoyed people-watching for a few minutes before I brought us back around to the purpose of our meeting.

"Mom has mentioned that the phone isn't working right, and Louisa and I both have tried to call her for hours at a time and just get a busy signal. We think she is not replacing the handset properly. She also said her remote control for the TV has stopped working. I suggested that she ask Elena to replace the batteries. I hope she hasn't pushed so many buttons that she scrambled the stations like a few months ago."

The laugh lines around Nora's eyes crinkled up at the image of our parents madly pushing any buttons they could to make "the blasted thing work."

When our laughter died down and the sun had taken the chill off a bit more, I said, "Mom is only eating cookies and orange juice unless Elena stays a little longer to prepare her lunch. It's no wonder that Mom complains of being weak and lightheaded. She just isn't getting enough food into her system, but Elena can't stay all day. Mom will not let her in spite of Louisa's insistence."

"Well, losing a sense of taste is only part of the picture. The planning and steps it takes to prepare a meal are probably becoming difficult for her. Getting up the motivation to think that hard is tiring and she may no longer have the initiative to cook for herself, plus the fact that operating a can opener or working the stove may be quite daunting," Nora noted.

A sudden wave of sadness washed over me at the thought of Mother simply sitting on the sofa all day staring at a blank television and watching out for the man peering in at her through the windows, a half-eaten box of cookies open next to her. I doubted that is how Mother envisioned her elder years. The sun began to set on that thought and I drove home lost in thought about my mother and her next birthday, wishing that I could be with her to share cake and ice cream.

I reminded Louisa that Mother's eightieth birthday was coming up in July, "Usually people have big celebrations for their eightieth, but I wonder if any of us are up for it right now. What do you think? She probably wouldn't be in favor of a party."

"Mom has alienated so many people that it would probably be an awkward affair. She loves to travel, so I am thinking of giving her a trip with us somewhere," Louisa suggested. "Would you like to go?"

"What a wonderful idea," I said with the first real excitement about Mother in some time. "She loves New Mexico and all the Native American history. Santa Fe would be fun. It's easy to get around and there are shops, museums, and restaurants everywhere. I would love to go with you, but it is so hot where you are right now that I don't think I can make it down. Would you mind taking her on your own?"

"Not at all, I completely understand. You can't afford to come down here and have an MS relapse. Stay safe, big sister. Charlotte can go with us and it will be fine," she said.

Louisa had rejoiced when my first marriage came to an end and I found myself moving to Dallas, where, although referred to as North Texas, the temperatures were no less extreme. I had lived with multiple sclerosis for eleven years at that point, and each year in the heat made it progressively more difficult to enjoy life outside of the confines of an air-conditioned house.

Thomas Babstock found me soon after I moved there, and following a fairy tale courtship, we married and started a new life together. My family adored Tom, and they made frequent trips to see us. We loved seeing them on a regular basis, but always had to look for indoor activities to keep the heat at bay. When the temperatures began to exceed one hundred degrees for weeks at a time, we heard the Northeast calling to us. Not only was the sixty-three degree average appealing, but we both longed for a faster pace and new horizons. Tom's business expertise lay in portfolio management, so the career options were not difficult to narrow down and an offer shortly came from a large financial institution in New York City. Working in "The Big Apple" had always been on Tom's bucket list; and just as anxious to see and experience new things, I gave him my endorsement, and we moved even further north.

Mother cried when we told her.

"My children keep moving further and further away from me," she told everyone.

My parents knew, though, that relocating above the Mason-Dixon Line was absolutely necessary. Tom and I had a constant stream of visitors from the South who joined us as we hiked the Upstate New York countryside, explored streams, went fishing, wandered through gardens, and walked along lakeside paths. I thrived in the mild climate and loved life. For the next nine years it was easy to forget that I had MS – until the holidays when a trip back down South was obligatory.

My sister was one of my strongest advocates and insisted that I keep myself out of warm weather situations. She never expected me to put myself in a compromising situation and, true to her considerate nature, understood why I could not go with them on Mother's birthday trip in the middle of July. That may have been just as well, for Mother and I still tiptoed around each other as if walking on eggshells, and it would not have been a joyous birthday for her. I accepted that, and felt badly about it, but knew that her experience was more important than whether I could join them for the outing.

"Mom, I am so sorry, but I cannot go with you for your birthday trip, but you will have a fabulous time with Louisa and Char wherever you go. Have you thought about what you would like to do?" I asked her.

To my great surprise, she answered very compassionately, allowing a glimpse of her former self to break through the cobwebs.

"I understand, sweetie. You need to take care of yourself. We will get together another time," she said.

Perhaps, she was secretly glad that I was not going on the trip, but I pushed any furtive motives aside and thanked her for her understanding, which had been a constant for so many years. Maybe she was not lost inside the world of dementia, after all.

"Thanks, Mom. That means a lot to me," I assured her. "Have you decided where you want to go? How about Santa Fe? You could go to the opera and enjoy the history of the pueblos. The stores are fabulous and full of pottery and paintings that I know you love."

But then, much to my surprise, the pleasantness of our conversation changed back to darkness as if a light switch had gone off in her mind, and she loudly exclaimed, "I hate that place. I don't want to go there. Don't I remember that Matt took Louisa to Paris last year?"

Stunned, it took me a few seconds to recover from her outburst, and to think, *"Go with it… go with it… don't confront her."*

"Yes, they went to Paris last year with Tom and me," I said, not mentioning that we had given them the trip in celebration of both of their fiftieth birthdays and their twenty-fifth wedding anniversary.

"I think that is where I want to go," she declared, and I was glad that a thousand miles separated us so that she could not see the look of consternation on my face.

I had no idea how Louisa would react to Mother's request to go to Paris. So many things about such a trip were prohibitive, not the least of which was Louisa's own physical state. I began to pray for the right words to turn Mother's attention stateside and to enthuse her about a smaller, more intimate excursion somewhere in the Southwest, hoping that she might soon forget her desire to travel abroad.

"On the surface, Mom's desire to go to Paris for her eightieth sounds so romantic, Nora. I just cannot imagine that she would really immerse herself in the experience, though. When she went to Rome about five years ago, she had no idea that there was anything to look at in the Sistine Chapel! It sounds wonderful to tell your friends that your daughter took you to Paris for your birthday, but I fear that she would fail to appreciate it, and Louisa is not really in the best condition to take a trip of that magnitude," I said excitedly over the phone.

Nora and I were meeting by phone, and actually I found the conversations to be freer, without concern for whether someone at the next table might overhear us. The familiar plum and sea foam green surroundings of our living room calmed my mind, and I opened myself up to new revelations and insights when talking to Nora from there.

"Louisa came up with a brilliant idea to suggest that they go to Brenham in East Texas close to where Mom was born and tour the ice cream factory there. Blue Bell Ice Cream is famous in that area. It is what Whoopee Pies are to Maine or Philly cheese steak is to Philadelphia. She loved the idea and soon forgot all about Paris in favor of the chance to get ice cream."

Nora and I laughed together on the phone, and Tom came strolling in to see what was so funny. He really hates to be left out, particularly at the mention of ice cream. Nora and I gradually stopped chuckling and the conversation turned somber once again.

"We return to the things we know best when our world begins to close in. At this stage she is the equivalent of a seven-year-old, and that is exactly how a seven-year-old would react if given the choice between ice cream and someplace far away, no matter how exotic that place may be," Nora noted.

The fact that Mother was happiest when enjoying the simple things slowly began to work its way into my mind, for it was hard to accept that there would be no more conversations about Notre Dame's rose window, the colors of the Painted Desert, or the fog moving across Loch Lomond. Mother's voice was never happier than when she was describing what she and Dad had seen on their latest excursion.

"I suppose her days of traveling for the thrill of seeing new places are behind her now. We probably could just take her down the street to the soda fountain and she would be just as content," I surmised.

Louisa made reservations for Mother to fly to Houston, and Charlotte would drive the three of them into the hill country to stay at a Victorian bed and breakfast. So, on the appointed day and time, Elena dutifully took her client to the airport. Not having the ability to check-in online ahead of time, Mother presented her credit card at the ticket counter, the only identification she had placed in her wallet that morning.

"Why did you take out your photo ID and your passport, Mrs. Adams?" Elena asked.

She replied argumentatively, "All I need is the credit card I purchased the ticket on."

"Louisa bought your ticket on her credit card, so they have no record of your purchase. Tell the agent your name and address and maybe she will let you through without a photo ID," Elena chastised.

Mother became silent, awkwardly clinging to the counter in front of the ticket agent. Her hands began to tremble. She looked up into the patient face of the young lady and haltingly told her that she did not know her name. Elena stepped in and began to offer the name to the agent, who stopped her short with the admonition that the passenger must verify her own name without any assistance from Elena. Mother's anxiety rose, and the more confused she became, the longer the line formed behind them. The agent recognized that asking for the passenger's name was an exercise in futility and told her that she must have a photo ID and she would be happy to provide her with a boarding pass if she could produce such. Elena led Mother, now shaking and sobbing, back to the car and quickly drove six long miles back to the cottage, hoping that she would be able to recall where her ID or passport were located. A frantic search of the desk in the bedroom expanded to her dresser drawer into which Mrs. Adams had emptied the contents of her wallet.

"Mrs. Adams, here is your medical insurance card and your photo ID. You need both of those for this trip. Do you have cash in your wallet – put some money in there, too," Elena directed without making judgment or chastising.

Mother obediently followed her instructions and the two raced back to the airport, triumphantly presenting her ID to the now smiling agent. As promised, the agent presented her with a boarding pass, ordered a wheelchair, and cleared the way for Elena to assist her through security and onto the waiting plane.

"Nora, Louisa explained away Mom's inability to remember who she was as just being flustered. I can't agree with that," I said.

"It may be that she has serious memory lapses when she becomes agitated, but one's name is pretty basic," Nora agreed. "I picked up a booklet at the health seminar for the aging last week and thought of you and your mother. She may be moving into a time when things will be very frightening for her, and consequently, her emotions will be much more volatile. Most likely she knows something is wrong, but can't express it."

I took in her words with a heavy heart and prayed for the day when Mother would not care that she did not know her name. It felt odd to ask God for a disease to progress, and, yet, short of her death, that seemed to be the only release for my dear mother.

Mother eventually arrived at the other end of the short flight, where Charlotte greeted her with a wheelchair, and for a few moments the world turned brighter and seemed less frightening. Mother, daughter and granddaughter were all joyfully reunited at Louisa's house before loading suitcases into the car and driving up into the hill country where the promise of ice cream awaited them. They toured the ice cream factory, and laughing and acting silly - because ice cream makes one do that - they licked their way through each free sample at the end of the tour. The remainder of the three days was spent driving through the gently rolling hills and the quaint little towns, and relaxing at the bed and breakfast in the afternoons before going out to eat dinner in a mom-and-pop restaurant somewhere.

Mother's account of the trip was simple, "...a very fine birthday present, as far as I was concerned." Louisa's gift had been met with approval, and Mother was satisfied that her eightieth birthday had been sufficiently celebrated. When I asked her about the trip, she couldn't recall many of the details other than the scrumptious breakfasts at the house and the samples of ice cream at the factory. She repeatedly told me what a fine driver Charlotte was... and how much pain Louisa was in.

Louisa was, indeed, exhausted from the three days with Mother and, much to my surprise, was not reluctant in the least to tell me that our elderly mother should not be living on her own. I wondered what had transpired to make Louisa say that, as she had been so opposed to it prior to the trip. Those three days were a pivotal point in my sister's acceptance of Mother's condition and it was interesting to note that Louisa's reactions were thereafter filled with anger and frustration at Mother's antics. I could identify somewhat with these emotions, having experienced them when she sat in our family room calling me names, absolutely refusing to act as the gracious lady I once knew her to be.

"Nora, my sister and niece had a hard time with Mom's toileting. Her legs are not strong enough for her to use a regular size toilet. None of them thought about this until they reached the bed and breakfast where she immediately needed Charlotte to help her stand up. That happened several times before they finally went to a pharmacy and bought a riser for the bathroom in their suite. Louisa was so put out with Mom for just not even thinking before she sat down that she might need assistance getting back up. Likewise, when they went out touring, my sister became so frustrated with Mom when she did not choose a handicap restroom over a regular one. Char had to come to her rescue many times before finally going with her into the restroom and directing her to choose the handicap stall," I told Nora. "To make things even worse, apparently, she did not shower the entire trip. Char bore the brunt of this when lifting her grandmother off the toilet seats. I felt so badly for her. She is so young to have to experience this. I'm really proud of her for stepping up and conducting herself in such a caring and gentle way. It would have been my inclination to react like Louisa did - with disbelief and disgust."

Nora replied, "I found it easier to care for Mommie when I put it in the context of the commandment to love our elders. Taking care of my parent when she could no longer care for herself was not only a way of showing my mother honor, but I felt was one of God's expectations of me. Allison, their frail bodies and aging minds are ours to nurture until He chooses to take them home. We can respond to that call with our noses turned up, or with a gentle and loving hand and attitude."

She encouraged me to read the material which she had picked up for me from the seminar, and I began to study more diligently what the Alzheimer's individual experiences in the several progressive stages of the disease. According to the many articles and books on the subject, I could expect her to respond more positively to quiet sounds... to soft touches... to a slower pace. Exuberant greetings and quick movements were off putting. Loud noises and surprises, even sharp contrasts in colors, could bring on an overly agitated response. I had noticed that Mother's reactions to something as ordinary as someone entering the room were exaggerated and alarming. She was fragile, like a piece of prized crystal, and desperately needed a gentle and loving hand.

The trip completed, but Mother's actual birthday still a few days away, the choice of what to give her for her birthday continued to hang over me. The search for a gift that would bring her joy and comfort had been ongoing for several weeks until I realized that she soon forgot items previously given to her, such as photo albums, jewelry, and books. Yet, she was able to remember experiences – licking on an ice cream treat, eating a rum-soaked fruitcake, or smelling the fragrance of her favorite flower, even if the did make her sneeze. All made lasting impressions on her, and although she did not always recall the actual flavor of the fruitcake or the kind of flowers in the bouquet, she did know that she was loved. That was my goal for her birthday – that she felt loved.

The fruitcake had been such a hit the year before that I decided to pull out all the stops and choose something truly decadent – a dozen chocolate-covered strawberries delivered by courier in a gold foil box. I tracked the progress of the delivery online and within thirty minutes of having reached her address, I dialed Elena's cell phone number.

With visions of melted globs of chocolate and sundried strawberries out on her doorstep, I was glad that she took the call and excitedly asked, "Mom, have you checked your front door for a package?"

"Ohhhh, yes! He rang the doorbell and then left it there before we could get to the door. I'm going to have one a day and they will be so luscious."

Mother cooed with delight at the thought and she smacked her lips in anticipation of tasting the next juicy morsel drenched in milk chocolate. Every conversation for the next few weeks contained details of eating chocolate-covered strawberries, and then... they were never mentioned again. But, for that short time period, Mother tasted love, and that feeling stayed with her. Her mind does not remember why, but her heart knows she is loved. With Mother, we must live for the moment - one moment at a time. Like a wave on the shore, it will only last an instant and then it is gone.

My conversations with Nora had taken on a more philosophical tone in the weeks following Mother's birthday.

"How important is the truth when Mom's reality is obviously somewhere else, Nora? She struggles to make sense of her world and to place events in neat little boxes that work for her," I noted.

"Let's take that question a little further. It may not be important where the real truth lies in your relationship with your mother, but I think the truth is important in your relationship with your sister," Nora conjectured. "How much do you want Louisa to accept *your* truth, as opposed to *hers*?"

"What is important to me is that she accepts that Mom is incapable of seeing reality as it really exists. She now knows that Mom's physical body is aging, but Louisa desperately wants to believe that she is still capable of rational thought," I answered. "My deepest desire is for Louisa to open her eyes and see that Mom's reality is clouded and smudged, and to acknowledge that Mom is really quite ill. Only then can we begin to meet her needs."

"So, it comes back to the fact that you feel you are many steps further along on this journey than Louisa," Nora suggested.

"Yes, you can't walk with someone on a journey if they are lagging behind. Walking with someone means elbow to elbow, arm in arm, ready to support them when they cannot do it themselves," I insisted. "Louisa probably sees me as someone who pushes Mom along a pathway that she does not want to follow, while I see her as having no choice and that the path itself is pulling her along. My vision is for Mom to walk this pathway with Louisa and me on either side supporting her and keeping her from falling. Unfortunately, Louisa does not even see the path, nor does she believe that Mom needs protection along the way. One of the greatest difficulties is learning how to communicate with my sister about the two different ways we are attempting to help our mother."

"What was the trip like for Charlotte?" Nora wondered out loud.

By Louisa's accounting, Mother was unusually sweet to the once-gangly teenager now turned beauty queen.   Charlotte's attentiveness to her mother had not gone unnoticed by Grandmother. We both marveled that Mother still had the ability to be that observant and rejoiced that she chose to praise Charlotte rather than tear her down, as had been her recent practice. Some of Mother's conversations, however, posed a big challenge for her daughter and granddaughter, for the sentences were dotted with nonsensical statements, subjects were wildly taken out of context, and fairy tales abounded. Mother found it increasingly difficult to recall proper nouns and became agitated at her inability to communicate. Getting her point across was frustrating for speaker and listener alike.   Charlotte noticed that most sentences were peppered with negativity, and she was appalled at her grandmother's use of very coarse language.   Perhaps most distressing to Charlotte was Grandmother's proclivity to lie, and she and her mother discussed it at length after the trip had come to a close.

"Allison, she just... she just... *lies*," Louisa said with disbelief. "Charlotte's eyes got so big every time Grandmother told an untruth."

In the year and half that we had been discussing the situation, I had never heard my sister acknowledge that Mother did not tell the truth.   Always the consummate professional and kindhearted supporter, I had never heard my sister even imply that someone was a liar, but to hear her express this newfound revelation about our mother was oddly heartening. I did not desire for anyone in our family to be a liar, but because the facts were indisputable, it gave me hope that Louisa might finally be seeing a bit of the cloud under which Mother lived.

"I just never knew that about Mom," she continued after a long breath. "After being with her non-stop for three days, it was so apparent. We had a suite where we could all be together. I wasn't about to put her in a room by herself, and I didn't want Char to be in a room alone. So, the bed and breakfast had the perfect solution. That's how we knew she did not shower, even though she insisted that she did. It's interesting that she had no concept of where we were staying. We drove up to this beautiful Victorian house and she said, 'This is where we are staying? Not a motel? Where is my suitcase? Did we bring my suitcase?' Her conversations were so odd. It isn't very hard, even for a stranger, to realize that something is wrong. Allie, her knee is really giving her problems. We had to help her over every little step – even the smallest rise in a sidewalk or threshold in a doorway was impossible for her to negotiate, even with her walker."

Louisa wanted to talk. The narcotics she took routinely dulled her ability to see our parent as she really is, and, yet, those three days were as if God had given her the gift of sight. I felt a sudden release of tension as Louisa finally saw Mother's new personage – a woman in desperate need of help, in need of guidance, in need of so much more than we were giving her. My sweet sister, no longer naïve, talked well into the night; and we comforted one another, for we knew that the long goodbye had begun in earnest.

Chapter 9

Our house was quiet except for the lowered sound of the television. Night had fallen several hours before and the moon made long patterns on the sheers at the family room windows. It was a perfect evening with the sweet smell of curry coming from the kitchen. Conversation had been easy and light between us, and Tom had fallen asleep in his recliner while watching his favorite show, which was not all that unusual these days. I smiled at the quiet sound of his breath going in and out; and turning off the television, I curled up beneath the blankets on the sofa and allowed myself to be lulled to sleep by the rhythm of his breathing.

We were both suddenly jolted upright by the sound of the telephone. Tom struggled to find his glasses and throw off the afghan before rushing to the kitchen to answer the ring, which had been set on the loudest setting in order to be heard throughout the three-story townhouse - and probably halfway down the street. The caller was Mom. Tom handed the phone to me while racing to pick up another handset from downstairs.

"I want Tom and you on the phone together," Mother was crying, and I had difficulty understanding her words.

My heart froze inside me. I had received such a call from her a decade earlier, and the news had not been good. Just as now, she had asked for both of us to be on the phone together before telling us that my father had passed. This call had the same urgency, and the lateness of the hour added to my anxiety. My immediate thought was that something terrible had happened to Louisa. Tom was the first to finally understand her words. I was so relieved to hear that it was not bad news about my sister, that I barely comprehended what she actually did say.

"I have cancer," came the words between her sobs.

"Oh, Mom, I am so sorry," was all I could say at the shocking news.

"Imogene, where is the cancer?" Tom, the more composed of us, asked when her sobbing had subsided.

"On my neck. I went to see Dr. Zachariah for my annual checkup and she did a biopsy. It came back today as cancer."

Tom and I glanced at each other, knowing that she must have confused the names of the doctors because she swore that she would never go back to Dr. Zachariah. I knew that she was going to see a dermatologist about a mole on her neck, so we believed that part of her story to be true, but then the story became more and more convoluted. It had become almost routine to listen to Mother's accounting and recounting of events and then to weigh the words carefully against accounts told us by Elena and Louisa before being able to dissect which parts were based on reality and which parts she had conjured up.

"Waverly Place was doing some tests and it came back positive for cancer. Two big burly male nurses called me on the phone and just blurted out that I have cancer. I have to go to the hospital to have it cut out," she said more calmly, beginning to enjoy the attention she was getting from Tom.

Feedback echoed over the two phone extensions making it difficult to hear, and as Tom was able to calm her down a bit, I hung up the phone on my end so that they could hear one another more clearly. I listened while he asked her leading questions about the type of skin cancer and where the procedure would be performed. He was familiar with squamous cell carcinoma, having had one removed from his own face the year before. Tom was the perfect person to reassure his mother-in-law and to let her know what to expect. Several members of our immediate family have been through this many times before. Mother's overwrought reaction made me roll my eyes.

"Oh, please," I thought. *"Get a grip, Mom."*

I was all too ready to belittle her hysteria over something relatively insignificant and to speak dismissively of the diagnosis when Tom reminded Mother of Aunt Goldy's success with the removal of a skin cancer, and that she need not be so worried. She could relax knowing she was in God's hands. Mother, however, seemed unwilling to give up her melodramatic stance and continued to tell everyone that she had cancer and would be undergoing radical neck surgery the following week.

I was glad to see Nora a few days after Mother's phone call.

"Nora, I'm not doing very well with Mom. I can't determine if she is blowing this out of proportion simply to get attention, or if she is really scared and concerned about the outcome of the surgery. The appointment is at a doctors' professional building, so it is not at a surgical center. Nevertheless, she called Sylvia and the pastor to inform them and to request that she be placed on the prayer list," I said over a chicken, walnut, and cranberry salad. "...and how could she know that it was 'two big burly men' that informed her over the phone that she had cancer?!"

"Your mother is not capable of taking things in stride," Nora noted. "Granted, her reaction to this is a little out of proportion because she does not understand there are different levels of severity of skin cancer, and she will probably never be able to understand that. Cancer is cancer for someone in her generation. It's all bad as far as she is concerned."

The conversation paused as we decided if we wanted dessert with coffee and tea. We opted for just coffee and tea.

"This is a major event when you consider what a typical day in your mother's life is like," Nora pointed out, directing the conversation back to Mother's reaction to the skin cancer diagnosis. "Medical issues are a major source of breaks from an otherwise monotonous routine. This is something important that she can talk about, and it could very well be something quite serious."

I felt sufficiently admonished and felt the need to explain myself.

"The problem is that we don't know when she is crying wolf. It is very difficult to gauge how to reassure her. I don't know whether to continue to try and redirect her or just go with it and justify her feelings."

"Whether you are offering words of assurance or trying to direct her focus somewhere else, you can still do it with love," Nora reminded me.

My prayers that night were for forgiveness – forgiveness for making my mother's feelings small and unimportant. Whether fueled by the need for attention or by fear over an unexpected medical issue, her feelings were real to her and my response as a daughter must be one of kindness rather than reproach, of acceptance rather than dismissal. She had held my small hand when I learned to walk on the hardwood floors of our little house in Nacogdoches, and now it was my turn to take her hands, gnarled with arthritis, and to steady her equally hesitant steps.

Elena sensed that something was bothering Mrs. Adams more than the impending surgery. The day before the appointment, Mother pulled out the family photo albums and the two of them sat side by side to flip through the pages. As they progressed through the years of school pictures and family vacations, she told Elena how proud she was of her eldest daughter. Elena was astounded that she could remember so much about my life and joyfully relayed to me that Mother said that she loved to hear me sing, admired my creations on the sewing machine, and was proud of my accomplishments in furthering higher education for women.

Then Mother asked Elena, "Why doesn't she want to talk to me?"

I was aghast because we had just talked a few nights before.

"What makes her think I don't want to talk to her, Elena?" I had quickly asked.

"She said that Tom talked to her, but that you didn't want to," Elena said.

"Oh, dear, she misinterpreted why I hung up the phone. The feedback on the extension was making it hard to hear her. She is really very sensitive right now, isn't she?"

"Mrs. Adams is easily upset. Lots of things are not clear and she can't always figure something out, so she makes things up," the caregiver explained. "I told her you wanted to talk to her and that you love her very much. She seemed happy to hear that."

I promised to call Mother that night and not to mention that Elena and I had talked. Any hint that her caregiver spoke routinely with her daughters would instantly put Elena's relationship with Mother in jeopardy.

When she finally answered the phone, I eagerly greeted her, "Hi, Mom. Are you ready for your surgery tomorrow?"

"Well, I think so. My suitcase is packed and I'm ready," she said. "I just want to get it over with."

"Good for you. I am so proud of you," I said as enthusiastically as I could. "Who is taking you?"

"Elena will take me, ...and Sylvia and my pastor will be there," she said slowly.

She sounded tired and small and troubled.

"Well, I think you will do very well, Mom. The doctor will probably just deaden the area and it will be like going to the dentist."

"I want to be put to sleep. I don't want to know what he is doing, and cancer is a lot more than just going to the dentist," she said indignantly.

"It's going to be alright, Mom," I said, not knowing how else to respond. "I will call you tomorrow night after you have gotten home."

"Oh, I will be spending several days in the hospital. You can call me there."

"Ohhh-kay, I will do that. Love you lots," I said before hanging up, pleased with myself for holding my tongue.

As we all expected, the procedure took place in the dermatologist's office. Mother's neck was deadened around the area to be excised and the procedure was completed in ten minutes, leaving her with five neat little stitches. She would get a complete report in a week when the stitches were removed.

Elena took her back home in less than an hour from leaving the house, and Sylvia went about her afternoon errands. The church pastor had other business to attend to and had not been present in the office waiting room, but called his parishioner later that afternoon to see how she was doing.

"Nora, I think the church folks have caught on to mother's cries for attention and help. Her pastor is very much in tune with his aging congregation, and I know that she is not the only parishioner for whom he prays daily. Mom and I talked that night and, of course, she didn't mention anything about staying overnight or going under general anesthesia. She primarily talked about going into the tiniest little operating room that was so crowded because of all the people that had come to be with her, none of whom she could name. Elena told me that the surgeon asked her privately if Mrs. Adams had Alzheimer's."

"Really, it is that obvious?" Nora asked.

"Apparently, it is. He also told Elena that Mrs. Adams should not be living alone, it is too dangerous," I related. "We all agree on that subject – well, maybe not my sister - but we are held up by legal issues of Mother's own doing."

"Any progress in getting her in to see the primary care physician?" Nora inquired as we stopped at the cash register before making our way out onto the sidewalk in search of an empty table in the shade.

'Well, yes, there is good news on that front. I almost forgot," I said as we found a spot under the wisteria-covered pergola. "She has an appointment next week to get a referral for a knee surgeon. Elena has planted in her mind that she has to see doctor in order to then see someone who can do surgery on her knee. It seems that Mom responds to opportunities for surgery and that is how Elena is coaxing her into the doctor's office."

"That is a great idea," Nora said in her charming soprano voice. "How does it make you feel to be…shall we say… sneaky?"

"That kind of thing used to bother me, but I got over it. Convincing Mom of something has proven to be almost impossible now that she has graduated from stubborn to just plain belligerent," I said blithely, beginning to accept the peculiar challenges presented by my aging parent. "Tom frequently reminds me that geriatric counselors condone the use of whatever tactics will work to get dementia patients to do what is required for their own care and well-being. One story a friend told me last week was about the woman who approached the neurologist's examining room with her elderly mother in tow, and pushing her through the doorway, said, 'She thinks she is here for a mammogram.'"

Nora threw her head back in a hearty laugh, probably recalling a similar scenario with her mother.

The day after the removal of the skin cancer from Mother's neck, my cell phone rang. I noticed that it was my mother calling, which startled me a bit, as she usually refrains from contacting me while at work. She started the conversation with a plaintive tone, which suggested that she thought we had not talked for some time, and that, indeed, proved to be the case. The next few minutes were a complete retelling of her surgical experience, as if we had not had the exact conversation the day before. I played along with the appropriate responses in the appropriate places, and she seemed quite happy to have spoken with me. She claimed that she tried to reach me the day before – "all day" - and that Louisa gave her my cell phone number. I knew then that she did not remember that all the family numbers were written down on the kitchen phone speed dial.

Mother's call worried me on several different levels, but of immediate concern was that she was slurring her words and speaking in a silly sing-song kind of voice. As soon as the call ended, I phoned Elena and asked her to drive over and check on her because she sounded... well, drunk... and Mother does not drink.

"Nora, when Elena got there Mom was acting very strangely, could barely talk, and was holding on to the walls to steady herself. She told Elena that she had taken a pill that made her 'feel goofy.' Elena searched in the kitchen and found an unmarked bottle that she knew did not belong to Mom. The bottle did not have a label on it, but the handwritten note on the cap read 'Painkiller.' Elena recognized the pills as Darvocet."

Startled, Nora looked up from her cup of tomato basil, "Darvocet - That is for major surgeries and really serious pain. Where did she get that?"

"Mom told Elena that Imelda gave it to her. There were several bottles of different things, including Nitroglycerin, which she was positive Mom should not have had. Elena had her drink several glasses of water before gathering up all the medications and putting them in her bag. When Mom was a little more coherent, she talked with her about the dangers of taking drugs other than those prescribed by her own doctor," I exclaimed. "It is just like those talks we had in school by police officers and their drug-sniffing dogs. Do you remember those? 'Just say No' wasn't around when Mom was growing up, but you would think she would know not to take someone else's prescription medications."

I was thankful that we had an Angel of Mercy in the form of Elena to intercede for us since Mother was not inclined of late to follow our suggestions. It was almost beyond my comprehension that my mother was abusing drugs.

"Elena also walked next door to talk with Imelda and to return the drugs. She also told her not to give Mrs. Adams any more medications," I added.

"Good for her. You are incredibly lucky that she cares so much for your mother," Nora interjected.

"Yes, but there is more…The next day when she was back at Mom's house, the pill bottles had all reappeared. Mom and Imelda had either forgotten or had ignored Elena's warnings," I said incredulously.

"No!" Nora exclaimed with equal disbelief.

"… and of course, Elena dutifully went through the whole process again."

"Your mother is a follower and Imelda is a problem for those who don't know how to 'Just say No.'"

"Louisa is so distraught. Being a parent, she had that very same drug talk with her children when they were in elementary school. Like you, she knows exactly what it is like to be the worrisome parent, except this time she is waiting for news of her parent."

"Allison, a parent has to trust that they have taught their child how to make good decisions."

"But, Nora, my mother doesn't have the ability to make good decisions. We *must* motivate her to accept around the clock supervision either in her cottage or in the dementia unit," I said with firm resolve.

Nora suggested that Waverly Place become involved in the situation with Imelda and contact Imelda's family who might be able to reinforce the dangers of sharing medications. In a brainstorming mode, we quickly came up with other ideas, including adding to Elena's hours, a topic that had been visited many times before.

"Mom is not able to readily distinguish the time of day, much less when her caregiver comes and goes. I think we can just ask Elena to stay an extra hour or two each day and gradually increase the number of hours without Mom realizing it. Louisa is in charge of Elena's hours. I will mention it to her the next time we talk," I said, seeing a small window of opportunity opening.

Following the episode with the drugs, Mother's support

system quickly kicked into high gear and worked behind the scenes to make small, but significant, changes in her life. Louisa and Elena agreed to quietly increase the time spent with Mother, while I fired off an email to Deborah about "Imelda's Pharmacy" now operating on Emerald Drive. For the first time we seemed to be making progress on behalf of our mother. She would soon be seeing her gynecologist, to whom I had already faxed a letter asking him to refer her to a neurologist. We would soon know if Dr. Lucas was completely in accord with the dementia diagnosis and willing to act on our request, even though Mother had not given permission for him to speak with us. Elena would be accompanying her to that appointment, and the lines of communication between Elena, Louisa and I were fully open. It felt exhilarating to finally be on the same page with my sister, and with the added bolstering which Elena provided, I felt hopeful for the first time in many months. I was proud of my sister and told her so the next time we talked.

"Louisa, you have accomplished some tremendous things with Mom lately...the car...taking over Elena's schedule... What can we do about her refusal to shower? I think the urinary tract infections she has are a direct result of poor hygiene. How do we talk to her about it? Is it something we can gently bring up?"

There was a long silence on the other end of the line before Louisa answered, "I just don't know. If Mom could have seen herself like this twenty years ago, she would be so embarrassed and horrified."

I thought of Nora's words, "Growing old is a gift," and struggled to embrace their truth when thinking of Mother. We want our elders to live on this earth as long as possible, and I wondered if that was not a selfish desire. When the mind and body begin to drift away from us there is such sadness, and sometimes anger, in seeing a life lose its brilliance. Finding new purposes for life, and new ways to love, challenges the strongest of spirits. Perhaps, the gift is in the opportunities for growth that these challenges present. Taking a single step can be precious because walking itself is no longer easy. The act of washing the body is not simple for a toddler, nor is it simple for my mother. The gift of growing old may be in the joy of learning to splash in the water again.

As if reading my mind, Louisa continued, "Mom doesn't know *how* to shower. I don't think it is that she doesn't want to, as much as it is that she can't remember all the steps; and who can get excited about doing something that you have to think about that hard? I told Elena about it after the birthday trip. Elena thinks she knows of ways to help Mom with hygiene that won't embarrass her. I think we have to completely trust her on this. God sent Elena to us, and now we have to let God work through her."

Mother had not talked about God in some time. More often than not she told me that she did not feel like going to church, and routinely mentioned weak legs, or a swimming head, or a favorite of late – diarrhea. Elena assured me that Mother was not having difficulties with incontinence, and that she had actually let Elena monitor her bowel movements. This came as quite a surprise to me, but the feisty Latin woman reminded her that she was a home healthcare aide and this was part of her job. Elena laughed when I asked if Mother was having problems with her bowel movements. It seems that diarrhea was the excuse Mother employed when she did not want to go somewhere because people generally did not ask questions if you told them you had diarrhea.

"Your mother is progressing rather quickly now," Nora gently said as she slowly stirred cream into her coffee. "How do you feel about that?"

Knowing that this beautiful lady had walked this way before me, I did not hold back, and we talked for the better part of two hours about our mothers and our families. Nora's mother had never been a happy person and this was made all the more pronounced by her husband's diagnosis of Alzheimer's ten years before her. Mommie had worn herself out taking care of her spouse and had no energy left to take care of herself, leaving the planning and decision-making following her own onset of dementia to her children. Her battle was a long-fought struggle until she finally passed away quite peacefully. Nora recalled what a blessed release it was to see her mother finally become calm and relaxed, but wished the feeling of peacefulness had come sooner.

"It is sad, Nora, very sad," I said. "However, there are moments when Mom still laughs out loud. The center of who she is, is still there, glowing vibrantly. I just have to find ways to bring it out and remind her that she is still a person of beauty and worth. I find it so terribly hard, though, because she has buried herself under such a cloud of negative thoughts. This part of the journey makes me particularly weary."

Nora, too, sensed that I was tired – not necessarily in body, but in spirit. It was not hard for her to see that my cup had been nearly emptied, and I was in need of refilling.

"Remember, caregivers need to care for themselves, as well as for their loved ones. I often had to just step back and leave things in someone else's hands for a while. That may be one of your biggest challenges – to realize that *you* need to take time to breathe for yourself," Nora reminded me. "Will you be going on vacation soon?"

"Yes, Tom and I are making our annual fall trip to Bliss to check on our property and to enjoy some lobster and rocky shorelines," I said with a bright tone. "That is such a rejuvenating trip, and I am ready. I need to go see Mom first. I sense that these days while she still knows who I am are very precious. Elena told me something very troubling a few days ago…"

Nora pushed her dinner plate away and sat back in her chair to wait for me to continue, her thoughtful eyes shining beneath her white bangs.

I took a deep breath and began, "Elena was finally successful in getting Mom in to see her primary care physician – the ob-gyn. She believed it was time for her annual visit and that she also needed to see him to get a referral for knee surgeon, so she went quite willingly. She let Elena go in with her and then, as the nurse was assisting her in preparing for the exam, the doctor interviewed Elena in his office. He asked Elena if there had been any changes in Mrs. Adam's life since he last saw her. She told him about the hallucinations and paranoia, her weakness, and that she forgets to eat and to take her medications. He said right out to her that Mom should not be living alone. Dr. Lucas admitted that as an ob-gyn he did not know very much about Alzheimer's, and would be referring her to a geriatric neurologist."

"That's fabulous, Allison," Nora said. "Don't you think so?"

"Absolutely! We are so thankful that he received and read our letters and is in complete accord that Mom needs medical help.

He told Elena, though, that he was very sorry he could not talk to either of Mrs. Adams' daughters because she had not given him permission. I laughed at Elena because she then said, 'Well, have you asked her?' So, when he went back into the examining room, he took the form and asked if she would like to indicate three people that he could discuss her medical issues with. Mom laboriously filled in two names – Elena's and Louisa's. Elena said the doctor wondered if she didn't want her eldest daughter to be in the third spot, and Mom replied, 'No, Allison is not a part of my life.'"

I almost choked on the words in the retelling. Nora remained still until the lump in my throat allowed me to talk again.

"Elena said the doctor looked over at her, but she knew that there was nothing he could do without Mom's permission, even in her current mental state," I said in a quivering voice, shifting slightly in my seat, no longer interested in the food and drink on the table. "You know, Nora, I am grateful that Mom at least put down two names and that we now have a link with Dr. Lucas's office through Louisa and Elena. It does not have to be me, as long as someone can discuss her case with him."

"You don't truly believe that she is spurning you, do you?" Nora's hand rested lightly on my arm. She paused as if to let the words sink in before adding, "Alzheimer's patients often turn on the ones they love the most."

In some strange way, that was meant to make me feel better, and I suppose it did. It is not the usual expression of love that one hopes for. Mother was living in a world driven by fear. She was afraid of losing herself. At times I wondered if she knew who she was. I recall that on my last visit to her cottage, she had a snapshot of herself prominently displayed on the filing cabinet on the way into her bathroom. Nora had warned me that it is common for dementia individuals not to recognize themselves in a mirror - and one entire wall of her bathroom was a mirror. The strategic placement of the picture of herself made me wonder if she wanted a reminder of who the person was looking back at her in the mirror.

"How can I possibly fault someone who struggles so with something as basic as her own identity?" I asked Nora. "Maybe she thinks I will take away the last bit of self awareness she has by institutionalizing her. Her autonomy has always been of the utmost importance to Mom. She believes that my sister is too ill and fighting her own medical battles to be of any threat. I, on the other hand, am perfectly capable of seeing that she has a fulltime companion, whether she wants it or not."

Nora chuckled, "Mommie wanted to make her own decisions, as well. After all, she had been doing it for eighty years and then to have her little girls running her life, telling her when to bathe, when to eat, how to dress – she just blew up. She was so mean to her caregivers at the nursing home, but they told us that is not all that unusual."

We both stared down at our plates, grateful that we had made our own decisions about the contents of the plates, realizing that someday we might not be able to make those decisions.

"The difficulty with Mom is that she wants to make decisions for herself – what to wear today, what she would like to watch on television, how much money to spend on a new pair of sneakers – but her brain doesn't have the ability to realize that it is hot outside and that a sweater is not appropriate," I said, looking back up at Nora. "Her brain can't figure out how to push the right sequence of buttons on the TV remote control to tune in to 'Andy Griffith'. As an adult, she should have the right to make decisions for herself, even the tiniest decisions, but her brain can't recall how to do those things and it makes her angry... and afraid. Who would not react in a similar way?"

"Caregiving is hardest when the person you are caring for not only doesn't appreciate it, but lashes back at you," Nora said with a faraway expression. "Mommie said some very mean things to me. It meant nothing to her that I flew across the continent just to see her. Mommie only knew that there were many blanks that her mind could not fill in, and it made her anxious and mean. I had to stay focused on meeting her physical needs and handling her affairs while pushing aside her hurtful reactions."

Her faraway gaze then focused and she turned back to meet mine, "It helped to think of it as a job, as a responsibility assigned to me by my boss."

My meal was cold, but the conversation was stimulating and it felt good to be talking to someone who understood the need to be more mechanical in approaching Mother's care plan.

Long distance caregiving is particularly difficult in that one does not get to know the ebb and flow of emotions, the already established routines, when one's parent is most tired or irritable, what triggers an angry outburst, or what calms and reassures them. I found that it was easier to speak with Mother after I had received a report from Elena about their day – was Mother rested, did she sleep well the night before, had she eaten, were there any visitors today, did they get out of the house to run errands, was there anything she might be concerned about. I counted myself fortunate that Elena could act as a barometer and tell me how to set my sails before calling the cottage. Mother's rebuffs landed more gently when I knew to expect them... and if she was in a sweet mood, I could plan to linger a bit longer on the phone with her.

"Nora, I think I want to go see my mother," I told her one hot Wednesday evening in late summer. "The time is coming when she will not know my face or recognize my voice, and I really need to be with her for as long as possible. Her outbursts and feelings have been so strong lately. I feel a change is coming very soon..."

"You are wise to see her now," Nora agreed. "It will only become more difficult. She will not get any better, only worse."

I looked across the little round table at her and detected tiredness in her eyes, as well. Nora's own recent knee replacement had been taxing on her and the pain of learning to walk on it was an ever present reminder that she was growing older herself. We often talked about the possibility that we would also face diminished memories, me less so than her, for both of her parents and all of her uncles had been touched by the disease.

Our conversation had taken on a sad tone, perhaps because Nora was weary and it took effort to smile through the pain of her recuperating knee, and because I was homesick my mother. It had been years since I had experienced homesickness. Home was always with my husband. Wherever his jobs took us, we had made that place home. This day, however, home was where my mother was – far away across many miles and shrouded in a fog of fading memories.

❖

Chapter 10

$\mathcal{M}$y mother did not hesitate for an instant when I asked if I could come see her. Tom's family just shows up on your doorstep and one is invited in like a lost puppy. Show up unannounced on my family's doorstep and the question would instantly be posed, "Who died?" So, I dutifully requested an invitation to visit.

"Yes, of course. I would love to have you visit. When are you coming?"

I told her that it would not be until the fall when the temperatures were a bit cooler, although, that would only marginally bring the ambient air temperatures down into the eighties. Still, that was better than the ninety-eight to one-hundred degrees they had been having. So, fall it would be - but for Mother, it was tomorrow.

Elena's weekly phone call revealed that Mother was expecting me to arrive quite literally "tomorrow." Whatever day it may be, it was always the next day that I would be ringing her doorbell. She excitedly told Elena that they must tidy up the guest bedroom and go to the grocery store. Yet, at the same time, Mother was worried. She was worried that I was coming to "fix her." Elena reassured her on a daily basis that I was not arriving for several weeks, as fall was months in the future. My sister had a similar tête-à-tête with Mother over my estimated arrival date and more importantly, my objective in wanting to see her. However much they reassured her, Mother did not seem to be reassured and held fast to the idea that my arrival was imminent and would be life-changing.

"Nora, Mom rarely calls me on the phone. It is usually something of huge importance to her that will prompt her to dial my number. She was so overwrought that I might be arriving right then, and urged – no, *begged* me not to come just then. She said it was much too hot for me - which I thought was rather sweet that she was concerned for my welfare, but I knew it was her way of saying 'don't come.'"

"Was that hard for you to hear?"

I smiled weakly.

"Yes, it is a bit hard to hear the fear in her voice. I love my mother and I believe that she loves me. But, it is such an unbelievably strange feeling to think that something has taken over her brain and her heart and literally turned against me. She must be in turmoil, and yet none of us can help her resolve those fears."

The little white-haired lady walking beside me had become my surrogate mother. When I needed my spirit lifted, her praise fell softly on my ears and brought calm to the churning inside me. God always provides when we take time to listen. Now, it was my turn to provide that same feeling of warmth and love for my mother. Labor Day arrived with only slightly cooler weather, but the time felt right to make a trip back home.

An uneasiness came upon me, however, as Mother still seemed reticent to greet me on the phone. There was always that tinge of fear and worry in her voice. Although never spoken directly to me, Elena and Louisa reluctantly shared with me that Mother's outbursts had become much more pronounced and pointed, and Louisa feared for my safety if I chose to make the trip to San Angelo. Mother had never been a violent person, and I found it hard to believe that she would take any such action, but... I would be alone with her in the house... at night... when her paranoia was deepest. Perhaps, she would feel equally threatened by my presence in her house without the protection of my sister to stand guard between us. I had not been alone in my mother's presence in many months and, no doubt, she did have many fearful thoughts which revolved around my pending visit. We both needed an interceder, someone who loved us both and was sensitive to the situation.

Tom was the first to offer to make the trip with me. After more than a year of surreptitiously listening in on the conversations coming from our living room, he had adopted a less "I can fix it" stance in favor of one that listened and validated my feelings. We laughed about the difference in the two approaches. While he was armed with a roll of duct tape - which he firmly believed could fix any problem - Nora offered a box of tissues.

"Louisa, my sweet husband has offered to go with me to see Mom," I told her on the phone a few days before the trip. "Both of us just feel that it would be beneficial in making a more comfortable visit for everyone since Mom is so uneasy around me."

"Oh, I so glad," she said with obvious relief.

I told her about the nagging sense of physical danger in visiting Mother alone, especially in staying overnight in a guest room that had no lock on the door.

"How awful," Nora exclaimed. "You really think she might harm you?"

I shrugged my shoulders before answering, "Nora, she is not in her right mind, if you will pardon the expression. Louisa confessed that she had the same thought. It gives me chills to think of such a thing, but Mom is really not at all the kind and warm person we once knew. Elena said that she keeps a 10" screwdriver on the bedside table in order to attack anyone who gets too close. I don't want to reach out to hug her and have her stab me with a screwdriver."

Chills ran through me as I described other precautions that Elena forewarned us about. It would not surprise me in the least to have her once again hiding all the kitchen knives in the trunk of the car, but most of Mother's preparations were innocuous and only served to point toward the battle she was mounting against the paranoia that pervaded her life.

"I have to see her, Nora," I said with determination.

Our flight to Texas a few days later was uneventful other than the nervous jittering of my leg and crushing grip on Tom's arm. We rented a car and drove three hours southwest across the still warm prairie. Approaching the Waverly Place security gate, Tom announced that we were there to see Imogene Adams. The gruff-looking guard in institutional gray barely glanced at his clipboard before waving us through. Every entrance after that for the next three days was met with a simple nod and a wave of the hand.

The cottage appeared just as I had remembered it with pots

of happy geraniums on the tiny front porch and a very brown ash tree struggling to grow in the rock hard front lawn. We pulled into the garage wondering if the door was up because she had once again forgotten to keep it closed or if she intended for us to utilize the shady darkness to keep the car cool. My sister had suggested that we arrive after Elena had reported to work, but in spite of the cool and nervous reception that I expected, I truly desired to greet my mother unencumbered by the influence of anyone else. Tom understood this desire and hung back as I got out of the car and approached the woman that had opened the door just enough to peer out.

Her beautiful hair was the first thing I saw as she slowly opened the door wide and looked down to take a tentative step toward me. She had been to the beauty shop and her abundant locks of now salt and pepper hair shown in the dimly lit garage. As she was wearing one of my father's pale blue dress shirts hanging loosely over a pair of khaki cotton duck pants and mismatched canvas shoes on her feet, I knew that Elena had not yet arrived to help her select clothes for the day.

My heart sank, though, when I saw that her face showed no spark of recognition, and she returned my enthusiastic hug with only a hint of a smile before promptly launching into a tour of the two-bedroom cottage. Tom and I glanced at each other over her shoulder, shrugged, and "oohed" and "ahhed" as if the last ten visits to her cottage had never happened.

"And that is more or less how the rest of the three days went," I later told Nora. "We sat in the living room or at the dining room table searching for things to say in response to old news and faded memories that just happened to come along into her head. My face ached from the smile I hoped appeared genuine while my heart was crying out for the mother that used to be the life of any party. She did not ask any questions about our lives and changed the subject each time we shared any particulars about ourselves with her. I grieved over the loss of high spirited card tournaments and noisy games of dominos or checkers. Those games are for children she said with great disgust, but I knew that her mind and hands had forgotten the moves.

Tom lavished attention on his mother-in-law every moment

that he could, and I truly believe he enjoyed being in her presence. He was unusually sensitive to both of us and devoted himself to making us find an uneasy comfortableness in each other's presence, a gift that I will forever treasure. Afraid to speak about mother anywhere within her earshot we saved our innermost thoughts for after bedtime when we could whisper intimately across the pillows. Even whispers could be heard, though, as we noticed the beam of a flashlight tracing the outside of the louvered door leading into the guest bedroom. We hoped that our tightly closed door ameliorated any of her fears.

On the last morning of our visit, she asked us what we thought of Waverly Place, and without thinking first, I told her very sweetly that we had seen it many times and were impressed with it each time. The look of surprise on her face gave way to red-faced apologies that she did not remember that we had ever been in her home. I tried to laugh it off and assure her that it didn't matter – we were there to see her, not the cottage. She was quick to remind me that only a doctor could make her move out of her cottage. No amount of assurances took away her fear that we were there to handcuff her and drag her away.

Mother never loosened her grip on the idea that she was in mortal danger because of our presence. We showered her with hugs and compliments and all manner of attention, but as the days slowly ticked by she became more and more sullen, until at our last lunch together, which included Elena, she would not meet my gaze or enter into any part of the conversation.

Any connection with my parent was gone. I was an orphan.

We drove the four of us back to the cottage and, quickly loading the car, said our goodbyes. I wondered if at that point she even knew who I was for she implored, "Please come visit me again. I don't get many visitors." This was a terribly odd thing to say in parting to one's daughter, and I said goodbye with one last hug and drove away, leaving her standing quite forlorn and confused behind her walker on the front porch. Elena told Louisa in a call later that day that as we drove away Mother asked who those people were that had come for a visit.

Dr. Lucas, Mother's primary care physician, had heard our plea to refer her to a neurologist, and set up an appointment through Elena with Dr. Forshey for the end of September. Mother had not wanted to make the appointment, but both Elena and Dr. Lucas told her quite matter-of-factly that he was the only person who could check her memory patch and renew the prescription. She asked Elena if that was the right thing to do – "Will it help me?" – to which the kind caregiver gently replied that it would. Louisa and I breathed more easily after hearing that the appointment was set and that Mother had been primed with the importance of keeping the appointment, but many things would transpire before the end of September.

A few days after Tom and I visited her, Mother was keeping watch out her front window for the man who prowled Waverly Place streets when she saw a red Cadillac speed down the street. It reminded her of the car that her friend Judy Wishner drove.

"Nora, Judy is probably Mom's most colorful friend and lived across the street from us with her husband and two daughters. She was a stewardess from the era when young ladies were chosen for these honored positions based strictly on their beauty and hospitality. Judy of course fell in love with a pilot, who was an equally eccentric, and married him. She went back to school and became a teacher and taught in the neighborhood school where Louisa attended elementary classes. Every morning we would watch Judy come rushing out of her house in high heels with her perfectly coiffed head of hair stiffly sprayed in place and a liberal application of make-up. Her arms were always full of papers - so full that she did not have a spare hand to shut the door on her bright red Cadillac and backed it out of the driveway at top speed with the door hanging open. Throwing the car into forward, she let the force of the car's speed slam the door shut as she aimed the car down the center of the street. She sped the six short blocks to school, with only one hand on the wheel, the other arm full of papers and folders, blazing a red streak through the neighborhood. Even now at a very advanced age with wrinkles that you could draw a plow through, her pancake make-up was firmly in place, as was the ubiquitous huge head of hair. In spite of her eccentricities, Judy was a kind and warm person. Her elementary students loved her, as did everyone in the neighborhood."

Nora was enjoying my tale about Mother's steadfast

friendship with Judy. The Wishners were our neighbors for many years, until Mr. Wishner died and their girls grew up and moved away, prompting Judy to downsize and subsequently move into an apartment. The neighborhood was quiet without her red-finned car zipping around. Judy and Mother continued to have the occasional lunch together, but more frequently, Judy would just suddenly show up at the cottage to go for ice-cream or to have a chat.

"Mom was positive the other day that she saw Judy's Cadillac at Waverly Place, all scraped up and dented on one side," I related to Nora. "And, then the story gets really garbled. Mom insists that Judy was murdered by her own grandson Jason, and that he is driving her car around Waverly Place. She is terrified by this and had Elena take her to the guard gate where she asked for name of person driving the car."

Nora wasn't sure whether to laugh or express concern. None-the-less, she was as dismayed by Mother's train of thought as I had been.

"Of course, the security guard declined to give her the name, so Mom marched, or probably more accurately pushed her walker over to the office to see Deborah Barnes. Deborah explained that she does not keep descriptions or plate numbers of cars that come in through the gate, to which Mom retorted that she wanted her to search for the murderer's name on their employee list," I exclaimed.

"Your mother has been watching too many cops and robbers shows on television," Nora quipped and leaned forward to hear more of the story.

"Deborah pretended to oblige and came up empty-handed for anyone named Jason on the employee list. Bless Deborah for her patience and quick thinking. They left her office and Mom had Elena drive them all over the senior community looking for an old beat up Cadillac, in the hopes of catching her friend's murderer. I get this image of my mother, the Miss Marple of Waverly Place, sleuthing through the streets with her walker and clip-on sunglasses, bent on solving another heinous crime."

Tom and I just shake our heads in dismay when we hear about Mother's latest adventures.

"You can't make this stuff up," Nora said.

"Well, Judy did one of her surprise drop-by visits a few days

after that. Mom reacted strangely because she thought her friend
had been murdered. Judy laughed at her and they fell into an
argument over whether Judy was dead or not. Judy is standing in
front of her and Mom is telling her she is dead!"

My shoulders shook with laughter.

"What did Judy do?" Nora asked, wondering how one
should respond to learn that one had, in fact, died and shouldn't be
standing there at all.

"Well, Judy laughed at the idea and tried to convince her
that she was very much alive. She assured her that the red Cadillac
had not been in an accident. Elena was there and said Mom began
yelling at Judy, screaming that she was dead and to leave her house
and never come back. Judy left, but called to check on Mom the next
day. Mom refused to speak to her, so Elena made a polite excuse by
saying that Mrs. Adams was on some new medication which made
her very confused. As far as we know Judy has not tried to contact
Mom again," I said, ending the story on that sad note.

"It is so mind-numbing to understand the thought processes
of a demented person. The things that seem perfectly clear to them
are so insanely bizarre to us, and yet ...," I let my voice trail off.

What had begun as a slapstick black and white movie had
been reduced to an accounting of someone quite literally losing
their mind.

After a few moments of silence, Nora finished my thought,
"...and you feel pain for your mother."

I smiled wanly and said, "A few months ago I would have
felt anger. I would have been like Judy and argued the point to no
avail. I might even have yelled at my mother."

Knowledge of the disease had given me a greater capacity
for compassion, a small step toward reconciliation – a step for
which I was grateful.

"Mother is very unforgiving of herself and feels her
mistakes acutely," I continued. "When the August maintenance
payment to Waverly Place was returned to the administrative
offices with a bold red stamp on it proclaiming that 'This account is
closed,' she made up an elaborate story about putting the wrong
checks in her purse - which is very believable - but she embellished
the excuse with her favorite fallback saying that she was in a hurry

because she had diarrhea that morning. She begged Elena not to tell us that she had bounced a check."

Tom and I had advised Mother several years ago to simplify her banking processes by paring all the checking accounts down to just one. Even in that early stage of dementia, she was easily confused as to how much was in which account and where the bank was located and how long it would take her to drive there to get cash should she need it. Branch banking was beyond her comprehension and putting a deposit in the mail was equally unpalatable, despite our pointing out that she put credit card payments in the mail.

Bouncing a check because she forgot where her money was located was an embarrassment for which she could not forgive herself. Unfortunately, the memory of it soon slipped away, and she remained adamantly sure that she was handling her financial affairs with perfection.

Catalog shopping presented other interesting challenges and resulted in the return of order forms and checks accompanied by letters which read, "Due to an insufficient amount to cover the taxes and cost of shipping, we are unable to fulfill your order at this time." Elena tried her best to explain that Mother's payment had to include taxes and shipping, but she just sat at the dining room table staring blankly at her caregiver, unable to comprehend the explanation. Instead, Mother called the vendor and, insisting that she had never paid taxes or shipping before, demanded that her merchandise be shipped to her immediately. The vendor's refusal to comply brought a torrent of angry words, and from that time forward Elena quietly confiscated any catalogs that arrived in the mail before they reached Mother's eyes. Strangely enough, she did not seem to miss them.

As autumn deepened, it became evident that Mother's knee had to be tended to. She was complaining of pain and limping more as each day passed. Although we suspected her weakness was due in part to dehydration, she repeatedly told Elena that the knee had "collapsed" and had caused her to fall several times. Mother herself told us rather emphatically several months ago that Sylvia had pointed out that she was tottering from side to side and wondered if something was wrong with her gait.

"She has difficulty lifting up her feet and putting one foot in front of the other," I described for Nora. "Louisa keeps telling me it is because of Mom's knee, but isn't there something unusual about the way dementia patients walk? Mother has taken on this characteristically awkward and faltering manner of walking. It is almost as if she is afraid to take a step. She looks at the floor and studies it before she moves her leg. It's like she has to mentally tell her feet what to do."

Nora reminded me that there are many manifestations of arthritis and other physical handicaps, including poor eyesight that can account for the different stances and gaits of the elderly. However, those with dementia do have a distinct way of walking, making me wonder how long we had missed this sign.

"On our last visit with her it was obvious that mobility had become an issue for her," I sadly told Nora, realizing that I should watch how I worded it. My dear friend was having her own difficulties with an arthritic knee and, perhaps, would feel uncomfortable with my description of my mother's declining ability to walk freely.

"Louisa placed a call to the orthopedic surgeon who, surprisingly, had no problem in speaking with a family member that was not listed on the privacy form. Mom's kneecap had become completely torn away from the top of her knee, most likely a result of one of her falls, and the kneecap was hanging loose under the skin on one side of her leg."

"Well, there is no wonder that she could not walk and was in such pain," Nora's natural caring and concern speaking louder than her words.

"Mom has always been in a hurry. She has such drive and determination to accomplish a task that she overlooks things like a chair leg or a wrinkle in the rug. I have never seen her fall, but have heard many reports about the bruises she acquires. The surgeon assured my sister that the procedure would be routine and, in the absence of understanding on Mom's part, explained how he planned to move the kneecap back into its proper position."

Louisa was not physically up to the trip or to looking after Mother – the birthday trip had taught her that – and I was so far out of her good graces that we felt my presence would only worsen the experience. With the assurance that it would be a relatively easy surgery, we once again relied on Elena to take Mother under her wing and see her through the surgery.

The day of surgery began with the usual struggle over taking the prerequisite shower and continued as Elena tried to convince Mother that she did not need to pack her oversized suitcase. She could not be dissuaded from packing all her medications, toiletries, nightgowns, and multiple changes of clothing. Elena finally gave in when the winter coat emerged and quietly loaded the heavy suitcase into the car for the short drive to the hospital. The two of them settled into the waiting room for Mother's turn to be called in. Her pastor dropped by for a prayer, as did her faithful friend Sylvia, neither of whom Mother remembered a few days later.

The wait to be admitted was longer than usual due to complications from an earlier surgery, during which time Mother became highly agitated. She demanded to know the reason for the delay and began yelling and cursing at the nurses and staff, who probably would have loved to take her in and begin the sedation right then. Soon enough, however, she was safely in surgery and gave all a chance to breathe a sigh of relief and take a respite from her seemingly constant bad mood. Sylvia witnessed the odd behavior of her dear friend and welcomed the opportunity to sit with Elena in the family waiting area, searching for the words to express her dismay.

Sylvia had been out of the loop for more than a year and was grateful for a one-on-one conversation with Elena, who gently explained that Mrs. Adams had become ill and was having serious problems with her memory. The two talked intimately about the woman they both knew so well, one as a friend from years past when she was vibrant and fully engaged in all that life offered, and the other as a dear client whose world was slipping away. They shared an understanding and a bond that comes only from having been drawn in by my mother's formerly sparkling personality and from loving her in spite of her failing mind.

The surgery over, she was wheeled into recovery where she was having a difficult time coming out of the anesthesia. Not one to take on any task quietly, her reactions to drugs had always been dramatic and she did not have an easy time awakening after the surgery. Eventually she was the last surgery patient to be moved into a room. She was so wracked with nausea that someone needed to be constantly at her side, and Elena and Sylvia took turns encouraging her with chips of ice. In spite of the calm and soothing attention of the women, she fought them and screamed to be let out of bed. Struggling against the safety railing around the bed and pulling on the numerous tubes protruding from her body, Mother made it clear that she wanted to get up and go somewhere – anywhere – that part was not as clear. She just wanted to go. When their friend and charge finally fell into a fitful sleep well after dark, the exhausted women went home, leaving her in the care of the understaffed and overworked nurses who had appreciated their presence.

Kindhearted Elena, in particular, had given all that she had to ease her client's pain, both physically and emotionally, but to no avail. During the night, Mother ripped out her catheter and IV lines, worked her way out of the bed, and tried to rush down the hall in an effort to "get away," before falling to the hard tile floor just out of sight of the nurses' station. An orderly found her in the darkened hall and called for help. She was lifted, struggling and flailing her arms and one leg, back into bed and sedated enough to keep her there while IVs and the catheter were reinserted. The surgeon was called and, upon examining the knee, found that she had completely undone his work and the kneecap was sliding back into its familiar spot on the side of her knee. In spite of her cries, he pushed it back as far as he dared and re-braced the joint, giving her strict orders to stay in bed with the brace, IVs and catheter in place. He was met with a haughty retort and Elena knew that she had to call Mrs. Adams's daughters.

"In spite of her own physical difficulties, Louisa made an emergency flight to San Angelo," I told Nora. "I waited for two days to hear news from Louisa about Mom's surgery before I finally called the hospital myself and reached Sylvia on the phone. Mother refused to talk to me on the phone."

Nora's eyes showed compassion as I poured out my frustration. She ordered lunch for the both of us, as I had not even opened the menu. When the waiter left us, she whispered, "...So, you called the hospital..." and I picked up my story.

"So, Sylvia filled me in as best she could while sitting at my mother's bedside. I read between the lines and came to understand that my mother had suffered another serious decline, not unusual for dementia patients after undergoing anesthesia. In hind sight, we would not have subjected her to the rigors of the surgery if we knew that, by her own bizarre behavior, she would reinjure her knee, and that her brain would experience another battle which it would not win.

Bless Sylvia for her joviality and lightness of heart in the face of her friend frantically trying to rip out another IV before reaching over to remove Sylvia's watch.

"No, no, honey. That's my watch. You can't have my watch," she said ever so gently.

I thanked Sylvia for being there and let her go to deal with Mother's anxiety, all the while struggling to gain control of my own distressed feelings.

"Where was Louisa during this time?" Nora asked, puzzled that my sister was not with Mother.

"The long hours of being by Mom's side and constantly working to keep her calm and in bed had exhausted Louisa's energies, and Elena drove her back to the cottage to rest," I explained after learning how truly difficult the trip was for Louisa. "I am ashamed that I was so quick to judge my sister when Mom was demanding so much of her. The stilted conversation with Sylvia told me that talking while in Mom's presence was impossible. Louisa did eventually call me on the second night. She took great care in describing every detail of the surgery, of Sylvia's presence, about Elena's support, and what is turning out to be a very fitful recovery."

Nora's smile was heartwarming and she shared with me that her prayers had been not only for my acceptance of Mother's new normal, if one could call it that, but also for a peaceful relationship with my sister. We talked quietly over a shared plate of apple pie ala mode.

"Sylvia and Louisa also had the opportunity to talk openly about Mom's condition for a few hours when Elena took over at the bedside. Louisa told me that Sylvia apologized profusely for not understanding that how seriously ill Mom is. She asked Louisa for the diagnosis and prognosis, and for the real story of what happened in New York. Sylvia was relieved to learn that I had not kept my mother chained to her bed in a cave in the basement and that there were no policemen standing guard at the hospital," I told Nora. "Sylvia made a promise to us that she would be a better friend to us all and would begin by correcting the slanderous stories Mom had spread about."

"How wonderful, Allison," Nora said excitedly. "I am so pleased that Sylvia is taking the initiative and time to rectify the wrong your Mother has done."

And then added much more seriously, "Sibling relationships can take a beating, too. This journey is as much about you and your sister as it is about you and your mother."

Nora's way of cutting through all the messiness in family relationships and reducing them down to the least hurtful denominator was always compelling. Her comment reminded me that Alzheimer's is a disease which the whole family must embrace.

I turned the conversation to a lighter tone by saying, "At one particularly trying moment Louisa told Mom, 'Don't make me call Allison.' Mom started screaming, 'No, no, don't call Allison.'"

Nora and I burst out laughing in the crowded bistro, drawing brief attention to our booth off in one corner. We didn't care. It was a rare moment of levity.

"Mom was moved to a room directly across from the nurses' station so they could keep a closer watch over her. Her bed was wired with a motion detector which beeped every time she moved. The constant activity and noise kept Mom in a continued state of anxiety and she yelled out every time her bed beeped. The IVs sound an alarm whenever they require attention and the ceiling loudspeaker goes off every time a doctor is paged. She was constantly screaming at every noise she heard. They had to move her roommate to another room because the roommate could not rest with all the commotion Mom made."

I swirled the soup around in my bowl and continued, "Louisa arrived at the hospital in the middle of all this agitation. She explained to me the tremendous stress of dealing with Mom's behavior, and I finally understood why she had not called until two days after the surgery. Louisa was just too exhausted, and I feel almost ashamed that I thought so harshly of her."

My sister was able to bring about some calmness in Mother, and in spite of her own fatigue and issues with her back, Louisa agreed with the doctors that she needed to stay until Mother was moved into a rehab facility. I offered to take her place, but she politely hinted that the very difficult patient would be even less cooperative if her eldest daughter appeared.

Sending Nora a halfhearted smile across the table now laden with food, I said, "It's alright, Nora. Someone has to be the favorite child and someone has to be the least favored one. My shoulders are broad and I can carry that burden. The load would crush my sister. Her body is collapsing, and I can at least spare her this pain."

Because of her totally uncooperative behavior, it was necessary to transport Mother by ambulance to the rehab hospital, conveniently located only a few blocks from Waverly Place. Mother screamed and fought the orderlies and the EMTs as they attempted to transfer her into the ambulance.

"She was terrified of what was happening. Louisa rode with her and tried to ease her fears by pointing out familiar landmarks as they passed by, what little they could see through the ambulance's tiny windows. She began to relax a bit as they left the concrete and steel buildings of the medical center and rode through the tree-lined neighborhoods to the side of town where the sky was open."

"It would not be unexpected for someone to feel that their life was completely out of their control under those circumstances," Nora said. "With your mother's tendency toward anxiety and the added confusion of dementia, her reactions are perfectly understandable."

"It's odd to think that being afraid and anxious is 'normal,'" I quipped, knowing that Nora was simply trying to put me at ease over my mother's distress.

Our conversation had run well beyond pie a la mode, and we continued talking over tea and coffee, my lunch hour long gone. My boss and coworkers knew of the difficulties in my personal life and gave me leave to take as much time as was needed. Even the gruffest of my colleagues who did not seem to have an empathetic bone in his body, offered words of concern on those days when he noticed my eyes were red. Somehow human suffering humbles us all.

The one who was, perhaps, the humblest of all my acquaintances spent the next hour sharing her wealth of information with me over the remnants of our lunches. One of the most interesting facts that she shared was the curious rate at which changes can occur in a dementia patient. While unbeknownst to any of us, my mother had apparently been suffering from the disease for many years. Because of her indomitable spirit to survive, she found ways to make up for any lapses in memory and had just naturally adapted behaviors to cover the fact that memories were slipping away and that it was increasingly difficult for her to manage her life. In thinking back, I was proud of her decision, quite on her own, to sell the Humboldt house and move to Waverly Place. We rejoiced together and it was the beginning of a happy time for her – until the memory lapses became so profound that none of us could continue to ignore them.

"The last few months have been terribly difficult for our family, but we can only imagine what Mom must be going through," I sadly told Nora, hoping that she could give me some glimmer of good news.

Nora put down her coffee and, looking right into my eyes with her own that had seen years of suffering, said, "There will come a time when she will not know what she has lost, and she will be happy. A kind of sweetness will descend, and although she will not recognize you, and perhaps not even know who she is herself, your mother will reach a time of peace..."

She pressed my hand as it lay still on the table, and with a smile as deep as the sky, said, "...and beyond that, you have the assurance that your mother believes in a place where she can peacefully rest forever."

Tears fell heavily from my eyes, but my heart found comfort in her words.

❖

Chapter 11

*W*ith Mother admitted to rehab for the next three weeks, I prayed that we would be able to make progress in having her examined by a specialist and maybe, just maybe, receive a formal diagnosis and plan for long-term care. It would simplify things a great deal if she could be moved directly from the rehab hospital into a dementia unit, and I had been pushing my sister for some time to follow through on this idea. Heretofore, Louisa had been reluctant, if not unmovable, telling me in no uncertain terms that our mother did not belong in a dementia facility. She was squarely set against the idea and as stubborn as Mother herself. Louisa was convinced that, with the proper medications, Mother's illness could be corrected and she could continue to live safely and happily in her own cottage. I suspect she had made this promise to Mother, vowing to fight her eldest daughter in my futile attempts to make changes in her living and care arrangements.

Mother's psychoses intensified, however, and what was to have been a routine recovery and physical therapy period turned into a struggle for survival. She visited every dark corner of her mind and found more and more of which to be afraid. Once again her bed was fitted with a monitor and, so suspicious had her nature become, that she refused to remain in group therapy sessions and hobbled back to her room to see who was wiring the bed in order to electrocute her. She complained loudly and often that her medications were not right, which led to the accusation of several nurses having overdosed her with murderous intentions in mind. Elena was no longer her ally, but rather a co-conspirator in these attempts to either lock her away in an insane asylum or to do away with her altogether. Normal voices and conversations in the hallway became whispered conspiracies against her, and she refused to eat, certain that the staff was bent on poisoning her.

Mother's antics were so out of control that the attending physician who was assigned to follow her progress made it clear that she could not go home without around-the-clock supervision. Relief washed over me when I heard this news, and much to my surprise, Louisa reinforced this order by asking Elena to suggest an agency that could provide additional healthcare aides for the next few weeks. Elena was adamant about using her own group of aides because Mrs. Adams already knew them, an arrangement we wholeheartedly endorsed. One or two of the aides had substituted for Elena in the past and were familiar faces to Mother and knew her routines, unusual as they were. Elena felt that the further disruption of new faces would not be in her client's best interest. So, a schedule was set up for Elena, her two daughters, and another trusted aide to rotate around-the-clock at the cottage once Mrs. Adams was finally released from rehab.

The rehab staff hoped that her release would be sooner than later, as Mother was like a very difficult and strong-willed child that had tried their patience and exhausted all of their people skills. The attending physician was nonplussed except to say that she had been the most challenging patient he ever hoped to experience. He was young and had many years of practice ahead of him, but this woman impressed upon him the desperate need for changes in laws regarding elder care.

I rang Nora as soon as I heard the news.

"I am almost ecstatic that a doctor finally impressed upon my sister the need for Mom to have constant care and supervision. For the first two weeks that she is home, she will have around-the-clock care, and I have my fingers crossed that we can continue that pattern indefinitely."

"What marvelous news, Allison," Nora replied. "You must be so relieved. It's been a long hard struggle for all of you, hasn't it?"

"Louisa's armor is beginning to show signs of cracking. Although the time she spent with Mom in the hospital and at rehab was terribly taxing, it was strong evidence that Mom is in trouble and she simply cannot ignore her needs any longer."

Sensing that there was still some animosity towards my

sister in spite of the positive turn of events, Nora reminded me, "Everyone comes into their own understanding and acceptance of what this disease can do at different rates. You have already taught your sister a great deal. She now knows that your mother ill - but knowing something in one's mind and accepting it in one's heart are two separate steps toward acceptance."

I realized the sad truth in Nora's observations and adopting a more compassionate attitude said, "You are right, Nora... This is so painful for Louisa. She and Mom are very close and I don't think she wants to truly own the decline in Mom's memory and ability to function. Mother was there for her when she got married, made a home, and had her children. She has been there for us at every celebration and every disappointment. It is now our turn to be there for her..., although it is not with the same feelings of joy."

Louisa's patience and tolerance for Mother's behaviors had run out, and her twisted body had reached the end of its tolerance, as well. She rejoiced at the news that Mother was to be released from rehab and took the opportunity to return to her own home for much needed respite.

Mother was discharged unceremoniously, all the while complaining and issuing verbal insults at the staff. She insisted that Elena take her home straightaway without stopping to fill the prescription for pain medication. It was also clear that she was not up to going to the pharmacy or to go grocery shopping, so Elena took her home without accomplishing either necessary task. She settled Mom comfortably on the sofa where she promised to remain until the caregiver returned with groceries and the prescription.

The petite caregiver should have known that Mother's promises are only as trustworthy as that of a preschooler in time out who jumps off the chair the instant her parents' backs are turned and begins playing with her dolls. Initially, Mother sat dutifully on the sofa staring at the blank TV screen and the vast array of green plants on the occasional table in front of the living room window. Perhaps, she thought the plants needed water, but for whatever reason, she managed to remove the protective brace from around her knee and push herself off the sofa to stand clumsily on two stiff legs. What happened next, Mother does not recall, but when Elena came back from the grocery store and the pharmacy, she found her limping along the sidewalk several doors away. She was crying from pain, as well as from fear, and chastised Elena for leaving her. "Where were you? I have been looking all over for you," she sobbed as her caregiver gently took her by the arm and guided her back up the walk to her cottage. Elena and the three other aides never left her alone again.

In spite of their efforts to give her as much space as possible, she highly resented being told to wash for dinner, to put on her knee brace, and to leave the laundry to be done by someone else. Her dictatorial eldest daughter may not have been there, but four other equally annoying women were. The home visits from the physical therapist were a further intrusion into her life and she vehemently declared that she would not cooperate, and in so doing, destroyed any chance of ever returning to full mobility.

Mother's ingenuity was really very creative, and I am certain that she learned some of her strategies from the soap operas she watched on a daily basis, which to this day she denies ever watching. Or, perhaps, the ideas came from her busybody neighbor Imelda. Some months ago, Elena had furtively listened in as the two elderly women sit around the kitchen table discussing ways to thwart the intrusions of their household help and children.

At the bidding of her misguided friend or following the lead of a fictitious soap opera character, Mother decided that she would have no more of these invasions and demanded that Elena leave her house. Elena assumed that she was making idle threats, and simply smiled and ignored the order to leave, which brought on a torrent of screams and finger pointing. The feisty caregiver remained unmoved and continued her household chores, all the while keeping an eye on her client to be sure that she did not harm herself. Her watchfulness turned to curiosity as Mother hobbled into the bedroom on her walker and closed the door behind her. Elena soon overheard Mrs. Adams talking to someone on the phone, but did not wish to intrude - something for which Louisa had always praised Elena and the other ladies - and she continued drying the dishes in the kitchen.

"They allow Mom to have her dignity and to keep her privacy. They know she is used to being independent," Louisa had said.

This time, though, Elena should have intervened in the phone call, for in a matter of minutes, a patrol car pulled up in front of the cottage and two policemen rang the doorbell. Still giving Mrs. Adams her rule of the house, Elena allowed her to answer the door and show the policemen in. In as stern a voice as she could muster, Mother demanded that they should make Elena leave her home. After asking a few basic questions, much to Elena's dismay, the officers agreed that she was within her rights to ask the employee to leave the premises and promptly ushered Elena to the door.

"They did what?" Nora said in disbelief. "What did she do?"

"Elena is so incredibly resourceful. She went to the security gate and told the guard what was happening. He hopped in his golf cart and the two of them zoomed back over to Mom's house where he stopped the policemen as they were getting back into their patrol car. I suppose he explained to them about the crazy resident, because they eventually smiled at Elena and left Emerald Drive. The guard promptly let Elena back into Mom's house with his pass key."

"Oh, my. Oh, my," was all that Nora could say.

I had never seen her at a loss for words and she continued to be dumbfounded as I told her that Elena quickly took control of the phone and called Louisa. With her pouty client on an extension, Elena explained to Louisa what had happened. Most likely for the first time in her life, my sister lectured Mother for failing to follow instructions and then for making the poor decision to call the police on someone who was trying to care for her. She ended the call with the final threat to call Allison.

Nora burst into laughter at hearing that once again Louisa had played her trump by threatening to call her sister. When we both settled back in our chairs spent from laughter, Nora inquired if the lecture had been effective. I supposed that it had not been, for when they went back to the surgeon for a follow-up visit, Mother's knee was still swollen even though it had been weeks since the surgery. The doctor was displeased that she had not been wearing the brace nor doing her exercises. He expressed concern that she was still on painkillers and seriously advised her to follow his orders in taking care of herself.

"The knee was in no better shape, maybe even worse, than before Mom had the surgery," I said. "I am hearing frustration in Louisa's voice for the first time. Last night I was so surprised to hear her agree that Mom needs to be moved into a care facility."

Nora gasped, "That is fabulous, Allison."

She beamed a contagious smile, and I suddenly realized what a tremendous step forward Louisa's attitude had taken. While just a few months before she had sided so strongly with Mother, almost to the point of hysteria, Louisa now did not hesitate to acknowledge that a change was needed. However, the exact details of how to bring about the change were still many months in coming.

I was impatient to make the change happen and took on the role of catalyst - but just as with any chain reaction, the timing had to be perfect. Little did I realize how minute the steps would be toward that end.

In the weeks that followed, Mother was plagued by a chronic urinary tract infection – the same one she had been battling since before her knee surgery. While there was a wealth of data supporting the fact that those suffering from dementia are reticent to bathe, there was very little on how to solve the problem. With Alzheimer's there is never really a cure for any of the symptoms, but somewhere there must be tips and techniques on dealing with this issue; and while searching I would also look for guidance in handling paranoia, bulimia, anger, and a host of other behaviors that were now presenting in my mother. The care she was receiving from her doctors had not touched deeply enough nor offered any real solace for her or those who loved her.

"Of course, the first place to search would be with the Alzheimer's Association," Nora sweetly suggested, and I smiled because that resource had long since been exhausted.

My search found a plethora of articles on the "Ten Warning Signs of Alzheimer's" and the many symptoms and stages that we would encounter, but found only a dismal amount of real life situations and solutions. The common threads of advice that ran through all the literature was to seek the advice of a qualified physician. Discussions with Louisa seemed to repeat themselves over the coming weeks as our frustrations with doctors mounted. None of them were willing to step forward and declare her incompetent – not that we really expected the ob-gyn to take this action, but he had been the one doctor that seemed to acknowledge that our mother was demented. He tried to assist in so far as his specialty would allow, but in spite of our frustration we had to admire his standing on medical principles.

Unfortunately, the neurologist he referred us to was equally unwilling to take a stand and with a robotic type of motion simply continued to reissue prescriptions for memory patches. Curiously, he would not allow Elena to be present in the exam room with Mother, which was a huge red flag in my opinion, but Louisa did not know how to circumvent this problem as Mother had not given permission for him to speak with anyone.

"How in the world does a neurologist, of all specialists, think that he will receive accurate information from a demented patient? How can he make a precise diagnosis without talking to a family member," I begged the question. "Louisa, he is not the right doctor for Mom."

San Angelo does not have a plethora of neurologists. In fact, the medical association listed only three, and one of them specialized only in pediatrics. We wondered how deeply Mother would have to fall into the cracks before some doctor somewhere decided she seriously needed assistance beyond what the home healthcare aides could provide.

A second bit of advice that every piece of Alzheimer's literature mentioned was to draw up legal documents to protect the individual's personal care and estate; including a living will, a directive for care, and a designation of guardian. Mother had all of these. Our father had wisely seen to these documents before his passing a decade prior, and Waverly Place required them for admission into the retirement community. The powers of attorney had been executed in Deborah Barnes' office with a notary as a witness to her wishes. In accordance with Mother's strong desire to remain fiercely independent, she selected Option B, which stipulated that the powers of attorney would not go into effect until a physician deemed her incompetent. And so, we found ourselves back at square one without a legal means to help our mother.

Louisa and I talked ourselves into circles discussing how to circumvent this all important detail; but without a physician to document the diagnosis and make the declaration that she could no longer make sound decisions for her person or for her estate, Mother would remain in her home indefinitely, a danger to herself and potentially others, exhausting all of her funds on home healthcare aides – an expense which she could not maintain.

I pushed my sister as far as I dared to act quickly to find another neurologist - one that would talk with the family – one that recognized her cognitive limitations – one that would actually provide a definite diagnosis, something we had yet to receive. Mother was a victim of a patient's rights system that does not take into account the imagined and confused stories of an Alzheimer's individual who is so adept at creating cover stories that her own doctor has difficulty separating fact from fiction.

It soon became evident to me that a vital piece in dealing with the hard realities of dementia was for caregivers, such as Louisa and me, to take a time out for ourselves. It was easier for me than for my sister. She had been on the front lines for many months while I worked behind the scenes to provide whatever support I could. My push to find a new doctor came to a screeching halt as I realized that my sister needed to take time out for herself.

Louisa had been juggling her own physical pain with that of Mother's, and with Elena and her crew settled into a routine, uneasy though it was at times, she turned inward. It was time for my sister to embrace her own needs and relinquish the burden of caring for someone else. I did not begrudge her that right, for the very biometric implant in her brain which was designed to interrupt the pain signals in her face, had also interrupted the signals going to the muscles supporting one side of her spine. Those muscles had received messages every few seconds to relax and to give way to the strength of the muscles pushing form the opposite side of her spine, curling and bending her shape until my sister was in severe and debilitating pain from not only her face, but from her back, as well. Unlike our mother, she received a diagnosis for adult-onset scoliosis within months of the first symptoms; but, like Mother, there was no one who could help her. And so, her body continued to collapse in on itself, sending ribs and organs into painfully awkward positions, compromising heart and lungs and making it difficult to breathe. Walking normally was out of the question and my fifty-three-year-old sister was stooped over like an old woman, relying on a cane to walk only a few steps.

"Nora, it was incredibly selfless of Louisa to fly to Mom's side in that condition," I said with a renewed appreciation for my sister's strength. "As frustrated as I am over the slowness with which things have moved along for Mom, it pales in comparison to Louisa's suffering. Without surgery, she will die."

She heard the despair in my voice and sat perfectly still to listen while the words and emotions spilled out. When I had spent all my tears and could find no more words, she quietly lifted me out of my emotional fatigue.

Beginning softly in her soothing way, she said, "God is with you. He is with you all – with your mother, with your sister, with you... He does not promise that all will end well, but He does promise that you will have the strength to endure it. Louisa has shown, as have you, a wonderful sense of determination and bravery to continue in the face of so many trials. I have every confidence that your family will be made stronger for this journey."

I smiled slightly, recalling one of the first questions I had asked Nora when we first began meeting two years ago. How could I show honor to my mother, as commanded by God, when my initial and almost instinctual reaction was to fight back and seek satisfaction from some personal desire to be right, in spite of the illness that had come into the family. By way of a very long and painful trek, I had finally come to know how to honor the woman who raised me. The answer lay in surrounding her with medical professionals who knew how to help her and in blanketing her with the invisible network of loving and supportive friends and family. She would never know of the battles we quietly fought for her every step to be healthier and happier.

"Mom forgot my birthday, Nora. Elena tried to persuade her to go to the mall for a walk and to buy a birthday card, but she refused to get dressed. She wanted to go to the mall in her pajamas," I said with melancholy bemusement. "It is so hard to wrap my mind around the fact that both my sister and my mother are suffering at the same time."

"Do you really believe that your mother is … suffering?" Nora queried.

Her question made me pause.

"I think she suffers from her fears. She is truly afraid of so much. But, then, she also enjoys attention and brings a lot of imaginary threats to bear on herself. Louisa's suffering is brought on by deep physical issues, and her pain is very real. They are both tremendous fighters."

We said goodnight with a prayer on our lips, and I sought out the warm and strong arms of my husband. I had already lost my father to death, my mother to the darkness of Alzheimer's, and I could barely stand the thought of losing the only other member of my immediate family. Tom gently reminded me that his family was mine as well, and I found comfort in his words.

Mother continued to resent and fight the women who supported her on a daily basis. In spite of her insistence that she did not need someone to assist her, I asked Elena and the team to continue staying with her around the clock, even though the two-week time period ordered by the rehab doctor had passed. Each time Mother insisted that the two weeks were up, Elena very sweetly said, "Oh, no, that isn't until next week." When the next week came, Mother had forgotten all about it, and so the live-in home healthcare became a permanent part of her life.

I had not asked Louisa before making that decision, but it was the right one. I thought, perhaps, she might fight me on it when she learned what I had done, but either her impending surgery had taken the punch out of her or she now fully embraced the need for continual care and that Mother should have companionship and supervision full time. Louisa did not protest and retreated back into the calmness of her own home to recuperate from her ordeal at Mother's side.

One morning soon thereafter, Mother called Charlie in a panic and instructed him to burn every document that had her name on it. She had pulled all the files out of her filing cabinets and was rifling through them to find and destroy anything bearing her name and signature. I had visions of a bonfire in the middle of her bedroom as she sought to do away with anything that could be used to commit her to whatever insane asylum she conjured up in her head.   Upon learning of Mother's latest intentions, Elena promised me that she had searched the house and confiscated all the matches and lighters that she could find. Mother's mind is devious, though, and Elena's assurances did little to calm my fears.

Feeling that Mother's pastor should know that one of his favorite parishioners was having difficulties and to ask him to continue to reach out to her, I called Pastor Art. I did not tell him that Mother no longer knew who he was and thought of him as a kindly gentleman from the neighborhood who came to visit every now and then. In actuality, Mother rarely remembered anyone from the church, and often asked Elena who "those people" were when they had gone. I thanked Pastor Art for faithfully shepherding his parishioner even though she no longer had the desire to seek God's presence.   In turn, he promised to stop by to visit Imogene and assured me that Mother was not lost. God knew where she was and would bring her home someday.

"What a lovely person he must be," Nora exclaimed. "It's curious how those with dementia do not feel the need for God."

"Mom recently told me that it was just such a hassle to get up and get dressed and get over to the chapel. For a couple of years now she has made up reasons for not going to church. I think it also has something to do with pulling away from social contact - and the church certainly is a social setting."

"We don't really know why they withdraw from society," Nora said thoughtfully. "I have wondered about that, too. Mommie just wasn't interested in being with people any more, and when she was, she was so spitefully mean to them."

We did not know whether to feel pity or to be amused at the thought of our sweet, gentle mothers becoming sharp-tongued old bitties that made movies like "Driving Miss Daisy" pale in comparison – although, our eyes now viewed Miss Daisy's story with a greater depth than when we first saw it before Alzheimer's came to live in our midsts.

"With each passing day, the healthcare aides tell me that Mom is continuing to change. Cajoling her into the shower has become an art form. They sort of dance around each other with each step moving them closer to the bathroom," I described with some delicacy. "Yesterday Elena managed to get her into the

shower and when she began to wash her feet, Mom grabbed the
sprayer head out of Elena's hands and sprayed water in her
caregiver's face, drenching her hair and shoulders. Mom snarled at
Elena, 'See how it feels to get all wet. Not so nice.'"

Nora's hand flew up to her mouth in surprise, "Oh, no."

"Well, like you, my first thought was how maddening that
must have been for Elena. Nora, she turned it around and told her
childish employer how refreshing it felt to have the water flow over
her head. Louisa and I guessed that Mom was trying to goad Elena
into a reaction that would get her out of having to take any more
showers."

Nora chuckled, her white bangs bouncing across her
forehead as she laughed, "It didn't work, though, did it?" She
paused, and pushing aside a now empty bowl of lobster bisque,
observed, "Elena is so cognizant of your mother's motivations and
is a genius in redirecting them in a more positive way. She is an
amazing woman - a good match for your mother, who is also an
amazing woman."

"Yes, Mom is a very accomplished individual, in spite of the
many obstacles to success that would have kept most women stuck
in a depressing spiral of monotony. She always wanted to be more
than she was and actively sought how to take the little that she was
given and make it into something special, something of worth,
either for herself or for her family... So many things have changed
for her now. Several months ago the social worker very sweetly
suggested that an apartment in the building might be easier for
Mom to manage. She hated that idea and told Deborah so in no
uncertain terms."

Mother vehemently denied that she needed to move into the
Big House, mistakenly referring to any other living arrangements at
Waverly Place as the dreaded Big House. There are actually all
levels of arrangements between the independent life of a cottage-
dweller and that of an advanced stage Alzheimer's patient in the
Johnston Center. For weeks to follow, Deborah's name could not be
mentioned without a torrent of obscenities describing "that woman
who wants to make me move out of my cottage."

"Sadly, Mom no longer even recognizes Deborah. The last
few times that Mom and Elena have seen her in the hallways on the

way to or from the hairdresser, Mom greeted her with perfect manners and then inquired who that lady was as they shuffled on down the hall. Elena wisely answered that Deborah was one of the nice people who works in the front office."

Mother fights so valiantly to keep up her image as the polished and sophisticated head of a family and a hard working civic leader, but persists in speaking down her nose at Big House residents who carried around dolls and spoke nonsense. "You don't want to know *those* people," she would say; and we would just smile, never dreaming of telling her that she was now one of those people.

Until lately, one of Mother's favorite things to do was to go to the beauty salon every Thursday for a wash, set, and comb out. She followed this routine for as many years as I can remember, and we knew that if we called her house on Thursday mornings the conversation was likely to be cut short as she rushed to collect herself and get to the beauty college.

Yes, my mother frequented the beauty college. Seven dollars was the going rate at that time, and she was very pleased to get a good cut and "do" for such an economical price. Neither Louisa, nor I, nor Dad ever dreamed of telling her that she received exactly what she paid for – a seven dollar helmet of hair sprayed to a stiffness that could withstand hurricane force winds. However, anything beyond a few days of wear on the "do," and holes began to appear in the ratted mass of hair which her little brush barely touched. Mother's idea of brushing her hair was to just pass the bristles over the top, skimming the stiffened hairdo at low altitude without actually touching the strands. Sleeping in a silk nightcap did nothing to maintain the shape, although she was most indignant that it did. We always imagined her head slipping off the pillow and landing with a thunk on Dad's shoulder. Tom praised my father for being a saintly man, never telling his wife that her seven dollar hairstyle, while very frugal, only held up for a couple of days, if that long.

Going to the beauty shop was one of the motivators for Mother getting behind the wheel of a car even after she had lost her license. The administration building where the salon is located is too far for her to walk and as every genteel lady needed to be properly coiffed, she simply had to keep her hair appointments. Elena took over the chauffeur duties and saw to it that Mother continued to visit the Waverly Place salon once a week.

Following one visit to the beauty salon, showing off a new "do," Mother and Elena made their way down the short hallway to the common dining room for lunch. This was a treat as Elena usually prepared something for the two of them to eat at home. They settled down at a table and turned their attention to grilled chicken and steamed broccoli, involved in light conversation about the nice color of the napkins and the servers' new uniforms. Munching on a carrot stick gave Mother's eye time to travel around the room and settle on her good friend Marge Tull who was sitting alone at a table happily enjoying the chicken and dumplings. Mother struggled out of her chair and shuffled over to Marge who greeted her enthusiastically. Marge was always a delight to visit with. She personified the perfect definition of chipper and had a smile on her face and a twinkle in her eye for everyone she encountered.

Mother's unannounced arrival at the table, however, caught Marge by surprise as her friend Imogene was armed with a napkin which she promptly wet with the tip of her tongue. Imogene reached over to Marge's face, and stating that she looked like a clown, began scrubbing a carefully penciled eyebrow off of Marge's shocked face. Elena, wondering what her client was up to, had followed her to the table and was equally chagrinned to see Mrs. Adams erasing Marge's hand drawn eyebrow.

"Stop that, Mrs. Adams," she pleaded. "That isn't nice."

Mrs. Adams retorted, "Well when people look like clowns, they should be told. Here, Marge, you put on makeup like this."

She pulled off her oversized glasses - for with Mother everything is oversized - and dramatically raised her eyebrows to show the stunned woman how it should be done. Elena admitted later that Marge did, indeed, look like a clown particularly with only one brow arching over the left eye and a blank space where the right one should be. Her dumbfounded expression alone would have played the part well, but being a proper Southern lady herself, Marge graciously said that she would take better care with her makeup next time and excused herself from the dining room.

Elena directed her to gather Mrs. Adams things from their own table and they made their way for the door. Ahead of them was a resident using a walker and Mrs. Adams loudly proclaimed, "Look at how fat her butt is."

Hearing someone speaking behind her, the resident turned back to them and said, "Thank you."

To which Mrs. Adams said in a stage whisper, "She thinks I am saying something nice, but I am not. She has a fat butt."

By this time in the telling of the story, Nora and I were almost falling out of our chairs with laughter.

"Nora, what in the world made her be so brazen all of a sudden like that - and, she just says the most contemptuous things to perfect strangers."

Nora assured me that near the end, the term "grouchy old lady" had applied to her mother, as well.

"We could not believe the things that would come out of her mouth," she recalled. "Even the nurses at the home were not accustomed to hearing language like that. Mommie could make them cry with the mean things she said to them."

"Mom has a problem with anyone who is overweight," I commiserated. "As the years have gone by she has become more and more outspoken and openly critical of anyone with the slightest bulge around their middle. For some reason she equates being a 'fat slob of a man' as being a 'no good person.' Before her knee surgery and the girls started staying around the clock, she was starving herself in order to avoid gaining weight. Louisa said that Mom would purposefully put her fingers down her throat to make herself throw up."

"So, between intentional bulimic behavior, simply forgetting how to prepare food, and forgetting whether she had already eaten," Nora conjectured that she must have lost a lot of weight.

"Yes, she looked gaunt and complained that her legs could not hold her up. Elena noticed that she was frequently shaking and feeling weak. She started preparing meals for her and bringing them over to Mom. She would sit with her to make sure that she ate and did not head off to the bathroom to get rid of it. Mom has slowly begun to gain weight and has some of her strength back."

"You must feel relieved, Allison, to have Elena so

conscientiously helping your mother."

I smiled and acknowledged that it did take a certain amount of concern off my heart, but the fact that my eighty-year-old mother was bulimic had caught me completely off guard. One expects to fight this battle with an acne-prone teenager, not an elderly person who was already frail. However, like any compulsive behavior, it would be a battle that Mother would have to fight the rest of her life. The urge to avoid becoming fat was deeply rooted in the belief that being overweight had cost my father his life - of course, when he died he was exactly what he should have weighed thanks to the strict low-fat diet Mother kept him on. When they married, my father was grossly overweight and the newlywed bride quickly marched her husband off to a doctor who put him on a low-fat, low-cholesterol diet, which Mother interpreted as low-taste and low-quantity.

With Elena now at the helm in Mother's kitchen, the fare was slightly tastier, but still lacked any suggestion of butter or meat fat for fear that Elena would receive a harsh scolding if she slipped a pat of butter on the canned green beans.

"Don't put that butter in there," Mom would say with a scowl on her face. "That's fat and fat killed my husband."

If she suspects that anything she has eaten contains the slightest amount of the offending substance, she puts two fingers in her mouth and declares, "I have to get that fat out of there."

Elena says Mother is changing so quickly now. When she first went to work for her just a year ago, she thought of Mrs. Adams as a lady.

"She had perfect manners and was demure and quiet. Now she goes right up to a table of strangers and introduces herself."

Louisa complemented her on wanting to make friends, but Mother hissed back at her, "I don't want to make friends. They need to know who I am."

We haven't quite figured out why she thinks they need to know her, but everyone from the security gate to the lawn maintenance crews to the maids to her neighbors knows Imogene Adams. Lately she has been approaching strangers, mostly men, and is soon arguing with them about whether they know her husband. When the victims of false identity contend that they do not know her or her husband, she retorts that they have been good friends for years and argues the point until Elena can pull her away or make her hang up the phone.

The phone in Mother's bedroom has long since been removed, but on one occasion she was overheard carrying on a lively conversation with some unknown person located in Chicago. Neither Louisa nor I know anyone in Chicago and are fairly certain that Mother does not have any acquaintances there either. That would explain the high phone bills that had been arriving the last two months.

The death knoll for the bedroom phone sounded when one of the aides who routinely took the night shift overheard her talking on the phone well past one in the morning. Upon investigating, the aide found Mother in her nightgown and bonnet calling an airline to make reservations to "fly home because Steve was waiting there for me." Wisely restraining from telling her that she was already home and that Steve had passed away ten years ago, the aide assured her that she would help her make the reservation in the morning as she deftly hid the handset in her pocket. With the gentleness of a parent giving a sleepy youngster a glass of water before tucking them in, she guided the confused woman back to bed and lovingly wrapped a blanket around her.

It wasn't long afterwards that the kitchen phone mysteriously ceased to function, as well. For someone who had become anti-social, Mother certainly seemed to be excited about using the phone. Like a child pretending to dial their first Princess Slimline phone, she pressed any series of numbers that came to mind, fully expecting Louisa or Sylvia to be on the other end; but the quartet of caregivers had unplugged the phone from the wall and let her believe that the fault lay with the phone company rather than in their client's inability to use a telephone.

Chapter 12

"*A*ccording to Mom, I am decades younger than when we last saw one another. Mom has been telling everyone – doctors, housekeeper, hairdresser, and visitors to the house – that I am twenty-seven years old. Not that I would mind being twenty-seven again, but it is strange to hear Mom refer to me as a young newlywed," I said, showing only the barest hint of a smile.

"What is so significant about your life at that time that makes her remember you at that age? Tell me about your life as a twenty-seven-year- old."

While Nora ate a salad topped with salmon, I told her who I was at that juncture in my life.

"I was beginning my first career as a music therapist for elementary aged school children. My music classroom was actually a metal portable building, and five hundred third through sixth graders streamed in and out of my door every few days. We made the trailer rock with music – literally."

Nora smiled at the imagery and asked me what music therapy classes entailed.

"Two of my classes were comprised entirely of students who had varying degrees of learning, physical, and emotional challenges. For the thirty or so minutes that they visited the music room, I hoped to transport them away from their isolation into a world where they could express their feelings and to resolve some of their negative emotions. However, reaching a seriously depressed and violent child on the same level as the student whose only challenge was that his legs did not work was a formidable task."

"So, regardless of their challenge, every child was put into the same class?" Nora asked with one eyebrow raised.

"Yes. The music touched only some of the children some of the time. A few of the children were in such turmoil that they could not process the emotions that music evokes," I pointed out, and then paused as a new thought entered my mind. "...which may explain why my mother has stopped listening to music. She puts her hands over her ears and screams that it hurts."

"Your mother loved music..." Nora led.

"Yes, she and Dad were my most faithful fans and were there for every recital from the time I was little until I graduated with my master's degree in music. She especially loved to listen to the big bands, and according to my Aunt Goldy, who moved with her from their little hometown into the city, Mom was the life of any dance party."

My dad must have seen that spark and feistiness in her character, and he, too, was attracted to her sense of self-confidence. Mother could play it prim and proper, though, and listened attentively to her teachers at secretarial school where they turned out not just typists, but young ladies who sat with straight backs and perfectly polished fingernails at the ready to take dictation or transcribe a letter. Mother took a position as a church secretary, and that is where Dad found her as he was visiting with the pastor regarding the church's Boy Scout troop. They were married only a matter of weeks after their first meeting, a fact they kept from Louisa and I for fear we might follow in their footsteps. It was not until years later that I learned of how quickly Dad had proposed and married my mother. Seeing the total look of dismay on my face at this well-kept secret, he simply said with that ever present twinkle in his eye, "Well, it worked out, didn't it?"

Like my mother, I had also ventured out on my own and found myself in a place far removed from the protective home life of my childhood. I rooted myself in the church where I found a sense of belonging and security, and that is where I met Scott Padgett. After a short courtship, not unlike my parents', we were soon married. Perhaps, my father looked back on his own brief courtship of his bride, and even though they had a wonderfully fulfilling marriage, he wished that I would take my time. However, I could not be dissuaded from marrying Scott after only a few weeks of courtship.

"At twenty-seven years of age, that is how Mom thinks of me. She sees me as that young newlywed on a fulfilling family and career path," I said, drawing my finger absently through the salt that had spilled on the table. "In spite of the fact that my marriage to Scott was ill-fated from the beginning, my mother's memory of me at that time was not tarnished. I suppose I shouldn't mind being young again. Mom's memory of me then was from a happy time, as if frozen in her mind."

Nora had finished her salmon salad, and delicately wiping her mouth on a napkin, sat back and said, "What a healthy way to think about it, Allison. You have a found a small bit of peace amongst all the turmoil in your mother's mind."

"You are right. I really don't mind being that young woman laughing and singing with the children," I said with a big grin and peacefully surveyed the room, as if imagining the happy faces of singing children.

I am grateful that Mother does not recall the years of heartache which followed. My students were the only children I was to have. The years soon thereafter were a blur of miscarriages, most of which I suffered through alone as Scott chose to run away from our heartache and was of little comfort at the loss of our babies. Instead, it was my parents who made the long drive down to be with me in my grief, both at losing another child and at watching a husband walk away. Scott spent most of his free time on his dirt bike, throwing up clouds of dust between us - both figuratively and literally. In retrospect, I don't want my mother to remember those times. I found solace in teaching emotionally disturbed children, furious with myself for not being able to mend my emotionally disturbed husband and make him fall in love with me again... and then the diagnosis of multiple sclerosis came to put the epitaph on the marriage.

Mother blamed herself for the MS. Like the rest of us, she didn't really know anything about the disease, and her thoughts ran the gamut from, "When will Allison die?" to "Is it contagious?" Dad could never pronounce the name correctly and got all tongue-tied and switched the "l" and the "r" sounding much like a Chinese translation.

A great yearning for my father suddenly overcame me as I

continued, "Elena says that Mom keeps a book on the pillow next to her at night because she is expecting Dad to come home from work at any moment. Dad could never go straight to sleep and read late at night to wind down from his day – murder mysteries, science fiction, and espionage among his favorites. There was always a warm glow from his reading light well past when the rest of the family was asleep. Mom is reliving that memory...except...for her is it not a memory. It is now."

"Does she talk about the grandchildren? How old does she see them in her mind," Nora asked.

I smiled before answering, "Yes, in her mind they are little tykes. Charlotte is seven and Charlie is four or five. They were absolutely adorable at that age, and it's easy to see why they are fixed in her thoughts at that specific age."

"It's as though a snapshot has been taken, freezing everyone in their own perfect time and place," Nora noted.

Dessert arrived at our table and the conversation quieted for a few minutes as we concentrated on the sweets before us.

"You know, I called Mom the other day to apologize," I hesitantly started and then quickly returned to dessert. I pushed the éclair around my plate a few times, and Nora let me take my time in bringing my thoughts to a head on my lips. "It seems that Elena and Louisa both believe the disease is moving along quickly now and that Mom is losing much of her capacity to recall things accurately. They encouraged me to make amends with Mom while I still could."

Many moments went by in silence before I continued.

"I had no idea what I had to apologize for, but they both felt it important to her well-being to free her from the angst she felt for me. So, I did. I picked up the phone and called the number for Elena's cell phone. Elena forced the phone into her hands, willing Mom to speak to me. I gently told her that I knew she was upset with me, but I wanted to know why. She couldn't tell me, Nora. She had no recall of anything specifically that was a barrier between us – she just thought I had done something to hurt her. In my mind, I think that her harsh judgment of me stemmed from that terrible hospital stay two years prior."

Nora interrupted, "Has it really been only two years? It

seems so much longer ago."

"That is when it became so clear that she was beginning to fade away. Alzheimer's warps the memory, but it also warps time," I offered. "Mom seemed to be holding on to images from that hospital room where the sitter at the foot of her bed had become an armed guard in her mind. The IV's in her arms to rehydrate her and pump her full of vitamins she interpreted as restraints tying her to the bed. The dementia diagnosis she heard as a statement identifying me as her only problem."

My words came faster and faster as emotions began to pour over me. Nora's bright blue eyes never left my face as she listened with her entire being. She was acquainted with my hurt.

"That is when my mother began to believe that she hated me, Nora. It is a blessing I suppose that she doesn't remember the why, but I had hoped that she would also forget the hatred and just wake up one day in love with her daughter again. I told her I was sorry - I don't know for what, but just that I was sorry. Mom started sobbing and wanted to get off the phone on the pretense that she had a doctor's appointment to go to. She cried so hard she couldn't breathe, Nora. It was like a dam had burst and all of her hurt feelings came tumbling out and the ugliness of the past two years just melted away."

Over the next few weeks, my mother's words slowly began to turn sweet again, as though she had been exorcised of the darkness which had hung over the two of us. I delighted in telling her how much I loved her, and for the first time in years she said she was proud of me. Perhaps, the spilling out of her soul had gone further back than just the twenty-four months since the hospital visit. She was emptying herself of years of bad feelings towards me, and I finally caught a glimpse of the woman who used to brush my hair while I sat on the floor at the foot of her bed.

My joy was to be short lived, however, as mother soon began to revert back to a state of paranoia and hostility, interspersed with only brief moments of sunshine when she still recalled our happier times together.

"Her mind swings back and forth like a pendulum between memories of family fishing trips and afternoons spent in her garden with the ghosts of horrible scenes that only she can see," I told

Nora. "Mom's dreams have turned to nightmares, and Elena tells us that she spends most of the night wandering back and forth from the living room to the bedroom to the bathroom, muttering to herself. Nora, that very tiny moment of respite has disappeared and Mom seems to be in more trouble than ever."

"Paranoia is part of Alzheimer's, as you know, but your mother has some kind of psychosis, as well. Allison, do you have a plan for helping her deal with these episodes? Is your sister prepared to consider taking her to a psychiatrist?" Nora asked very delicately.

"No, Nora. Louisa actually proposes to cut down on the cost of twenty-four care by reducing the aides' hours! Because evening and nights are more tumultuous, Louisa is contemplating letting Elena off for a few hours every afternoon and then returning to serve Mother her dinner before the night girl arrives. How in the world she believes that it is safe for Mom to be alone is beyond me, Nora," I exclaimed, shifting around uneasily on the leather cushioned bench seat. "Louisa is so concerned about the money. True, we do not currently have access to anything other than her checking account, but we must find a way to keep her money flowing and continue around-the-clock care."

Raising my voice, I asked, "How can she even give the slightest thought to leaving Mom on her own? I sent her an email and suggested that she is letting her fear of having Mom declared incompetent stand in the way of her safety, to which she replied that she was not afraid, although she could see how I might think that. Louisa was considering asking the doctor for stronger sleeping pills so that she would sleep through the night and, therefore, could be left alone."

Nora gasped, "That borders on abuse. You didn't let her do it, did you?"

I shook my head, "She quickly dropped that idea when I reacted much the same way you did. Louisa has not mentioned the sleeping pills again and the night aide is still going. I heard a report from the aid that Mom put on her coat and gloves to go down to check the mailbox in the middle of the night. She has also been putting her clothes into plastic baggies to keep them dry on a canoe trip that is coming up. Mom seems to be quite busy at night, so I assume that she is still receiving twenty-four hour care."

With the smallest of smiles, Nora said, "That is a new behavior isn't it?"

"Yes it is. She was doing so well there for a while. It almost seemed that she had become herself again," I said with a note of apprehension. "She just finished another round of antibiotics for that ongoing bladder infection. Elena is still puzzled as to why that keeps happening."

Nora assured me that most geriatric patients, not just Alzheimer's individuals, tend to have chronic infections.

"It could be something as simple as not drinking enough fluids, or a lack of good hygiene."

"I am not certain which of those causes it might be, most likely a combination of both," I said. "Although Elena insists that she is cleaning her thoroughly after each visit to the bathroom."

"It seems that incontinence is also a symptom of this stage," I wearily noted. "Toileting and taking care of herself has become a major focus. The higher levels of fulfillment and self-actualization have crumbled, and she is struggling on a much more physical level to survive... and just a few weeks ago she was eagerly approaching strangers and introducing herself."

We finished up the last bits of cake, and not wanting to end our discussion, I reluctantly said goodnight. There was still so much that Nora could offer me. I couldn't begin to tell her how valuable - and comforting - she had been to me.

"It is so hard to see my mother growing away from me," I thought as I walked across the parking lot to my car. As I slowly made my way home, Nora's first words echoed in my head.

"Growing old is a gift... but, not one that we always know what to do with," she had said.

How true her words had been. Every day, Mother presented new and surprising aspects of growing old, few of which were easy to understand. One afternoon, Louisa followed through with her idea to give Elena a few hours off, not only to afford her a break in constant caregiving responsibilities, but to cut down on the cost. Mother's reaction was immediate and, although Louisa did not expect it, I could have predicted it with one-hundred percent accuracy. As soon as Elena left the cottage, Mother locked all the doors. She flatly refused to answer Elena's repeated knocking on the front door, followed by the back door, followed by each of the windows around the front of her little cottage. Elena chuckled, in part because it was funny, as the elderly woman followed her movement from window to window, closing the blinds in her caregiver's face as she tapped on the glass asking to be let in. Mother's lack of patience could not stand up to Elena's persistence, however, and Mother finally and reluctantly unbolted the front door, admitting her barely ruffled caregiver.

"Mom told Elena that she was in the bathroom and didn't hear the knocking," I burst out laughing. "Can't you just see Elena smiling through the glass as Mom scowls back with that persimmon face and closes the blinds in her face – and then has the audacity to claim she was in another room altogether?"

"It reminds me of the ostrich trying to hide its head under the sand," commented Nora, chuckling as she pictured the scene. "I presume that is the last time Louisa tried to leave your mother to fend on her own..."

"Yes, that did it. We have agreed that Mom will never be left alone again," I said with a deep heartache, for I knew how much Mother longed for independence and for the right to be alone with her own thoughts and activities.

Sadly, I have to accept the new person she has become. Our conversations on the phone are still limited pretty much to the weather and whatever she had for lunch. I'm not sure that she really recalls what she had for lunch or even if she has even had lunch. It really doesn't matter because she wants to talk, and we enter into a somewhat lopsided dialogue. Her responses to my questions, intended to draw her into deeper conversation, are somewhat nonsensical and lacking in substance. "Oh, I don't know about that," or "Well, we will see," – phrases which could mean anything or nothing.

"Nora, something that is so unexpected is Mom's lack of emotion when speaking. For the most part, there is no change in the pitch or tone of her voice except to emphasize a word by speaking it very loudly. Her personality doesn't sparkle like it used to. She just exists in an all-beige world," and then I laughed. "Beige has been her favorite color for some time now. I would characterize her personality twenty years ago as brilliant orange with flashes of red and pink depending on whether she was laughing or trying to press her point. Occasionally, she would descend into a black mood and just shut down all communication. It's like that a bit now, but more... well, beige."

"Colors are very important in influencing an Alzheimer patient's state of mind," my friend reminded me.

"Mom is telling everyone that at Christmas I kept her in a cave in the basement," the dismay could not be mistaken in my voice. "I thought she would like the powder blue bedroom on the bottom level. She had her own bathroom and plenty of privacy. We placed wedding pictures of her and Dad on the bookcase where she could easily see them."

"Oh, how lovely," Nora's eyes twinkled as she relaxed with a cup of espresso, which I think she ordered more to warm her fingers than for the strong flavor.

"We also put photos on the bookcase from their forty-fifth wedding anniversary. That was such a wonderful reception. I think Mom knew they would not make it to their fiftieth because of Dad's failing health. How could she look at those photographs and feel the lace on the pillowcases and cuddle down in the oversized comforter, and not know that she was being pampered. She said the room made her vomit."

I was not only dismayed, but hurt by her crass comments.

"Only after Tom reminds me that it is the disease speaking, and not my mother, can I release the frustration and move on to happier thoughts."

Nora put down the tiny cup, traced her finger along the rim, and quietly said, "That must be terribly difficult to bear."

I loved Nora for justifying my thoughts and feelings, for the simple acknowledgement of them made them sting less. I had every reason to be sore at heart, and yet, my heart still reached out to Mother with a longing only a daughter can have for her mother.

My dear Pollyanna of a sister still believed that Mother knew what she was talking about the majority of the time. I am certain that is not the case, but stopped trying to convince her otherwise. As long as Louisa stayed on track to seek a declaration of incompetency, I did not protest too loudly. Pushing that viewpoint serves no purpose, and I have learned to pick my battles carefully. Engaging in a verbal war of words with my sister would have been detrimental at this point, and it really was not advantageous for me to always be right as Louisa repeatedly points out.

Chapter 13

$\mathcal{M}$other's antics, if you will, would have been quite laughable, if they were not so bizarre. Nora and I met at the usual little restaurant - such a quaint English place that I am tempted to rename it as "The Sandwich Shoppe." I took a big breath before plunging into a monologue to bring Nora up to date on my family's collective journey.

"I have been reading about a shift in the treatment of Alzheimer's individuals. We used to try to force them back into a pattern of conventional behavior, probably because the medical profession, caregivers, and family members are so caught off guard by the odd needs of the memory-impaired mind and we insist on pointing them back along the way they have just come, back towards our definition of sanity. And, I ashamedly counted myself as part of that group that wanted my mother to return to some state of normalcy. This is her new world now, and she will never be going back to the old life we knew together as mother and daughter. I finally know that and embrace it."

"Allison, think about how far you have come in your understanding of this disease. Some people never grasp that their loved one has permanently veered off course and are creating a heretofore undiscovered future all his or her own. You, on the other hand, not only seek to educate yourself about it, but you truly know that you are in partnership with your mother and that you must walk together in the direction the disease takes you both."

"It's really tough, though, not to limit how many pieces of cake she has, or to want her to wear matching socks, or to restrain her from wallpapering the rooms with sticky notes," I remarked.

"Sticky notes!" Nora almost choked on her drink. "Tell me about the sticky notes."

"Well, apparently, it started in her bedroom. For some unknown reason she removed all the files and folders from the two filing cabinets in the office area on one side of the bedroom. Elena said I would not recognize it. She has strewn papers all over the bed, the dresser, the bookcases...everywhere. Elena started to straighten them and get them back into some semblance of order with the thought of refiling them, but Mom slapped her hand," I paused as a vision of my mother striking someone like a four-year-old at play. "She told Elena that she was not to touch any of her papers. Mom took her by the hand and led her into the kitchen where she pointed to various areas of the kitchen counters that were free for Elena to touch. There is one end of the kitchen counter where she keeps her phone – now disconnected; calendar and address book –neither of which she can read; and an assortment of notepads and pens. She said that was also off-limits to Elena, and then began searching through the kitchen drawers in search of a marker."

"Okay...what was the marker for?"

"Well, she wanted a marker to draw a line on the kitchen counter showing Elena which space was for her use and which space the aides could use. The following day when it was Elena's turn again at the cottage, every room in the cottage had sticky notes on the walls with lines drawn on them to differentiate where the caregivers could go and where they should leave Mom's possessions alone. Elena laughed when she saw them, and Mom immediately started yanking them off the walls. 'Some crazy person got into my house and put these on the walls,' she told Elena."

Nora and I chuckled over this very unusual way of literally marking one's territory.

"She is really in a mode of survival, isn't she?" Nora asked, not really expecting an answer, but making more of an observation than asking a question.

I, on the other hand, wanted to reach out to my mother and to ease her mind – calm the suspicious thoughts which, no doubt, raced through her head and literally drove her crazy.

"She is willing to have me visit her again, although she believes it would be my first visit since she moved into Waverly

Place. I made the mistake – again – of reminding her that I had been to her cottage many times before. It was a very gentle reminder, but she took offense at it anyway," I said with a frustrated sigh. "After we hung up, she couldn't tell Elena who she had been talking to – just that one of her 'lovely daughters' had called. She later told Elena that it was the daughter that wants to put her in a cage."

Nora choked upon hearing those words, and when she had recovered, sadly said, "I guess that is an idea in her head that will never go away. Isn't it so odd how she bounces back and forth between such conflicting thoughts?"

"No matter how hard Louisa, or Elena, or I work to assure her that I am not going to put her in a cage, she simply will not shake that image from her head. I think she knows that inevitably she will have to move out of her house, and the options of where she would go make her afraid. Mom lives with such fear," I said, unable to really grasp what that would be like.

Our conversation died away. Neither Nora nor I wanted to pick up the thread and chose to devote our energies to acorn squash soup and avocado sandwiches. As we polished off a raspberry torte between the two of us, Nora asked a leading question.

"Does she recognize your voice on the phone? Dorothy and I are fairly certain that Mommie knew who we were right up until the end...or at least, we wanted to believe that."

"I'm not certain, Nora. Something about the disconnected things she brings up, and the strange way she sometimes answers my questions – I don't really believe she does. The last time Tom and I went to see her, I am certain that she did not know who we were at times," my voice lowered to a whisper. "I believe we are getting close to the threshold beyond which she will not know us."

"I am so sorry, my friend," was Nora's gentle consolation.

"That is really alright. I have been preparing myself for this dark doorway. We are nearing the end of what was and entering a new and unknown what will be."

There was little more to say, and we bid each other goodnight.

The center of Mother's soul, which at one time I believed to still be burning brightly within her, had cooled to only a glowing ember. I wondered if she knew how much of her world she had lost. At what point does the mind shrink to such a diminished state that the heart does not care? I am told that someday soon she will forget people who have been so prevalent in her life, and moreover, she will not realize that she is supposed to remember them. It will not bother her and she will relax into a happier, although much smaller world of her own imaginations. I prayed that day would come soon. Mother's constant state of confusion was breaking my heart.

Several days went by before Nora and I reconnected.

"Last night Mother did not sleep well. The aides reported that she spent most of the night packing suitcases for a trip that she and Charlotte were going on together. Tom questions whether the caregivers who stay with her at night are actually awake and tending to her needs. He wonders why Mother should be allowed to stay up packing suitcases instead of sleeping in her bed. He protests that the walls should not be covered with sticky notes that weren't there the evening before, and that she should not be up trying to dial the airlines for a ticket to Nacogdoches to see Dad. I tried to explain that stopping such behaviors is detrimental to her thought processes, no matter how bizarre and convoluted they may seem. Although, I have not witnessed it nor even heard a report on how the night time caregivers are dealing with it, but I would hope they might cheerfully help Mother pack the suitcase before gently encouraging her to get some sleep and finish the packing in the morning."

It was actually my brother-in-law Matt who first pointed out that attempting to correct or confront the odd behaviors of an Alzheimer's patient achieves the opposite effect and worsens their condition. Matt had been witness to my first angry outbursts toward a "stubborn woman who does not listen." I am now deeply ashamed of that verbal assault on my mother where I placed my own need to be in the right before her need to maintain a feeble grasp on her world. My confrontation, no doubt, added to whatever darkness was already happening in her brain.

"It is terribly difficult to put aside one's own needs to humor someone that seems a little off," Nora reminds me in almost every visit we have together. "This is as much a learning process for your family as it is a journey for your mother. Don't be so hard on yourself for the past. Learn from it, forgive yourself, and move on with a renewed intention to behave differently."

Nora describes repentance so eloquently – learn, forgive, and adopt a renewed intention to do good. Sounds simple, but when lifelong habits and attitudes get in the way of unconditional love, repentance is not an easy bedfellow. Learning from one's mistakes implies that one acknowledges a misstep. For many months I refused to see that my confrontational ways were damaging to my mother. She could not correctly administer her own medications. She could not balance her checkbook. She could not operate the controls on her car dashboard. She could not... and the list grew as the months passed, as did my anger and frustration. Not only was my mother incapable of learning anything new, but I was incapable of absorbing that simple fact. I had to accept that she could no longer learn.

In the future, Mother would not be exploring anything new, and would, in fact, have difficulty performing tasks she had been doing for her entire life. Things such as organizing a box of pills or adding and subtracting a row of numbers or turning the right knob to get heat in the car – these things would evade her from now on – and my getting angry with her would serve no purpose other than to give evidence to my own shortcomings. I had to learn new ways of loving her.

This lesson was learned the hard way, and I vowed to be more watchful of Mother's changing abilities and needs and to find ways to make the transition from a vibrant life to a more beige one a little easier for her. I lament my negative and harsh reactions to her floundering ways and for finding delight in her failures.

"Nora, why is it that when someone has hurt us, we react with childish glee when they themselves are hurt or fail at something? Is that the definition of a bully?" I exclaimed over the phone.

She surprised me by laughing at my questions before reassuring me that I could never be perceived as a bully, and, yet, it still bothered me that I had secretly wanted my mother to feel pain... like the pain she had caused me. Mother's suffering was more like that of a fearful and bewildered child who was trying to understand a world that changed around her every day. The child would be excited about all the newness in her ever-expanding world, while Mother was lost in a maze of jumbled up trails that no longer made sense to her. Perhaps, if I had understood dementia more completely, my words would have been more patient and my actions more loving. The word "*if*" is a convenient way of saying that one understands one's faults and would have acted differently given better information or different circumstances. "*If*" is a mournful word, lamenting what could have been, but was not.

"Al-li-son," Nora's elongated pronunciation of my name was not derived from her Southern upbringing, but from her frustration with me. "Forgive yourself. You are not perfect. You have done remarkably well in dealing with a terrible, terrible event in your family. This is like watching someone walk off into an abyss from which there is no return. It is a horror show. You are so courageous and loving to stay by your mother in spite of the way she has treated you," and her voice, which rarely rose in pitch or volume, reached out and grabbed me.

After a long silence, Nora's voice dropped to a whisper, "*This* is agape love - sacrificial giving of one's self without expecting anything back. You have grown to completely love a woman that most would turn away from. Most people don't understand what it is to lose your mind- but *you do*, and you love her anyway."

I was humbled by her words and simply said, "Thank you, Nora, thank you."

"Mom's difficulties have actually taken a back seat for now," I explained to Nora. "While she inches her way through this confusing haze, my sister's condition is quickly moving toward..."

I could not finish the sentence, as if saying it out loud would make it so. After weeks of diligent searching, Louisa's doctor had located a surgeon who specialized in correcting adult onset scoliosis. Louisa's case was particularly intriguing to him as the spiraling and collapse of her spine had taken only a few months - rather than the typical span of years - to turn her body into a corkscrew. The extreme rate of her decline, combined with the fact that she had electrodes implanted in her brain which emitted tiny shocks every few moments in hopes of interrupting the pain signals shooting through her face, most likely made her the only patient in the world with these exact circumstances.

Winning a spot on the surgeon's calendar usually took up to a year, but she was bumped up to the top of the waiting list. We all waited for a cancellation which might come too late as her body continued to implode. At the rate of collapse, Louisa would be gone in a matter of months. She was number one on the waiting list and, as the days went by, that wait seemed to stretch out longer and longer while the days we would have her with us seemed shorter and shorter. Finally, the call came for her to be at the surgical center in Cleveland in three weeks. They had a cancellation, and Louisa was given the spot.

"Are you going to Cleveland?" Nora asked.

"Not yet," was my quick reply, hoping to hide my cynicism. "Louisa and her family are really strange in how they deal with extreme family situations. Matt prefers to be alone whenever Louisa is in surgery. I don't know what kind of coping mechanism one could call it, but he would really rather read a book than visit with friends and family. Many years ago when she had one of her first brain surgeries, I assured him that no one expected to be entertained, but he still refused to invite us to be there in the family waiting room. Most of the time, he and Louisa did not even tell my parents that she was having surgery until she was already back home recuperating."

Nora was nonplussed and sat back in the booth for a few moments before commenting.

"That must be very difficult, Allison."

Her eyes said much more and I appreciated her unspoken support, although neither of us really knew how to wipe away the hurt of exclusion.

I stared down at my cup of clam chowder for a long time before slowly forming the words which my ears did not want to hear, "There is a good chance that Louisa will not survive the surgery."

"Do you want to go?" Nora asked after our eyes met. "Would Matt turn you away if you just showed up?"

"Probably not, but Louisa would be very angry with me if I put such an imposition on Matt. She has told me before that she doesn't want me at any of her surgeries because Matt is uncomfortable with chit-chat. I have wanted to ask her what about the feelings of her mother and sister who are always shut out and must sit at home or at work wondering if the latest surgery was successful."

I paused, and looked away.

"The surgery is supposed to take over nine hours."

"How does all this make you feel?"

"Pushed away," I said numbly. "But, I truly do understand that for Matt and the kids it is difficult enough to deal with their own thoughts without having to deal with someone else's emotions, as well."

We let the evening draw to a close, acknowledging that the individual needs of family members often do not run concurrently, but strong in the belief that a collective faith would sustain each of us wherever we found ourselves that day.

I reached out to Aunt Goldy the day before Louisa's surgery, in part to update her on Mother, but also to tell her about Louisa. I felt the need to share my burden with someone in my family, to reach out for support from my aunt - because I could not call out to my mother. It was an empty spot in my heart that only another woman with a sister in peril could understand, and my aunt would know that feeling as someone who also longed for her sister.

"There is a danger that Louisa might not survive the surgery, Aunt Goldy," I said softly. "Her heart is already damaged from the pressure of her ribs constantly pushing on it. It would be much appreciated if you would let all the cousins know that she needs the prayers of her whole family."

The reply was so quick and reassuring, that my heart immediately found ease. We talked with the closeness of a niece and aunt, assuring one another that the strength of the Hickson family would hold us up when we felt that we could no longer stand. My cousins and I sent the usual greetings to each other once a year at Christmas, enjoyed catching up in an occasional phone call across the miles, and still felt the close ties we had as kids playing in each other's back yards. I knew my aunts and cousins would be vigilant as Louisa and Matt and their children faced the difficult days ahead.

We also talked about Mother, which in many ways was

more difficult than talking about Louisa's challenges. Aunt Goldy had been surprised that her sister had not called in some time, but was coming to realize that the disease would be affecting us all as she slowly forgot the ties to relatives in distant places. I shared with her the circumstances surrounding the knee surgery, Mother's rehabilitation, and the unexpected side effects of the anesthesia. She was troubled to hear about Mother's recalcitrant and ugly moods and wanted desperately to see her, but for their own physical reasons, she and Aunt Minnie were no longer able to travel. The remembrance of sweeter times weighed heavily on our hearts and the call ended abruptly with both of us in tears.

The next call was to Aunt Minnie, who is very down-to-earth and was not surprised to hear that Imogene had reached a point where she did not easily recognize friends and family. Both aunts kept saying, "That isn't Imogene" as I described their sister's screaming and uncooperativeness. I did not tell them that she thought she was in her own home and demanded that the nurses and doctors leave her house, or that she believed the bed was wired with the intention of electrocuting her to death.

"Nora, it was so terribly sad for me to tell them that I had already said goodbye to the person that I knew as Mom," I managed to say.

Although the words stuck in my throat, I told them it was time for them to say goodbye to their sister.

"You have a sister, Nora. You know how horrible that is – to say goodbye. I truly hated to tell them, and coupled with the news of Louisa's surgery, these were terribly difficult phone calls to make."

"Allison, you did what a loving family member does. This was probably even more heart wrenching than when you will have to call and tell them that their sister has died," Nora consoled me. "At least with death there is closure. This kind of conversation will continue for some time into the future, and you are carrying that burden faithfully and with a great deal of love."

The day of Louisa's surgery arrived like any other for tom and me with the ringing of the alarm clock, a quick breakfast of cereal and juice, and the mad dash through traffic to our offices in Manhattan. Tom sent out updates on Facebook and received many supportive and encouraging messages throughout the day. We later learned that many of our friends and colleagues had stood vigil with us, offering up a constant melody of prayers for my sister.

My boss and I rarely shared our private lives with one another, but I sat down in front of his desk piled high with music scores and ventured to tell him everything that preoccupied my mind that day, and somehow just in the telling I found solace. His concern was genuine, and he kept me mercifully busy editing and tweaking scores for a Broadway show. At the end of the day, he expressed his well wishes for my sister and urged me to go home and get some rest.

The surgery took well over the anticipated nine hours and extended into the early evening. I received one update from Char during those long, long hours of waiting. The surgery was halfway completed and Louisa was doing well. Her spine had been straightened, one vertebra at a time, and the team was ready to encase her spine in a steel cage that would be its source of support for the rest of her life.

After work, Nora picked me up at the circle drive in front of my office building and we went for a quick bite to eat at a nearby diner. The waitress was overly cheerful, something that would ordinarily have made my toes curl from all the sugary sweetness, but somehow that night it washed over me harmlessly. Distractions were welcomed, and Nora and I talked about her new sweater, how her knee was taking the cold, and whether or not the Specials were good. As we watched the people wrapped up in layers of scarves, with coats drawn tightly about them, my cell phone rang. I fumbled about in my rush to retrieve it from the depths of my purse and was relieved to hear Matt's voice on the line when I finally pushed the button.

"She is out of surgery and in recovery," were Matt's first words. "It was longer than usual because he had to straighten her pelvis, but everything went well."

He sounded tired, but very optimistic that the next critical twenty-four hours would go without any problems. Louisa would be in a drug-induced coma for several days and would be monitored closely by the ICU staff before they would slowly awaken her to begin the long recovery. It would be a full year before the bones knit themselves together with the man-made materials inserted into her back. Pain medications would be a constant topic with the surgeon's assistants, who really did not and could not comprehend the amount of medications she already took to make her life livable. The next few months would be a struggle, even more so than before, to find the right cocktail of painkillers that would allow her to remain awake and pain free for even short periods of time.

Thankfully, Mother was at a point where she had no real understanding of her daughter's surgery other than she hoped it would take away Louisa's pain. When Matt called to tell her that the surgery was over, he did not receive the expected response. She just recited the usual rhetoric, "Oh, that's good," before launching into a tale about Elena poisoning her with bacon.

"I don't want bacon. That's what killed my husband," she told him. "He ate bacon and doughnuts, and that is what killed him."

"Matt must have felt very strange and bewildered to hear Mom say that," I told Nora. "It is hard to comprehend how someone could be so out of touch and so wrapped up in themselves. I pray that he knows it is the disease and that his mother-in-law truly does care for Louisa. She has just forgotten how to show her love."

Out of deference to Louisa's still fragile recovery, Tom and I elected to spend Christmas at home rather than visit Louisa and her family in Cleveland. Although it felt odd to be celebrating Christ's birth without family around, we enjoyed the opportunity to stay up beyond our normal bedtimes, sleep in, and remained in our pajamas all day. I hung closely to the phone as Louisa's progress was faithfully reported by Charlie and Charlotte. She progressed slowly, but steadily, awakening from the drug-induced coma, and was taken off the respirator and began breathing and eating on her own. On the last day of my winter break from work, she was strong enough to talk in person on the phone for the first time. Perhaps because I was still enjoying a bit of eggnog, or maybe the sheer joy of hearing her voice strong and clear in the headset was to blame, but we giggled our way through the brief call and hung up after wishing each other a very happy – and healthy – New Year.

"What kind of impact will Louisa's surgery have on her ability to handle your mother's affairs?" Nora asked a few weeks later as she eyed the piece of strawberry pie and whipped cream waiting in front of her.

She must have sensed that not only was I concerned for my sister, but the timing could not have been worse in our pursuit to seek an incompetency ruling for Mother. Neither Tom nor I truly believed that Louisa was up to the task. However, as Mother had designated her as the guardian when the time came to appoint one, I thought it best not to rock the boat too much for it wouldn't have made a difference. I had no ready answer to Nora's question.

Abandoning my half-eaten soup, I described the last time the four of us had traveled together – Louisa and Matt, and Tom and I – a couples' get away to the seaside town of Bliss, Massachusetts, near our retirement property. We were joined by Tom's sister, Cindi, and her husband, Jay, who had flown in from California for our annual spa weekend in an historic home along the tree-lined main street of the old harbor. Whether sitting lazily on the front porch with a glass of lemonade and the local paper or riding the waves at sunset aboard a schooner, we always enjoyed our time together and managed to squeeze every magical moment out of the visit - except for my sister, who spent most of her time slumped over in her chair at the breakfast table or asleep with her head on my shoulder as we drove along the rocky shores looking for secluded alcoves to explore. Louisa relied heavily on narcotics to ease the pain which remained after the bio-metric implants had done as much as they could to give her a sense of normalcy. Rather than a shot or a pill or a patch, this particular narcotic was stronger than morphine and was rapidly delivered through what she called a lollipop because of its rounded shape on the end of a stick. The lollipops were intended to be consumed orally every eight hours, but Louisa unwrapped and sucked on stick after stick until she had ingested more than twice the normal amount in order to erase the ice-pick pain jabbing through her face.

The pain inflicted by trigeminal nerve neuralgia is reported to be worse than that of childbirth, although the pain of TNN never goes away, and the unwavering perseverance with which my sister dealt with her debilitation caused me to pause many times when I complained of a paper cut or bumped my knee on a desk drawer. The closest discomfort that I have experienced personally would be that of a gallbladder attack or the passing of a kidney stone, both of which were alleviated by a surgical intervention. The mind-numbing medications afterwards had been welcome, but fortunately I had the choice to stop taking them and return to life with my eyes open and mind alert to the brightness and vitality of my world. Louisa does not really have that choice and every day she has to take more and more of the drugs to feel relief.

More than once, as the group was seated at dinner learning how to crack open a lobster or fishing delicacies out of a mussel shell when Louisa's hands would be frozen in mid-air halfway between the plate and her mouth. We all understood her stupefied state and took turns gently nudging her awake so she could finish routing the fork to her mouth. As friendly chatter went around the table Louisa made an effort to chime in. With her head bobbing, eyes closed, and hands suspended in the air above her plate, she muttered some nonsensical combination of words, slurring them through her lips.

"Nora," I said, hearing my own words as if echoed from a distance. "My sister is drug dependent. Not because she wants to be. Not because she even has a choice; but rather out of an effort to survive – to just to get through the day…"

The din of glasses clinking and utensils on plates grew louder as my words faded away. She probably did not even hear my last thoughts, but after an appropriate silence between us Nora once again posed the now familiar question, "So, how does this affect your sister's ability to be your mother's guardian?"

The implication of her query was obvious and meant to drive me toward the cloud looming over the entire family; that being the inescapable fact that the one person Mother had chosen to lean upon could do little more than that for herself.

After many weeks in rehab, Louisa returned home, and the tasks of learning to live and function in her newly modified body began in earnest. She tackled each daily task bravely and with the same determination that made all three Adams women stubbornly persistent, learning how to accomplish simple things like brushing her teeth and putting on socks without being able to bend over. As

Louisa learned new ways to put on shoes, do the laundry, and load the dishwasher, our mother was continuing to forget how to do those same tasks.

The holidays soon passed and January came, bringing with it the blizzards – three of them back-to-back within a week. Life in the Northeast came to a complete standstill, enshrouded in a four-foot blanket of wet snow which was soon frozen into mountains of ice. After three days, the power came back on, phones were restored, and life slowly resumed its steady and reassuring rhythm. Over the next few weeks, the sun gradually emerged and helped to melt the forty-eight inches of snow and ice encasing my car.

Only then did Nora and I attempt to get back into the comfortable routine of dinners and phone calls. We picked up right where we had left off; Mother was still fighting the presence of around-the-clock care, and Louisa was fighting to remain upright and alert. There was one bit of significant news, however, to share with Nora.

"I spent last week in Texas with Louisa. It was the first time she would let me see her after the surgery the first part of December. It was fabulous to see her standing straight and almost as tall as I am. It was really evident, however, that even though the curve in her back had been corrected, the pain in her face remained unmercifully constant. She still described it as an ice pick stabbing at her jaw and cheek and running through her eye," shivering as I described it.

"The three-hour plane ride gave me a lot of time to think, maybe a bit too much time, because I hatched the ill-conceived idea that we move Mom to a facility near Louisa. After spending that week with her, though, it was very obvious that that was a bad idea, Nora. Straightening Louisa's back did nothing for her facial pain, not that any of us really expected that outcome. She still relies on the lollipops, which just numb her mind and slur her tongue. More than once she reiterated that she could not have Mom living close to her, much as she would like to," I spoke with despair in my heart that was echoed in my voice. "I actually came to agree with her, Nora. I now admit that moving Mom to be near my sister would be a mistake. Even if Mom were in a long-term care facility, ongoing attention would be needed by someone outside of the facility - and

Louisa is not capable of providing that level of attention."

"In fact, when I arrived at their house, her study was filled with stacks of papers that she rustled through every few minutes when her head fell to one side and jolted her awake. She couldn't stay awake long enough to complete a task. She just didn't have the strength and concentration to finish paying a bill or even look up a recipe. I felt badly for her because she tried so hard."

Nora had slowly continued eating her chicken and apple salad while nodding that she understood the difficulty of the situation. She had the unique ability to finish a meal all the while making me feel like she was totally engaged in the conversation. I never seemed to finish my entrée and found that to be the case as my soup had long ago turned cold and filmy on the top. Nora was a listener, a guide, a seeker of options – all qualities I admired and needed.

In spite of Louisa's difficulties, to my way of thinking there did not seem to be any other options than to go forward with our plan for her to seek guardianship of our mother. Mother had already signed a Designation of Guardian form to be presented at the appropriate time for some judge in some court to declare her unable to make financial and medical decisions for herself and to appoint my sister as her guardian. The judge may very well see Louisa sitting in front of him in a drug-induced stupor claiming the right to make decisions for Mother, and under those circumstances he would be in the right if he denied her the petition and appointed someone else completely unknown to our family as Mother's trustee.

Nora gasped, "What would you do if the judge awards the guardianship to someone else?"

"I suppose I would have no choice but to file my own petition, which Mom would most likely resist, given her fear of me," I shrugged my shoulders as I spoke, not knowing any other answer to give.

I had intended to only spend a weekend in The Woodlands with Louisa, but while she was standing straight and tall again, the improvement in physical stature was not reflected in her mental stature. She and Charlotte met me at the bottom of the escalator next to baggage claim where my niece and I had a reunion complete with the requisite squealing with delight which generally made Tom shake his head with amusement. We were typical women who had not seen each other for some time and reveled in each other's presence once again. When we had finished exchanging compliments on hair and choice of shoes, I turned my attention to my sister who was standing patiently behind the safety of her walker. Louisa's face was thin, punctuated only by the hint of a smile and eyes that used to shine like the sky on a sunny afternoon, but now matched the grayness of the sweater she wore. She was tired. Her body was slighter than I had seen her in years, although I did have difficulty keeping up with her as she zoomed along with the walker. No... Louisa's body was not tired - her spirit was tired. As we made our way from baggage claim to the handicap section of the parking garage, her words came tumbling out.

"Mom is not doing well," she hastily said, as if there was much to tell and she could not speak the words quickly enough.

Forever the sister who saw the good and the positive in any person or situation, this declaration was a shock to my ears. Louisa never spoke ill of our mother, but chose her words carefully, always giving Mother the benefit of the doubt. To hear her sharing bad news was startling.

"What happened?" I asked, fearing what I would hear next.

She did not answer as Charlotte cautioned her to be careful because the crosswalk still had patches of ice. The walker slowed to a crawl as Louisa chose her footing carefully and conversation stopped until we reached clearer sidewalk on the other side of the street.

"While we were waiting for your plane Elena called and said that Mom doesn't remember anyone at all. She showed her family pictures in the living room, and she could not identify anyone - not even me," Louisa said, her voice trembling. "I want to call Mom when we get home. She needs to close the Security Bank checking account and have it transferred over to her primary bank. We may have to go there."

"That is really hard, isn't it... I mean, when Mom doesn't recognize you?" I asked rather rhetorically, not meaning to be insensitive, but relieved that my sister was finally experiencing firsthand the inexplicable emptiness of losing one's mother to this soul-robbing illness. Perhaps, she would now understand and forgive me for the persistent pressure I had placed on her to have Mother committed.

After lunch, Charlotte delivered us safely to their home in the countryside outside of Houston. I settled into Charlie's room, and after a quick freshening up, joined Louisa in her study downstairs. Louisa's face was in pain, but she was set on making two calls - one to Dr. Lucas's office, her ob-gyn, to ask for a Certificate of Incompetency and the other to Mom. Neither call went as hoped.

Dr. Lucas's nurse had always been responsive to Louisa's calls regarding Mother, who was one of their oldest and most challenging patients. Dr. Lucas and his staff were experts at dealing with pregnant young women and their myriad of physical and emotional needs. An octogenarian suffering from dementia pushed their medical skills to the limit. The head nurse had a soft spot for Mrs. Adams, though, and reached out to Louisa anytime she requested it. Louisa left a message and the return call was quick to come. She explained to the nurse that we desperately needed the doctor to sign a Certificate of Incompetency which had been faxed to their office earlier in the day before Louisa and Charlotte left the house for the airport. The nurse's reply was not what Louisa had hoped to hear and she began to explain, quite in vain, the need for the doctor to help us. The nurse apologetically held her ground and truly regretted that the doctor was not willing to put himself in the position of declaring someone incompetent. His specialty lay in bringing new life into the world, not in preventing its decline.

To our dismay, the nurse directed Louisa back to Dr. Forshey, the neurologist who refused to allow anyone in the examining room and declines not communicate with the family. Louisa slowly chose her words in expressing our dislike of the neurologist's methods and his subsequent inability - or outright unwillingness - to help our mother. I hastily jotted down a few words on a piece of paper and put it in front of Louisa who read it with a frown, but soon changed her expression to one of hope as she asked if Mom could be referred to a neuro-psychiatrist whom we had heard was effective in dealing with Waverly Place patients. Louisa was placed on hold for what seemed like eternity as we struggled to get over the disappointment.

"I can't really blame him, Louisa," I whispered as we waited. "He is an ob-gyn and dealing with forgetful old ladies is not his thing. He and his staff have really bent over backwards to help her with any strange symptom that she has presented, but they are not specialists in memory loss."

Louisa nodded her agreement as the nurse came back on the line. She listened intently and began taking notes before asking, "That is the earliest that Mom can be worked in? Six weeks from now?"

I was troubled that we had lost on the first front to declare Mother incompetent, but understanding the ob-gyn's position, was relieved to hear that he was more than willing to use his influence in the medical community to arrange an appointment with a doctor that could assess her situation and act on his findings.

"Thank you," I heard Louisa say. "That would be wonderful to be on the waiting list. That will be so helpful. I appreciate all that you are doing for us."

Louisa clicked off the phone, leaned back in her chair, and reached for a lollipop. Her hands were shaking as she tried to open it and soon handed it to me to slit with my fingernail. She leaned back and closed her eyes, sucking hard on the round knob of narcotic-laced medicine on the end. I let her rest and quietly continued the alphabetizing of files she had asked me to help her organize. Concentrating on whether Mother's hospital records should be filed under Hospital or Empire General, I was startled to hear Louisa saying hello to Elena.

"Can I talk to Mom?" she asked. "I need to give her instructions on closing a bank account and transferring the money.... Oh, really.... she is not having a good day.... well, could you please try.... the checking account only has enough in it for one more payment to you."

I turned my face away and hid it behind the folders containing Mother's EEG results. My face is far too expressive for me to hide my displeasure.

"Nora, this just infuriates me. Louisa absolutely does not get it. Weeks ago I had warned Louisa that the account would soon be depleted and that she had to convince Mom to move the funds over," the angst in my voice caused several nearby diners to turn their gaze in the direction of our table.

"Granted she is only a few weeks out of a major, major surgery, but I guess I really wasn't aware of how unwilling she is to act on things when it might mean falling out of someone's favor."

"Well...," Nora offered. "By procrastinating, it is also easier to avoid conflict and confrontation. She knows that your mother will not receive any of this news kindly."

She paused, and then continued with a pointed gentleness, "Your sister is hurting, both physically and emotionally. She may not have the energy to do what is required."

Giving her thoughts serious consideration, I admitted, "When I have a headache, the last thing I want to do is anything that requires effort, and certainly not anything that will get a strong reaction. You are right, of course, but we still cannot ignore what has to be done. She promises me that she will accomplish certain things and then... she lets me down."

"Does she let you down, or is it your mother she is letting down?" Nora gently asked, redirecting my misplaced feelings.

Turning red in the face, I laughed halfheartedly, "Louisa says I am too impatient. I maintain, however, that when dealing with doctors or attorneys, nothing is ever accomplished by those who just sit back and wait. Even when she feels well, my little sister just does not have the sense of urgency that gets results in time to avert a disaster."

"Was your mother able to transfer the funds and put money back into the account?"

"No, she was not able to do it on her own. Louisa called Mom to explain what needed to be done. I could see from her face that the conversation was not going well. Louisa talked to her like she was a four-year-old, which is pretty much how my phone calls with Mom have gone. Louisa looked at me and shook her head. She put her hand over the mouthpiece and mouthed that Mom didn't know who she was talking to."

Louisa kept talking in spite of the now evident fact that Mother had forgotten who she was. My sister moved through the step-by-step instructions she had rehearsed, advising Mother on how to close the account at one bank and move it over to another.

She explained in the simplest of terms on a very elementary level, but shook her head at Mother's detachment and distance. There was no recognition or excitement in her voice. She only said yes or no, and then they hung up without exchanging the usual rhetoric of "I love you and miss you."

"Nora, it was so sad. It tore Louisa apart to feel a terribly black void between them. There was nothing there, she said - just emptiness. She cried and cried, and I held her until she pulled away to get a tissue."

Nora and I sat in silence and finished chasing salad around our plates. There was really nothing more that Nora or I could say. It was the same song as before, just a different verse with my sister singing the words instead of me.

My dear friend finally took a deep breath, and smiling across the table, said, "It seems that time has taken the three of you a step further along your mother's journey. Alzheimer's is especially painful because it takes its time in emptying the mind. It is not a disease that happens suddenly, and every slow step she takes will seem like forever."

She leaned in close and her eyes conveyed as much as her words, "You and your sister need each other now more than ever, but the two of you are not alone in this. Remember all the friends and family that you both have. They are holding you close in their hearts and sending prayers for you to have wisdom, to be strong, and to hold fast to that love that is so much a part of your family."

With her gentle word, I let my mind relax a bit and reached into the depths of my heart and did, indeed, find strength to forgive my sister for her unwillingness to see the truth, and to, instead, love and support her as she climbed her way out of the darkness of denial. I had already made that climb and knew it to be steep and difficult.

Chapter 14

*A*s Louisa and I sat in her study that week sifting through the stacks of papers, we talked quietly and easily, as only sisters can. As different as we are in temperament and interests, we enjoy being together. Louisa has a refreshing way of turning the less perfect into a thing of beauty. Although annoying at times, she habitually praises and edifies everyone she meets. She always sees the good in someone, even if it means stretching the truth a bit.

As we waited for call from Elena with confirmation of their trip to Mother's bank, Louisa stopped shuffling papers back and forth across the desktop and swiveled her desk chair around to tell me that she was considered a shut-in by their church. The term struck me as odd because Louisa's age did not meet my definition of a shut-in, although everything else about her did. It was shocking to think of my younger sister in such a way, but the reality of it had escaped me until then. Once her back healed and the brace came off her body and the walker found a spot in the attic, the truth of the never-ending pain in her face and her reliance on drugs remained as unavoidable and irreconcilable facts.

With her eyes half closed, a lollipop dangling out of her mouth, and a medical statement suspended in mid-air between two stacks of documents, Louisa asked, "Where is Mom's soul right now? Does she still remember who God is?"

As her head began to lean back against the chair in sleep, I answered, "Her soul is resting right now, waiting for her body to pass and to let her soul go. God has not abandoned her. She is still His beloved child."

Louisa was asleep before I finished. I took the paper she still held suspended above the desk, and gently lowering her hand into her lap, prayed that she would awaken refreshed and free of pain, even if for a few hours.

The dogs kept me company while I slowly worked my way through the piles of papers. One sat quietly at my feet and followed my every movement from the piles to a folder and into the file drawer, while the other paced back and forth between the window - searching for squirrels to bark at - and the trashcan full of interesting smells like Scotch tape and liquid paper. The time was not wasted as it gave me an opportunity to read and ponder the two or more years of Mother's medical history since her dementia had become so obvious to us. I relived the four days at Empire General as she struggled to deal with all her medications, to the weeks following where pervasive paranoia set in prompting her to write one of the strangest wills her attorney's law firm had ever witnessed. The next few months were spent keeping up with Mother's frantic change from doctor to doctor in search of a physician who would treat her imagined ailments while ignoring the ever growing and real loss of cognitive skills. I shook my head in disbelief at the lengths she went to in order to remain independent and the efforts I had gone to in convincing my sister that our mother needed help and supervision.

Weary of sorting and filing papers, I glanced over at my sister as she slept in her chair next to the desk piled high with folders. Louisa was still very much in recovery from the surgery and needed help in the simplest of things, like reaching for a file in the filing cabinet and drying her hair after a shower. Emotionally, she was struggling with the new realization that her mother no longer knew her. I had walked over that bridge already and knew the loss she was feeling.

"It took my breath away to look at her. I just didn't know what else to say to ease her pain. There isn't enough air in the world to express the heaviness of being shunned by the person who gave you life. It's like her very being was deflated," I said and shuddered slightly, as if from a sudden chill. "Louisa needed me, and I could not leave her. So, I asked my boss for the rest of the week off and took Family and Medical Leave to help her continue to recuperate from surgery and to prepare for taking over Mother's affairs."

"Tom supported you in that decision?" Nora asked.

She had shown such concern, not just for me, but for everyone with whose life mine meshed.

"He is a very understanding and compassionate person. Not all wives can say that about their husbands. How did he fare with you being gone?"

"It's interesting that you ask that," I noted. "In his family, the elderly relatives were brought into the family to live out their days. They weren't sent to long-term care facilities. Tom saw three of his grandparents age in various ways and has taken all this in a very matter-of-fact fashion; whereas my family becomes so emotional that we short-circuit our ability to deal with the situation. He has been so incredibly good for me and has taught me how to balance my emotions with the reality of Mom's illness and to do the same with the added dimension of my sister's incapacity. His guidance, and yours, have been important in helping me be patient with Louisa. Now that I am here with her, I see how conflicted she is. Louisa is handicapped by more than just physical issues. She continues to struggle with the idea that something is seriously wrong with Mom."

"Overcoming denial of an illness is the first step toward a healthy life, not just for your mother, but for her family, as well," was Nora's wise comment, spoken from the heart of someone who knew.

Nora's words never fell on deaf ears. I was grateful for any comfort she could offer for I realized it was honed in the fires of personal pain and loss. She continued to listen intently to the recounting of the visit with my sister.

Louisa stirred and awoke in pain and headed straightway for her medicine cabinet. I knew we would only have about twenty minutes before the drugs kicked in and she would become loopy again. I was torn between the necessity to discuss Mother's dwindling funds and the desire to pass the time happily reminiscing about when her kids were little. The choice was made for me when Louisa wheeled the walker back into the study bent on looking over the online bank account to see if the funds had been transferred, yet. They had not, and we sat there studying each other trying to determine the next course of action.

We had become experts at making suppositions and creating

all manner of scenarios to explain our parent's action or the lack thereof. In light of her noncommittal response to Louisa's instructions on how to close the one bank account and shift the funds over into another, we doubted that the transfer would actually take place. Louisa put in a quick call to Elena to review what needed to happen and to stress the fact that Mother only had enough money in her checking account to cover Elena's fees for one more week and that, in turn, meant making a late payment to Waverly Place.

"Sometimes we aren't quite sure if the message has been received because of Elena's accent or the poor reception on her cell phone," I explained to Nora. "It seems that something did happen to prevent the money from being transferred, but it was not because of a lack of communication with Elena. Mom did not understand what Louisa asked her to do and was convinced that her daughter had asked her to give the caregiver all of the money in her checking account."

"Oh, the poor dear," Nora exclaimed. "She must have been terribly confused."

"Well, she was. Believing that everyone was bent on stealing her money, she flatly refused to go to the bank for any reason; and Elena, even with her patient and caring way, could not convince her that going to the bank was absolutely necessary. Louisa and I checked the online banking every few hours throughout the rest of the day until we realized that the cutoff time for deposits had come and gone. We needed a Plan B, but without the legal power to access any of Mom's other accounts, the reality of the situation finally hit Louisa."

Nora and I were seated on stools at the high top counter, elbow to elbow, as I described the week with Louisa. The sandwich shop was fuller than usual and we could not find sanctuary in our usual spot among the high backed upholstered booths. Speaking within earshot of other diners, I felt exposed and somewhat uncomfortable, until I realized that they were just as absorbed in their own conversations about their child's ear infections and getting the car detailed. I relaxed a bit and concentrated on talking between sips of tomato basil soup.

"We truly did not know what else to do," I sighed. "By now

you realize that Louisa really struggles to keep up. Her mind is in such a fog the majority of the time that she has great difficulty focusing on a task until it is completed. Trying to manage the financial affairs of someone with dementia is truly more than Louisa can handle. She takes her task very seriously, but is in much the same situation as Mom."

Nora glanced sideways at me and asked, "What do you plan to do?"

"By the good grace of God, Elena talked Mom into going to the bank the next day. She apparently told her that whatever Louisa had asked her to do was the right thing and she needed to do it 'to protect her money.' Then Elena pulled out that old threat – 'If we don't go to the bank this afternoon, we will have to call Allison.'"

Nora and I burst out laughing at the image of my mother's reaction to this imaginary threat. Whatever misconstrued idea Mother had in her head about my intentions towards her continued to be a powerful motivator, and Elena had played that card well.

"And it worked," I cried out. "I suppose that school teacher image with the ruler in my hand will always be in Mom's head. She is afraid of me because she knows that I am capable of bringing about changes in her life that she is not ready to accept."

I stopped breathing for a moment, and looking far into the distance, said, "I don't think she will ever be ready to accept the changes that are surely in the near future."

Repositioning my purse in my lap so it would not slip onto the floor, I continued, "Louisa and I waited all the next day for an indication that the money had been moved, until very late in the day, the magic words 'deposit pending' appeared on the screen. Elena called later in the evening to say that they went to the bank where Mrs. Adams promptly told the clerk that she wanted to take all of her money and give it to her daughter Louisa, pointing to the Latin woman beside her as she said this. Elena quickly jumped in to clarify the request and told her that she was *not* Louisa, that the account was to be closed, and the money transferred into Mrs. Adams' account at another bank. Mom never understood that the funds were still hers and just stood dumbfounded while the bank authorities grilled her caregiver. Elena was asked to present a photo ID before they fingerprinted her and took her picture."

Louisa and I relaxed a bit after seeing a fresh replenishment of funds clear through the bank the following day. A silent understanding passed between the two of us that Mother would never again be able to complete a financial transaction, and that we had truly entered that stage where obtaining legal access to all of her financial dealings was an undeniable necessity.

We then turned our attention to filing for guardianship and moving Mother into the Johnston Center, the very place that she had chosen to be when the time came – and that time was now upon her.

"Nora, it's so sad to think that Mom chose the Johnston Center, but doesn't want to even look at the people in the beauty shop and the hallways who will soon become her neighbors."

The sorting, stacking, alphabetizing, and filing of all Louisa's papers had been a valuable exercise. Not only would she be able to quickly locate a document or notes on any subject relating to our mother, but I had verified that we, indeed, did not have the originals of the Durable Power of Attorney nor the Medical Power of Attorney. However, among the assortment of handwritten and typed notes there was a letter written two years prior to her "Family, Friends, Physicians, Church, and Waverly Place" in which she reiterated how productive and independent her life was – none of which was true even at that point – and that Waverly Place was her home and it could provide her with any kind of care that she might need in the future. She had no intention of leaving Waverly Place.

Louisa and I marveled that just two years earlier she wanted to be in whatever level of care was most appropriate, but now, well into dementia, staunchly denied that she wanted to be anywhere other than her cottage – a complete turnaround from her original intention when she moved into the senior community. It was sad to note that the diminishment of her mind had skewed her perception of the very place she had chosen to be for the remainder of her days. Mother had no idea of the burden she had brought upon her family in her struggle to deny proper care and appropriate housing. I could only shake my head in frustration at our efforts to care for someone who refused to be cared for.

Charlotte thought her grandmother's reversal of thought very strange, as well. One evening after work she curled her long legs under her on the sofa beside me for a chat. I had some of Grandmother's writings in my hands and it appeared to Char that I had been crying, which I had. I read her a line in a letter addressed to her brother Charlie, "Allison has been civil to me lately. I hope that lasts."

Char let out a little guffaw and exclaimed that Grandmother was crazy for choosing her brother as the executor of her new will. Charlotte could not understand why, as the eldest grandchild, Grandmother had passed her over and given that duty to the youngest member of the family. We talked for a long time, sharing how painful it was to hear slanderous comments coming from someone we loved and thought loved us. I understood her dismay and assured her that Grandmother truly did not know what she was doing. We shared a supportive hug which somehow took away part of the hurt.

"Why does one person's illness have to affect the whole family?" Charlotte asked rhetorically as we each went to dress for dinner, feeling somewhat better knowing that we were not alone in our sadness. I suspected that she was not just asking about Grandmother, but included her mother in the question.

"Louisa's progress that week was very slow. One morning when I came downstairs for a bowl of cereal, Matt had not left for his iron works shop," I told Nora as we eyed the dessert menu. "This was really unusual as he was always up and out of the house by six a.m. He has a deep love for working in his shop and takes all the tasks of overseeing his team of craftsmen very seriously. He creates some gorgeous gates and garden benches. Tom and I dream of someday having his handiwork in our house in Massachusetts."

Nora's eyes brightened, "He must be very good."

"He is. His work ethic is very high, and that is what surprised me so much when I found him still sitting in his recliner drinking a cup of coffee. He was waiting for me to get up and come downstairs before he left because Louisa had fallen in the shower and hit her head."

I cringed a bit as I explained that she had managed to get her brace on, but then slipped on the tile floor and landed flat on her back, cracking her head against the hard surface. Miraculously, other than a few bruises, her back seemed to be unaffected by the fall. It was firmly supported by four twenty-one inch steel rods screwed into each of her vertebrae and crossed at the top and bottom with T-bars attached to the hip bones and cervical collar.

Her head was another matter. Matt was shaken by the fact that she had hit the floor so hard that she nearly lost consciousness and was speaking in garbled sentences. He was over a foot taller than my sister and easily picked her up from the floor as if she was a pillow. Matt had a muscular build, and Louisa's eyes smiled with admiration every time she saw him coming across the lawn or in the door. They adored each other, and Louisa's pride in her husband was matched by his concern for her welfare and safety. After her fall that morning, he toyed with the idea of staying home, but I assured him that I would keep a close eye on her, and he reluctantly backed his diesel F-350 out of the garage after promising to be home early. I moved my reading into the easy chair in their bedroom and listened to Louisa's rattled breathing through slack jaws. Unable to concentrate on my book, I sat and watched my only sibling, softly speaking a prayer that someday she would know what it is like to be free of pain.

Missing my husband very much at that moment, I dialed his number at work, hoping he was not in a meeting. He must have heard the sadness in my voice and silently listened as I told him how our day had begun. Tom is a fixer by nature. Some things, though, cannot be fixed, and my sister's illness is one of those things. Nevertheless, after several minutes Tom sensed a lull in the recitation and jumped in with a flurry of questions.

"Why did she slip? What was she wearing on her feet? Why wasn't someone with her holding her up? Are her eyes dilated? Can she raise both arms evenly? Is her speech still garbled? Why doesn't Matt want to call the doctor or take her to the emergency room?"

For every question I had an answer, generally not an acceptable one, which then brought on a flurry of new questions. We volleyed back and forth for a while until I tired of thinking and begged him just to offer me encouragement, which he did with a gentleness that comes from a caring soul. Tom's soul is old, loving, and true. He has a depth that is surprising and an exceptional thirst for knowledge. We have traveled together through more joys than disappointments, reached for new adventures while fully exhausting old ones, and have now entered the sad chapter of a parent who is not aging well. Experienced with elderly grandparents, Tom provides the plumb line against which I can measure events along my mother's journey.

Nora chuckled at the image of Tom the Fixer. She knew him well from his work as head usher at the church. He jumped in with both feet and picked up the disorganized pieces of well-intentioned volunteers and turned them into a well-oiled machine of hospitality and efficiency, guiding worshipers to their seats, ringing the church bell at precisely half past the hour, and providing emergency aid for the occasional member who had passed out in their pew, fallen down the church steps, or run their car into a sign post. Nora's husband, Mark, was also an usher and gave her firsthand accounts of Tom's heroics while Nora and I, blissfully unaware of all these events, sang our high notes in the choir loft.

"Unfortunately," Nora wistfully began. "Alzheimer's is not something that can be fixed. With baby boomers like you and me, it will be a common occurrence among our own generation, as well. We are only a decade or so away from any first signs of the early onset type of the disease."

Conversation stopped as our number was announced and we picked up our desserts at the pastry counter and climbed back on to the stools, cradling bowls of chocolate mousse layered over ladyfingers drizzled with chocolate syrup.

"Well, if we keep eating like this, we won't make it to that age," I laughed as we dug in.

For the next few minutes we precariously perched atop the stools and turned our full attention to the decadence of the chocolate desserts before us. Whether because of the laughter or the chocolate or both, the conversation seemed easier as we licked the spoons and ordered the usual cups of coffee and tea.

"There was nothing more for me to do at Louisa's than to help her finish out the week. Her strength had improved slightly and every day we noticed small improvements in her mobility and flexibility. We came to the end of any further actions that we could accomplish on Mom's behalf, and with the weekend before us, we decided to call a Mom-free evening and just enjoy each other's company before I flew home the next day. "

Nora, always quick to point out the positive, summed up the week.

"It sounds like your visit was very special and that you spent precious time with you sister and her family. You accomplished so much for your mother – or at least, it seems that you know what you need to do next. Was Tom glad to see you?"

I smiled as I recalled him standing at the top of the escalator above baggage claim, with a single red rose in his hand anxiously awaiting my return. "I know I looked tired, Nora, but you should have seen the grin on his face."

The conversation with Nora ended happier than it had begun with a promise to get together again in a week, unless something happened sooner and I once again needed the support of my good friend.

Mother's bizarre behavior continued on its unpredictable course with ever-increasing speed. Perhaps in her effort to clear out the house in preparation of "moving back home," she removed all the paintings from the walls and placed them under her bed for safekeeping, except for one. This particular piece was of the Painted Rock Scout Ranch, which my father had been so instrumental in developing into a world-class experience where boys could come from all over the country to backpack the rugged terrain. "This painting is *mine*," and she placed the fourteen by sixteen-inch painting with its ornate wooden frame under her pillow. I just shook my head as Elena described how she had tried to convince Mrs. Adams that the newest pain in her neck and back was due to the sharp edges of the frame, but she insisted on keeping it under the pillow where no one would find it and steal it from her.

Alzheimer's had been stealing Mother's memories for some time, however, and the one heirloom picture that she should have saved above all others was haphazardly thrown into a box bound for the church garage sale. "They can get something for the frame," she declared, completely failing to realize that the photograph was of her husband as a baby. The file folder label affixed to the frame identifying the baby as Charles Herbert Adams, born February 12,

1927, did not clear the fog from her mind. The family heirloom had no meaning for her.

Elena spied the photograph in the garage sale pile, and wrapping it in sheets and a towel, hurriedly hid it in her car. The picture was the one item in the house that I truly wished to have and had expressed that to Mother on previous visits there. Whether out of spite or from a failed memory, she did not honor my request. The next day Elena packed up the picture and shipped it to me. I now look on the picture of my father with a heightened appreciation, not just because of who he was, but because of the manner in which I had come to possess the picture.

"I don't think I have the desire to call my mother anymore," was my sad revelation to Nora during our dinner the following week. "There were a few brief months where a glimmer of recognition was in her voice when I called. At the time, I had much more of a need to talk to her than certainly she had a need to talk to me. Mom has not initiated a call to me in months. I think I told you that she missed my birthday."

I looked up at Nora with slightly moist eyes.

"Crossing those bridges is so difficult isn't it?" she replied gently. "Think of the bridges as a means for continuing. Her life goes on and so must you. This is not the end, but just a passageway to the next part of her life."

Nora's words always seemed to focus on the very thing I needed to hear, and I smiled and thanked her for her refreshing way of looking at things. It was ironic that crossing bridges was not something which Mother did easily. Like elevators and escalators, anything which transported her to another place was eschewed. Mother fought every inch of the way and created her own obstacles. If one must grow old, one should at least try to be a lady about it. After a recent acting out episode in a local pharmacy, Louisa observed that "Mom knows how to organize her dying, but she doesn't know how to organize her living."

"One of the letters in Louisa's files was from Mom to Charlie," I chuckled as I told Nora about the contents of the letter which Mom had instructed to be placed in the safe deposit box. "She told him that, upon her death, he should clean out both of her refrigerators and divide the food evenly among the family members, and to be sure and purchase Styrofoam ice chests ahead of time."

Nora's delicate face broke out in a grin. She had never met my mother, but had a keen understanding of the generation that had lived through the Depression. I doubt that either Nora or I had ever gone a day when we were hungry or found ourselves without clothes or a home or a job, should we want one. Our minds could not easily comprehend the value placed on every morsel of food, even to the point of wanting to save the leftovers at one's own wake.

"Heloise and my mom were best friends, Nora. On more than one Christmas I received the latest book written by the housekeeping queen. I can still picture Mom sitting in her rocking chair next to Dad's in the evenings reading through *100 Ways to Pickle Anything*. Did I tell you that Mom was so thrifty that she invariably offered to bring a frozen turkey to whichever daughter's house was hosting Thanksgiving or Christmas? One year she even seriously contemplated how to pack the turkey in her suitcase so that it would not drip all over her clothes. Mom pointed out that it would be nice and thawed out by the time her plane arrived."

Nora was laughing so hard she could barely catch her breath. Our laughter suddenly abated, however, as Nora and I returned to the gravity of the situation.

"Things are different now, Nora. Mom's world is now very, very small and she is afraid of almost everything, including the doorbell. The sound of it sends her into near hysteria. Elena says that she begins to tremble and look toward the door with fear on her face," my heart was heavy as I described the intenseness of her paranoia.

"She is afraid to eat for fear that she will be poisoned. One day last week one of the aides made banana pudding. Mother told her it looked really good, but refused to eat it. As soon as Elena arrived the next morning, Mom led her to the refrigerator, exclaiming how good the pudding looked. Elena asked her why she had not had some to eat and Mom told her, 'I have already had breakfast, but you can have some,' so she did as she was bid and ate some of the dessert. For the next hour Mom kept checking on Elena to see if she was short of breath, or dizzy, or sick at her stomach."

"Oh, dear, she wanted to see if Elena had been poisoned," Nora conjectured.

"Yes, and Mom loves banana pudding. Elena said that she won't even take a drink from a juice glass unless Elena has tasted it first," I explained.

Perhaps by the power of mere suggestion, my dinner no longer seemed appetizing and I boxed it up to go home with me. Our conversation continued for another half hour as Nora expressed her concern over where Louisa and I should go from there. We had convinced the ob-gyn to make an appointment for her with the only other adult neurologist in town, which was a major advancement in our year-long struggle to enlist the professional assistance of a specialist who could be the turning point in Mother's care and living arrangements.

"Is there anything you can do that would be helpful to your mother, to your sister, or for yourself, while you wait for the appointment with the neuropsychiatrist?" my friend asked. "That must be terribly difficult to be patient when you know your mother needs help right now."

The wait was, indeed, difficult. Every day brought more reports of Mother packing her clothes in little bags to go on an imagined camping trip; or of her insistence that the caregivers are lazy and that they must sit next to her bed and watch her sleep; or listening to tales about her husband designing and building Waverly Place. I am certain that the last story is a confabulation, a cross between Dad having developed the Scout camp and Mother's residency at Waverly Place.

On days when her neighbor comes to visit, things are particularly difficult. Imelda opens the door and walks right into the living room without so much as an invitation or welcome. She shuttles Mother back into her bedroom where they talk in hushed voices for extended periods of time. For some curious reason, the caregivers are not able to hear the conversation over the room monitor, but when they emerge, Mother seems more determined than ever to issue orders to the ladies, even going so far as expressing a desire to fire all of them for being so lazy. My consternation over Imelda's visits could not be missed in talking over the unwelcome intrusions with Elena. How she could simply walk in through the front door revealed the fact that they were not keeping the door locked.

"Well, lock it," I implored. "When she knocks on the glass door tell her Mrs. Adams is not receiving visitors today and close the main door. I thought we were limiting her visitors to Sylvia, Judy, and the pastor."

Elena could not have overlooked the annoyance in my voice. I was finding long-distance caregiving to be taxing, and as much as I admired and needed Elena, wished that Mother lived closer to us. The physical distance between us made me heartsick. Elena told me that the last time Sylvia came to visit she brought a bouquet of flowers for the table. A few minutes into the visit Mother asked Sylvia what she thought of the beautiful flowers that her husband had given her. Elena tried to tell Mrs. Adams that it was her friend who had brought the flowers. Mother heatedly told her to mind her own business and insisted that Sylvia was not her friend, but a cousin, and that her husband had, in fact, brought the flowers. Sylvia soon left, hiding tears over the friend she was losing.

My annoyance with Elena melted away as she also described visits from Judy, which had become very abbreviated. Perhaps, like Sylvia, Judy found it too painful to see her lovely friend fading away into the shadows.

Mother's pastor, Art, also came to call, always with two other female parishioners in tow. He wisely told me when she began this journey that he does not visit females in his congregation without other women in the room. Elena said that his visits did not go terribly well, as Mrs. Adams would become overwhelmed and confused by too much chatter in the room. It was observed that she would often just stand up, with a great deal of assistance, and then wheel herself on the walker to bed, without so much as a goodbye or a thank you for coming. I promised to call Art and let him know where we were in the process of finding appropriate care and housing for Mother. I trusted him, and she needed his prayers.

Normal every day activities that most people perform without much thought were becoming fewer and fewer in her new world. Once very diligent in keeping several to-do lists next to the kitchen phone, she no longer planned out her activities, probably because inventorying the pantry is now well beyond her abilities and ordering her thoughts enough to put them on paper is but a fleeting moment in time. A list maker for as many years as I could think back, it seemed odd that little scraps of paper no longer lay on the kitchen counter. Elena makes the lists now and keeps them in her head.

A few months ago, going to the grocery store and the pharmacy were big events for the two of them. However, treks out to the department story, going for groceries or to pick up prescriptions have fallen off the radar as the experience is overwhelming for Mother. Elena finds it easier to do the shopping on her own and quickly rounds up all the needed food and supplies, avoiding public arguments with Mrs. Adams at the checkout. The credit card balance increased by several hundreds of dollars whenever Mother won the argument and Elena gave in to the random piling of things into the grocery cart. This pattern continued for several weeks before Elena just stopped taking her along. Mother's world instantly became smaller.

"Nora, it is so sad. The only time Mom gets out of the house is to go to the beauty shop or the doctor," was the statement I led with as we sat deciding whether to have soup, sandwiches, or both. "The things we can talk about on the phone are so limited. I feel like I am losing what little connection I had with Mom. We used to talk about the price of cantaloupes and whether West Texas cantaloupes were sweeter than those from Arizona. It is a good day now if she can describe what she is wearing."

The conversation paused because Nora sensed I was still working something out in my mind. Breaking out of our usual soup and sandwich routine, we each ordered pasta before I picked up the threads of my thought.

"It's troubling now to hear Mom struggle so much with words," I softly explained, more to myself than to Nora. "It is troublesome to wait while she gathers her thoughts to form sentences with words she can no longer remember. I know she gets frustrated because of the nonsensical things she comes up with and I feel as if my calls are...."

My voice trailed off as the realization hit me that Mom and I were losing the last delicate thread that connected us across the miles.

"It would be different if you were there, Allison," Nora reassured me. "You would be able to just sit beside her and hold her hand even though she can't express herself."

"But, I am not there," I was quick to point out, speaking with a tinge of anger, not at Nora, but at the ugliness of the disease that once again was crowding in on my relationship with my mother.

Nora let my anger simmer for a moment before saying, "Then go. Go see your mother."

Her words were simple, but there were many things holding me back, not the least of which was the cost. How often would I need to be away now that Mother needed my physical presence more than ever? Having worked for the music publisher only a few years, my vacation time was precious and every absence from work was already planned. As a schoolteacher many years ago I enjoyed long winter and spring breaks, as well as three months off in the summertime. However, with the change in careers, my vacation days were very few in comparison, and the extra days I stayed on with Louisa had depleted my vacation days down to but a few hours. I felt ashamed that money was coming before family, but like many who were struggling with the recession, Tom and I did not have many dollars to spare. I filed for unpaid leave and found some solace in the fact that my boss did not even give it a second thought. He supported my need to be with my mother."

The tone in my words began to tighten.

"Taking an unpaid leave right now puts a burden on us. I am having a difficult time accepting that we have to bear the burden of Mom's financial mistakes and my sister's lack of action. Mom's accessible money will be depleted in a matter of days and I can't impress upon my sister the seriousness of that fact..."

My anger and frustration continued to well up, and Nora chose not to interrupt as I worked it out in a rambling torrent of thoughts. I silently thanked her for knowing when to speak and when to listen. I consider listening to be a virtue even though faith, hope and love are the most widely thought of virtues, all three of which require listening, not just with one's ears, but demand the heart's full attention. Nora listens with every ounce of her heart and is not afraid to tell me when I should steer my course back to faith, hope and love.

This was one of those times. I was angry at the recession; angry at Mother; angry at Louisa; and most of all, angry at Alzheimer's. My pasta was thoroughly tossed when I finished talking, as my hand had not stopped running the fork around the plate, arranging and rearranging the chicken and sundried tomatoes. In some very small way, the physical activity helped to diffuse the heat of the moment, and I was able to gain enough control to stop and catch a cleansing breath before finally putting the fork down.

Nora just smiled and said, "You have every right to be hurt."

I relaxed a bit and smiled to myself as she began the intuitive process of justifying my emotions, placing them in their correct context, and redirecting my thoughts into a more positive vein. In spite of the fact that I knew exactly what she was doing, it was still comforting and certainly more constructive and healthy than continuing to seethe about a situation that never seemed to have an easy solution.

She continued, "Do you know, yet, how much it will cost to file a petition for guardianship? I assume that is what you and Louisa have decided to do…"

"It seems that at this point a guardianship is the only action that makes sense. Going the power of attorney route still gives Mom full control of her medical and financial decisions," I said with conviction. "The first step toward guardianship is to acquire a physician's certificate of incompetency."

"And, how is that progressing?"

"As you know, neither her ob-gyn nor her current neurologist is willing to do this, so we have an appointment with a neuro-psychiatrist for a few weeks from now. Elena has agreed to take her,… but, you know, Nora," I stopped as a lump was starting to form in my throat.

Forcing the lump aside, straightening my back, and squarely meeting Nora's eyes, I spoke with resolve and determination.

"Mom needs her family to be there with her. This is not a time to sit back and let someone else take responsibility for her healthcare. True, in the past she has slammed the door on my participation in her life, but this appointment is much too important to give in to Mom's tantrums."

We talked for a long time about my mother's reluctance to include me in her life, as well as Louisa's diminished physical and mental capacity to handle Mother's unpredictable behavior. I left the restaurant with a new resolve to go to San Angelo, with or without my sister.

Louisa was strongly against my proposed trip. She agreed that this was a transitional time for Mother and that family needed to be with her - but just not me. I was dumbfounded. What other family was there? Louisa was not in physical condition to travel alone so soon after major surgery and there was no other family but the two of us who could legally act on Mother's behalf. There was something about the hesitancy in Louisa's voice that told me she was not telling me everything.

"I'm hoping that Charlie can get off from school for a few days and go with me. I think Mom will react better if he is along," she said.

I took a very long and deep breath before answering, "No, Louisa. Not this time. Going with Mom to see a psychiatrist that has the medical knowledge to examine and declare her incompetent is our responsibility – not Charlie's. We are her children and it is our responsibility to help her through this and see that she is cared for properly. He does not have the skills or the knowledge to make that happen. Mom is not ever going to react favorably to being moved out of her cottage. Charlie's presence will make absolutely no difference in her fear of going to the Big House."

Louisa is the younger of the two of us, but I usually let her take the lead because...well, it's just easier that way. I am amused to recall that my aunts said the exact same thing about my mother – it's just easier that way. Matt and her children would agree wholeheartedly on that fact, as well. I had spent the last two years finding ways to preserve Louisa's sense of control when there was little else she could control in her pain-ridden life; to maintain our mother's dignity without taking away control of her own life; and to protect them both from themselves. We could play those games no longer.

"I am going for Mom's appointment at the end of this

month. You can go with me if you feel up to it," I told Louisa, the tone in my voice left no room for negotiation.

The line between us buzzed with white noise, but was silent otherwise.

"But... you see, 'Allie," Louisa began very hesitantly. "Mom has put a restraining order against you."

"She did *what*?"

"It's legal and everything. She had a restraining order filed against you, and you can't get in to see her," Louisa repeated.

My breath suddenly left me body, and I felt nothing but empty space where my heart should have been. The surroundings of my office dissolved in front of my unseeing eyes. I could only sense the hot moistness of the earpiece against my head.

"That is the first time I have heard that," I said in a very unsteady and halting voice.

As the emptiness grew deeper it became impossible to talk, and I closed the cell phone abruptly ending the call, and rising from the chair at my desk, I found my way into an empty conference room down the hall. The waves of emotion rolled over me, and under me, and through me.

"Mother, what have I done that would cause you to do this?"

I didn't care if my co-workers could hear me scream.

"How can you cease to love the one you cradled in your arms?"

Grief enveloped me and, like a child, I rocked back and forth as waves of hurt and disbelief poured out leaving me gasping for breath.

"Will you ever let me hear your voice or hold you again?"

There was no answer - only the sound of my own cries. The smiling faces of men and women in business suits looked back at me from the walls, searching for understanding of my pain. I leaned back into the webbing of the chair and let the stillness of the room slowly calm my sorrow before getting up and returning to my desk. I wiped any remnants of despair from my face and gradually began to feel in control again.

"Louisa, I am sorry I hung up on you. It just took me by such surprise," I said upon calling my sister back.

"I thought you knew that she had done that," Louisa replied. "Don't you remember when she went over to see Deborah

Barnes and had you removed from all the documents?"

"But, Louisa, that is very different than filing a restraining order," I began. "A restraining order is so final. I can't believe that she never wants to see me again. That just hurts so much."

My throat became crowded again.

"She didn't say she never wants to see you again," Louisa protested.

"That's what a restraining order is," I cried out, about to lose my patience and not in the mood to argue over Mother's misconstrued actions.

"Oh, Allison, I am so sorry. That is not what I meant. No, she didn't file a restraining order. She just had Deborah remove your name from any contact with the Waverly Place office and from getting past the guard gate. I chose the wrong words. I am so sorry," Louisa said over and over. "You know me – I have trouble with the right words these days."

Louisa had become very much like Mother, who could not find the right words because dementia had stolen them away from her. Louisa could not find the right words because medications clouded her mind. Matt privately told me during my week's stay with them that his wife was becoming more and more like his mother-in-law every day that she is on the painkillers. He hated the narcotic lollipops and what they had done to her.

A sudden rush of relief came over me, and rather than chastise my sister as she struggled to find the right words, I found it easy to forgive her. The bite of Mother's actions was still raw, however, and she had done what in her mind was in fact tantamount to a restraining order. Although her requests at the administration office carried no legal weight, she believed she was safe from whatever imagined threat I could pose. The more Louisa and I discussed it, the more I understood that my little sister was wary, as well. She feared Mother's reaction upon seeing the daughter that might have the strength to move her out of the cottage.

Louisa had one foot in reality and one foot still in the doorway of uncertainty. I sensed that she had many questions about taking control of Mother's future, as if it violated her and left Mother impotent to make decisions for herself, little realizing that

Mother had long ago crossed the point where she could even distinguish one moment from another.

Louisa was a staunch believer in the dignity of every individual - particularly that of the parent she loved so dearly. She and Mother had always been close, and Louisa firmly defended her against any and all criticism – except for comments regarding her cooking. They shared a bond made strong by the fact that they had both borne and raised children, had been active as leaders in the community, and had suffered so greatly the loss of my father. Louisa's persistently positive outlook on life balanced Mother's need for attention, and she readily responded to Louisa's never-ending showers of praise and encouragement.

"Mom has really done remarkably well, Allison," she would say to me should I point out one of Mother's bookkeeping errors. "When Dad died, she had no knowledge of their finances before she was forced into taking over all of their investments. She has also tried her best to understand the medical insurance issues. I am very proud of her for what she has been able to accomplish."

Louisa's praise of Mother did not fall on deaf ears, but her defense of Mother even in the face of blatant errors and misjudged steps, was wearing thin on me.

"Did I tell you that Mom canceled her major medical insurance?" I asked Nora. We were talking on the phone one evening when a late spring snowfall had prevented us from meeting face-to-face.

I heard a gasp on the other end of the line and described how the recent change in retirees' major medical insurance required Mother to complete a new application form and signify her choices in coverage. Louisa completed the form for her, but the insurance carrier needed to speak directly to the insured to verify the choices. The call came in and Elena, having been prepared and prompted by Louisa as to what Mother needed to do, handed the phone to Mrs. Adams. She answered all the pertinent questions, but stopped the agent in the middle of the explanation of benefits to ask, "Will this cost me anything?" Of course, the answer was yes, for there are premiums to pay – to which Mother promptly replied, "I don't want it then." The agent ended the call, completely unaware that she had been talking to an individual suffering from dementia who did not know the difference between an insurance premium and a Premium cracker.

"Dear soul," Nora sighed. "She cannot be faulted for being frugal, but she really is her own worst enemy."

I wholeheartedly agreed and explained that Louisa was miraculously able to reinstate Mother's insurance, and at the same time convinced the agent to skip the verbal authorization. In retrospect, it seemed that we were always reacting to something Mother has done, rather than taking a proactive stance to protect her. It was my heartfelt opinion that we had to take bold steps in advance of whatever new escapades she might present to us.

"Louisa does not want me to go to San Angelo, Nora," I said somewhat wearily. "I am going, though, with or without her blessing. My mother needs at least one of her daughters next to her when the psychiatrist asks her questions to which she will not know the answers. She will be lost and confused, and I cannot let her go through that alone. I want to hold her hand as the doctor pushes her to recall long forgotten details of her life."

And then Nora asked the question that had been hanging in the air, "What if she will not allow you to come into his office? What will you do then?"

"I will sit in the reception area and pray that he sees a demented elderly mother in need of her daughter," was my quiet and simple reply.

"My prayer will be the same."

It became a struggle of will to convince Louisa that, contrary to Mother's wishes or not, I would be there on the appointment date. However, my sister's staunch desire was to be there with her son, whom she deemed to be the one person that Mother would follow anywhere.

"No, Louisa," I said firmly. "Mom's daughters need to be there. Not the executor of her will, but her daughters. Charles only has authority to act upon Mom's death. We have authority by our birthright to act upon her living. This visit is crucial in preparing her for the end of her life. *We must be there.*"

Louisa and I were typical siblings growing up side by side in a middle class home with two adoring parents who carefully watched over our every step until we were young adults on our own. Other than the relationship we shared with our mother and two aunts, our sisterhood was the longest relationship either of us had known. I loved my sister dearly, but as adults we rarely lived in close proximity to one another and actually preferred the distance between us because we still desired to lead very independent and self-sufficient lives, traits we probably inherited from our mother.

We are alike in many ways, but also had traits distinctively our own. Louisa is blonde and blue eyed; I am a brunette with brown eyes. She is slender; I am round. Dad always said Louisa played the piano better than I, in spite of the fact that I was the music major. Perhaps, that is why I switched to the pipe organ. Louisa is a people person; I am task oriented. While I am the more critical, she is the more optimistic and positive. I am impatient and Louisa is content to sit back and wait for time to weave its spell.

We shared much that only sisters would understand, and yet I am unable to take away the burdens she now bears. It is difficult for me to discern whether to offer to take the load of Mother's illness, or to push Louisa to stay awake long enough to fill out another form and to make another phone call. At this moment, Mother's needs outweighed those of my sister, and so I pushed Louisa to the point of tears. Although I felt badly that she was so reticent, it was the right thing to do.

"I am going and will arrange to get to Mom's house just before she has to go to the appointment," was my plan. "She won't have time to sit and think about why I am there. We will just get up and go, and I'm hoping that in the confusion, she will allow Elena to just lead her willingly to the car."

"But, you don't even know if the doctor will allow you in with her," Louisa protested. "Mom may put her foot down, and with all the privacy rules, you might go all that way and be turned away…"

Louisa continued giving argument after argument to curtail my travel plans, each of which I countered with the same quiet, yet firm response, "Nothing is certain with Alzheimer's. I must try."

My stubbornness and unwillingness to budge on my conviction eventually prevailed and pressed Louisa to acquiesce, and together we made plans to go to San Angelo, unsure of whether

Mother would recognize and welcome us, or if we would be facing the rage of a woman who would fight us with every ounce of her being.

Chapter 15

The plane touched down smoothly on the short runway and quickly taxied to one of four gates, a fact about which the little regional airport boasted. The sun was burning through the expansive sky unimpeded by trees or hills or anything else on the windswept plains. The air smelled gritty as the plane was depressurized and fresh air flooded the cabin. We were among the first to deplane and an attendant quickly settled Louisa into a waiting wheelchair and rolled her up the causeway, into the elevator and over to the first baggage carousel while I raced for the rental car desk. Our plane had been delayed due to thunderstorms, leaving us with only a few precious minutes before Elena would be loading her elderly charge into the car for the ten-minute ride to the psychiatrist. I quipped to Louisa that I would need the psychiatrist if we did not make it there in time. The rental desk dealt quickly with three gold members who had pushed ahead of me in the line, and finally turning to me, was irritatingly thorough in asking all the necessary questions regarding insurance waivers, upgrades, and if the car would be returned to a different location – all questions I had already answered when making the reservation online. It was soon apparent, however, that the reservations agent was not to be dissuaded from repeating the questions and I gave my answers with lightening speed after which another question was presented in an agonizingly slow West Texas drawl.

"God, give me patience – and give it to me now," was my unspoken prayer.

The airline agent, having successfully retrieved our suitcases from the baggage carousel, wheeled Louisa to the exit just as I ran past her with the car keys. I raced to the parking lot, located the jet black sedan in space #21, threw my carryon in the back seat, and briefly studied the foreign shift pattern before lurching to a stop at the handicap ramp. We had twelve minutes to reach Waverly Place before Mother and Elena were to depart. Louisa's cell phone, which she had just turned back on after the flight, promptly rang. Elena was on the other end speaking very urgently, but softly from the guest bathroom of the cottage. Mother, being highly suspicious of any conversations which she could not readily hear, always assumed that every conversation was related in some negative way to her and that she was in imminent danger. Elena had learned early on to conduct phone calls on her cell phone from the safe confines of the guest bathroom which was hidden away behind two doors. So anxious was Mother's reaction to phone calls that I wondered, if at times, her aide even stepped into the bathtub and drew the shower curtain for extra soundproofing.

Some months prior I asked my aunts if something might have happened to Mother when the three girls were growing up together, and both soundly put that thought out of my head by telling me that they were actually somewhat spoiled by a very loving father and family members who doted on the girls. Aunt Goldy admitted that her older sister had always overreacted to situations and that, of the three of them, was the most easily spooked.

"Cricket was always on guard against what might happen to us," she said. "She constantly lived in a 'what if' kind of scenario."

The abysmal recovery and rehab in the hospital following her knee surgery was the perfect example of a lifelong fear for her own safety, but this time it was amplified through the paranoia of an old woman with dementia. Our appointment with the psychiatrist was vitally important. Mother needed professional help that none of us, including the home healthcare aides, were trained to provide. We weren't even certain that she would know us, for in the latest phone conversations with us she showed no signs of warmth or recognition. Elena was our greatest ally in helping Mother hold on to what little threads of memory of her daughters that still remained; and we were moving now with great purpose to capture the last bits of our mother before she disappeared behind a cobweb of names and faces that she could no longer connect.

Louisa assured Elena that we were racing across the last ten miles as quickly as safety and sanity would allow and that we would be there within minutes. Fortunately for us, Waverly Place is located on the west edge of the city and accessible from the airport by a straight shot down a four-lane highway to the city limits, where we took one left turn followed quickly by a right turn into the gated entrance of the senior community. The security guard waved us through the gate with barely a glance and I broke the five miles-per-hour speed limit as we wound our way through the sedate streets lined with little cottages. Not to arouse Mother's suspicions, we left our bags in the car and made our way up the short sidewalk to the front glass door, desperately hoping that she would know us and receive us with an open heart.

She did. The look of joy on her face was a precious sight as she motioned for me to join her on the sofa and allowed me to place my hand on hers. She did not speak anything other than "This is such a surprise" before tears started to run down her soft, wrinkled cheeks. Louisa filled up the empty space with her words of cheer as she always does, and the five or so minutes we had before Elena announced that they had an appointment to keep went by very quickly.

"Oh, well then we will go with you," Louisa said and began to gather her purse and organize her walker.

Supported by her caregiver's strong arms, Mother slowly and painfully rose from the sofa and tangled the legs of her walker in Louisa's. We laughed as the pretend dueling of the walkers continued for a few moments before everyone made their way to Elena's car parked in the garage. Getting settled in took more than a few moments, and Louisa and I looked anxiously at one another as the minutes ticked closer to the time of the appointment. We kept up a lively stream of chatter with Elena and did our best to engage Mother, but had little success. She laughed when we did and made a few sounds of approval or disapproval - all in slow motion. To the casual observer, it may have seemed that she followed the conversation, but for those of us who knew her, the responses were only forthcoming after she observed the responses of others and mimicked them as if on a five-second delay.

As we pulled into the circle drive of the medical complex,

Mother admitted that she was thoroughly lost and did not recognize where we were. None of us responded, but made busy with the preparations of getting two walkers out of the trunk.

She looked around puzzled and slowly asked, "Which one of you has the doctor's appointment?"

Louisa cheerfully answered, "You do, Mom," to which she replied, "I don't need to see the doctor."

Louisa and I had decided that we would be as honest as possible without scaring Mother about visiting a psychiatrist. To her generation, seeing a psychiatrist was a mark against one's mental capacities that could never be removed. We did our best to direct her attention elsewhere as we neared the door to the psychiatrist's office. She wheeled the walker up close to the names etched on each doorway we passed in an attempt to read something familiar and to ascertain where she was. Fortunately, she could not read a single word and we passed safely by an endocrinologist, a psychologist, and an addict recovery center before reaching the psychiatrist's office where Louisa stood holding the door open for her while conveniently blocking the name and title on the glass.

We looked at each other with great relief, having made it through the gauntlet of arriving on time for the appointment and keeping the doctor's identity from Mother. Now came the next hurtle in this journey of uncertainty – would the doctor allow us to accompany her into his office or would we be prisoners to the laws preventing us from participating in conversations between doctor and patient. We exchanged another look tinged with comingled hope and dread.

Our fears were turned aside when Dr. Owens emerged from the hallway and swept us all into his office before we had a chance to position ourselves uneasily in the waiting area. As far as the doctor was concerned, there was never a question about whether he would speak with Louisa and I, and Elena very quietly stepped back and disappeared into the hallway beyond the glass door as we had previously discussed.

"Nora, I think Elena was glad to finally act as just the limo service for one of Mom's doctor appointments," I told Nora at our appointed dinner spot. "It seemed fine two years ago when we started the home healthcare for a caregiver to take her to routine appointments, but the further she declined, the more important it became for either Louisa or I to be with her. Unfortunately, for most of that time I was not in Mom's good graces, and Louisa was not physically able to go. So, the burden became Elena's by default."

"I still get the impression that Louisa didn't think it was necessary to go with your mother to the appointment with the psychiatrist," Nora almost retorted, but catching herself, changed her tone of voice. "She was still very much in denial, right?"

"Yes," I sighed. "She always wants to believe the best in someone, but it gets in the way of reality. She was still uncertain of the diagnosis until the three of us sat together for the first time in the presence of a specialist."

"That certainly was not easy. Tell me about that visit," Nora urged.

After a bit of jostling with the two walkers, the doctor visit began quite comfortably with the usual chit-chat and small talk to establish each of the characters in the play. I sat on the sofa behind Mother, just in case she should glance over and suddenly remember that she didn't like me and fall back into a mire of accusations. She seemed to remain calm, but I could see her arms and hands shaking as she clutched the arms of the chair. I reached forward and placed my hand on her arm until she quit trembling.

Dr. Owens took a comprehensive medical history and asked the magic words that Louisa and I were waiting for as a cue to hand him not only Mother's list of medications, but a summary of the last two and a half years. He read through the list and the summary while continuing to take her history, never letting on that we had just communicated her history to him. Had Mother heard us tell him the details of the last two years, she would have protested and denied it all, but most of all would have been embarrassed to hear us telling a stranger about her greatest fears. Louisa and I had accomplished all that we could at that point and relaxed in the faith that we had finally found someone who could help us provide the best care possible for our parent.

It was obvious to the three of us listening to her answers that most of Mother's memories were lost to her, and although she had been able to carry on in the past by making up stories to support whatever truth she imagined, she could not do so in the presence of Dr. Owens. He was gentle and kind, but thoroughly quizzed her on our family. I did not have to hide my reactions sitting well out of sight behind her; while Louisa, whom Mother could see sitting in the next armchair, kept her face completely emotionless during the questioning. Nevertheless, the psychiatrist could see the worry on my face as Mother could not recall that the year was 2011, if she had any living relatives or what profession her husband had been in for over thirty-six years of their lives together. Mother valiantly struggled to spell "world" backwards and could not; nor could she perform the math to figure out how many years she and Dad had been married. I gave her hints to the questions when she called out my name and asked for help. In retrospect, we both thought it interesting that she did not seek out Louisa's help.

"From a very selfish perspective, Nora, the very fact that she looked back to where I was sitting behind her and reached out to me for support was like a balm to my heart," I said as a wide smile moved across my face. "Somewhere – somewhere deep inside her mothering spirit I was still her firstborn."

Nora looked deep into my eyes, which were sparkling with joy.

"You prayed for one last time for closure as mother and daughter. God is indeed merciful."

I took in a deep cleansing breath of fresh air, "He is indeed. The roles between Mom and I were reversed, though. I was the parent helping the child. She was not afraid to seek out my help, and that is what felt so… so comfortable. My mother wanted me. She needed me. She knew that she loved me, even when her mind was struggling to remember my name."

Nora and I sat quietly just letting the warmth of those thoughts penetrate the silence. There were no other words to describe the peacefulness – not that any were needed, for we both knew the sweetness of what had transpired.

With a final outburst from Mother regarding the "big, fat clerk" at the motor vehicles office who noticed that she lived at Waverly Place and consequently refused to renew her driver's license, Dr. Owens concluded the session by asking if there was anything else that needed to be covered. The interview had been almost exclusively a volley between doctor and patient, except for a brief interlude where Louisa and I took the floor to very gently confront Mother with the fact that she could no longer manage her finances. She had made the statement during the exam that she handled her own affairs and paid all of her bills on time.

Louisa broke her self-imposed silence and gasped, "Oh, Mother," which resulted in me waving her off with my hand well below Mother's eye sight.

She took a measured breath and asked, "Mom, do you even know where your checkbook is?"

Mom indignantly answered, "Yes, it is in the second drawer of my dresser."

My sister began shaking her head and I leaned forward off the sofa to tell Mother what had really been happening to her bills. The psychiatrist listened intently without saying a word, observing, no doubt, the interaction between mother and daughters. I did not care what he thought of our relationship, I only wanted him to know that Mother had no idea that she was not and could not manage her money.

"Mom," I began in a quiet, non-accusatory tone. "I'm sorry, but that is not true. You have not paid any bills since October. You have been throwing all your mail into the trash saying that it was not important, even the Waverly Place invoices. Elena has been retrieving the bills out of the garbage and sending them to Louisa who has been paying them for you."

She slowly shook her head, and I fully expected a torrent of heated words exclaiming what an evil daughter I was; but there was just bewilderment on her face. She could not find words to express whatever emotion she may have been feeling. I turned my attention to the doctor and explained with as many ambiguous and multi-syllabic words as I could in order to speak over Mother's head, thereby telling him that the funds to which my sister and I currently had access would be depleted in a matter of weeks. I stated very directly and to the point that a change was immediately needed in her living arrangements and the handling of her personal affairs. In the absence of any semblance of understanding on Mother's face, Dr. Owens looked at me pointedly and said that he would fill out whatever paperwork was necessary to ensure that this happened.

It seemed inappropriate at the moment, nor did I really have the energy to celebrate, but we had just crossed a monumental threshold. The long sought after medical diagnosis and willingness on a doctor's part to help Mother in spite of her own objections, had finally taken place. The three of us rose and thanked the doctor, and he showed Louisa and his new patient to the reception desk to set up the next appointment and gave them a prescription for an additional medication which, while he promised it would not reverse or stop the constant forward movement of the disease, it had helped other patients for a short time. Elena was called back in to assist with the making of the appointment, and the doctor quietly pulled me back into his office.

"You need to see an attorney immediately and start proceedings for guardianship of your mother," he said quite earnestly.

I almost stopped him short, anticipating what he would advise, and assured him that we had already begun that process and would be seeing an attorney the next day. He reiterated that he would be more than willing to provide whatever kind of documentation was needed, but that we should not delay.

"So, just in the short time he saw your mother, the doctor knew that she was essentially incompetent?" Nora did not sound overly amazed, but spoke as if just confirming what we both knew to be true.

"Yes, I asked him if we needed to correct any of the information that she had supplied to him. He had already assumed that almost everything Mom told him was a fallacy," I said, expressing great relief that we had finally found a medical professional who was not only willing, but almost insistent, that specialized care and supervision of her affairs was necessary for Mother's future well-being.

Nora's words of assurance and understanding at our having reached this milestone were gratifying. Our conversations always lifted my spirits and gave me additional energy to keep going - to keep trying - to keep the faith. None of us will ever be able to fully answer that question that all God-fearing hearts dare to ask at some point in their journeys, *"Why did you allow this to happen?"* However, we all have the simple and peaceful choice to believe that through the grace and mercy of a loving God, we do indeed have the strength and wisdom to walk difficult pathways. Nora's unshakable belief in this truth was a beacon that I had followed through the dark fog, and I strove to, in turn, be that beacon for my sister and my mother.

"It was such a struggle to open Louisa's eyes to the idea that we had to intervene in Mom's care," I told Nora over a plate full of angel hair pasta and marinara sauce. We had ventured to an Italian restaurant several doors down from the sandwich shop after deciding that soup and salad would not be sufficient for the conversation.

"I just do not know why she has been dragging her feet so hard on this. Perhaps, she has made a promise to Mom to keep her in the cottage as long as possible, but that is so unfair to her. That is just dragging out the inevitable. Maybe she can't get her thoughts together enough to step in because she herself is in so much pain," I conjectured.

"Could it be that Louisa is also afraid?" Nora stopped my rambling sentences with a hard question that had the solid ring of truth.

Perhaps, Nora was right, but, regardless of Louisa's motivation or lack thereof, we had now made headway in formulating a diagnosis and a long-term care plan. In anticipation of this outcome, I had already made appointments with Waverly Place personnel to explore what was required in moving Mother out of the cottage and into the Alzheimer's unit. Just as important, I sought the advice of Deborah Barnes in recommending an elder care and family law attorney, and had subsequently made an appointment with a highly respected attorney who specialized in setting up guardianships.

Fully expecting my unilateral decisions to bring about another outburst and reprimands from my sister, I hesitated to apprise her of the appointments, but tired of secrets and manipulative behavior, I chose the direct route of disclosure. To my great surprise, Louisa greeted the news of the appointments with enthusiasm, and I began to wonder if my judgments toward her had been too hasty. The day after the psychiatrist visit we sat at the breakfast table at the hotel discussing the plans for the day.

Louisa's thoughts kept wandering from one topic to another as she tried to wake up from another fitful night. She found it hard to focus, not only from the lack of sleep, but also from the sleep-inducing narcotics she had already been taking into her system before I awoke. Hot cups of tea, for neither of us had ever acquired the taste for coffee, helped revive our spirits.

As she tackled the waffle-making machine at the breakfast bar, Louisa asked me to help her stay on track for the tasks that lay ahead that day. I agreed unconditionally, and we shared a laugh as the batter overflowed the waffle iron and made shapes that looked like zoo animals. As silly as it was, it felt good to concentrate on something outside of ourselves and our mother.

The day was to begin with a visit to Waverly Place's front office, where we hoped to meet up with Deborah to review the file, which in a few short years of Mother's residency had become quite thick. Neither of us were quite sure what documents were still intact in the file, however, as Mother had told us so many times that she had changed this, removed that, or added some condition to her living arrangements.

Nora laughed at the mention of the confusion over the documents. Her mother, too, had made a jumble of her personal papers and had not been able to remember all the legalities of keeping an orderly life. My mother was no different, and in her effort to appear to still be in control of her life, made blustery claims about editing this or that document, visiting her attorney, and filing court orders. We found no proof of any such claims in the Waverly Place files and once again dismissed her stories as just that – stories that she had pieced together from facts she believed to be true or stories she made up to protect herself from all manner of perceived intrusions upon her person, real or imagined.

Deborah, accustomed to hearing from Mrs. Adams's daughters on a regular basis, was pleased to see us and offered her assistance in even the smallest of ways. Because of the contractual agreement with Waverly Place to live unencumbered in an independent cottage, there was usually very little that Deborah could do for her residents.

"She must have been relieved to hear that you were making progress with the doctor's appointments," Nora interjected.

"Absolutely! She said that Mom had some sort of psychiatric issues going on and needed attention. You know, in many ways, it must be hard to see a senior trying so valiantly to live independently when you know they need assistance, but you are tied by a legal agreement not to interfere. The only intervention that they can give is in the event of a physical accident or something gone awry with some aspect of the house. Just because she is in a senior community, the fact that she is in independent living, is really not much of a safeguard. The only real benefit is that she will not have to make an additional deposit to move into a higher level of care in one of the medical units."

"I am so sorry that you have to walk the thin line between protecting her privacy and assuring her safety."

"Thank you, Nora. I know you understand the delicate balance of power between parent and child. It will be easier when we have passed through this transition time and all find ourselves with clearly defined roles once again. Mom is hurting so deeply – her identity is being stripped away and she does not know her purpose or place in the world anymore," I said with growing concern.

"Her soul knows who she is, even if her mind has forgotten," were Nora's simple, yet poignant words.

We finished what was left of our pasta dishes and awaited the dessert menu before I continued with my story.

After leaving Deborah's office, Louisa and I pushed on through the various hallways until we found ourselves at the Johnston Center, the specially designed facility for those suffering with Alzheimer's and other severe forms of dementia. Leslie Porter, the director and head of nursing, greeted us warmly and we soon found ourselves pouring our hearts out to the kindly, yet efficient woman on the other side of the desk. We described changes in Mother's behavior, cognitive abilities, and daily living skills before I hopefully asked if the Johnston Center was an appropriate place for her. Leslie assured us that our mother did meet the requirements and pulled out a brochure to walk us through the medical, housing, and social services of the center. After hearing a very informative description of life as a resident there, I found myself uplifted by the positive approach of caregiving provided to the special people who lived there. Mother had always steered us away from this part of the building when we accompanied her to the beauty shop or to the front office.

"You don't want to see the people who live there," she invariably said disdainfully, as if the inability to remember how to tie one's shoelaces made one a leper. "They carry baby dolls around and talk to themselves."

As we listened intently to a typical day of activities for a senior at the center, I told Leslie, that according to Mom, Waverly Place had been designed and built by our father in 1960. She laughed, knowing that Dad had been influential in the community when we moved there in the '60s, but had not been a part of Waverly Place's history. She quickly responded with a smile, "Oh, well then - we need to update our history."

The director of admissions verified that there was a vacancy and explained the admissions procedure to us, beginning with the diagnosis by a medical doctor who was willing to write orders for her admission. I held my breath and waited for my sister to answer, and was pleased to hear her say that we could meet those requirements. Much to my surprise, Louisa seemed quite willing to follow through with the doctor's orders to seek alternative living and care arrangements for Mother, in spite of any promises of independence she may have made to her.

We accepted Leslie's invitation to tour the Johnston Center once again – the third time that I could recall since Mother had moved to Waverly Place - but this time with a different eye, that of a daughter seeking a place of refuge for her mother. Recalling Mother's disdain for her lack of privacy while living at the YWCA when she first left home as a young lady in search of a career, we selected a private room for her over the dorm-like feel of a shared bedroom. The private room felt good as soon as we walked in. The spaciousness was surprising, but our excitement on discovering it had two windows and a private entry hallway was slight in comparison to Leslie's surprise when we all noted the room had its own private bathroom complete with walk-in shower. Her tenure as director of admissions' was going on ten years and she had never known that this particular private room was indeed a suite. Without further hesitation Louisa said, "This is the one. Please put

Mom's name on it," as if the room would suddenly become occupied by another before our very eyes.

"Nora, my sister's impulsiveness was heartwarming because she rarely makes such decisions lightly or quickly. I was thrilled that she was willing to take a step forward in what had become a somewhat static attitude to this whole process," I exclaimed. "As we were driving away from the Johnston Center toward our next appointment I asked her what had made her come to such a conclusive decision. She said she looked around at the residents who were involved in various levels of activity and saw that some were just sitting alone in rolling recliners and staring off into the distance with no expression or movement in their faces. A few were gathered around tables engaged in some secretive form of conversation that only they understood, while two women were snuggled together on a loveseat stroking a cat sitting across their laps. Louisa simply said, 'Mom fits here.'"

It had been a long hard fought journey to that point. All of us – my mother, my sister, and me – had walked different routes to arrive at the same point. Our journeys had paralleled one another, with Mother's being the one in the middle driving the course and momentum of the other two. Louisa had walked much more slowly, often trailing behind; while I tried to keep abreast or even slightly ahead of Mother, who shuffled steadily along, rarely looking up, completely unaware of our presence.

"I think of families that are torn apart by this disease," Nora said, leaning her chin on her hand. "Not everyone is as sensitive to the needs of all family members as you are, Allison. I was fortunate in that Dorothy just let me handle everything – which in one sense made it very easy, but it was a huge weight to make decisions alone. Brother had already died and I think Dorothy just did not want the responsibility."

"I understand that it is common for adult children to literally run away from their aging parents and refuse to take up the responsibility for their safety and well-being," I said, shaking my head. "How can someone not think about the parent that spent over twenty years raising them, caring for them, teaching them…"

Nora filled in the silence when my voice trailed off, "…loving them." She paused before continuing, "Not everyone is nurtured by their parents. Not all adult children had happy childhoods and perhaps don't feel that responsibility so keenly. Caring for an aging parent is as difficult as caring for and rearing a small child, more so when we consider that the parent is an adult and has rights protected by law."

How painfully aware of that fact Louisa and I would become when we sat down that afternoon with the family law attorney. There were still questions to be answered at Waverly Place, however, and I quickly drove us a few blocks over to the marketing office. We were greeted by a receptionist who promptly left to call the marketing director out of a meeting to talk with us. I glanced over at Louisa and frowned, wondering if they had lost track of our appointment, and when the director practically flew in the front door and announced that she had another meeting in fifteen minutes, I realized that we would have to make the most of the abbreviated appointment. Louisa had popped a lollipop into her mouth as we left the Johnston Center and was beginning to get that glazed look in her eyes which meant that although free of pain, she would soon not be able to form a cohesive sentence. It was my turn to take the reins and move us forward.

The director of marketing answered a rapidly fired set of questions regarding the terms of the contract for her cottage, the process for notifying Waverly Place of the move, the condition in which the house should be left, how much money she would receive upon vacating, and when we might expect the funds to reach her checking account. Mother had signed a forty/sixty contract and having fulfilled the occupancy tenure for a forty percent refund, we could expect several tens of thousands of dollars to be deposited into her account approximately four months from the date she gave notice. The founding philanthropists had wisely created a process that made difficult transitions between living arrangements as seamless as possible.

"Once she is in Waverly Place, she is ours," Leslie quipped, and at the time I thought that sounded rather threatening. I soon relaxed, however, with the realization that she was free to move from one type of residence into another, and more importantly, her name would be placed at the top of the waiting list. It took Louisa most of the next several hours to comprehend the math involved in computing the monthly cost of the cottage, plus the cost of the around-the-clock care, versus the cost of the Johnston Center. The figure for the Alzheimer's unit initially scared her, and she almost backed out entirely until Tom emailed a graph to her comparing the costs of the two care and living arrangements. Not to my surprise, but much to Louisa's astonishment, home healthcare was nearly three times the cost of the Alzheimer's unit.

Not to be overlooked, the aides, as loving and attentive as they were, had reached the end of their expertise in dealing with a stubborn elderly woman with psychotic episodes. She had become verbally abusive and very difficult to motivate in recent weeks. Never physically abusive, the constant attention that she required was no less exhaustive than that of caring for a toddler. In the Johnston Center, Mother would receive immediate medical attention by a staff of nurses and doctors that knew she could no longer accurately identify or describe what hurt. She would still need to be taken to outside psychiatric and dental appointments, but all other medical needs could be taken care of onsite by individuals trained in the needs of the severely demented.

"The Alzheimer's unit also gives Mom a social structure," I explained to Nora excitedly. "She was once very active in interacting with others and loved being a part of the social scene, sometimes leading the activities herself. The center has a calendar packed with opportunities to experience music; going out on the town – which I think is something like a closely supervised field trip to a mall; and meals taken in a family setting. She would not be alone like she is at her house. There will be others to talk to on whatever level she is able to communicate."

We were grateful that Mother was not terribly ambulatory, as our morning's rounds of appointments had taken us within mere blocks of her. We were fairly certain that we would not accidentally meet her out on the sidewalk taking a stroll, but we had kept to our timeline and eventually found our way to her house for lunch. I hid all of the pamphlets and materials we had picked up along the way in the trunk of the rental car on the off-chance that she would see them lying on the car seat. Louisa suggested that we put our notebooks and folders in the trunk, as well, and we headed for her house almost empty-handed.

The previous day's visit with Mother and the surreptitious visit to the psychiatrist had left us wondering if she would greet us as warmly as she had the day before. There was some doubt that she would even remember that we had been there or if she would return to that stage where dark paranoia made her suspicious of our presence. Our fears soon dissolved as she was only too eager to hug our necks and accept the invitation to go out for lunch. She chose one of her favorite places to eat, which served up a fare somewhat nostalgic of the foods she grew up on. On the drive past the department stores, gas stations and office buildings, she repeatedly asked where we were going, having completely forgotten the answer given just a few minutes before. Each time either Louisa or Elena or I would sweetly tell her we were going to her favorite place where fried chicken, cheese grits, buttermilk and cornbread adorned the menu. The ride was pleasant in spite of her lapses in memory and we all giggled and chattered like schoolgirls glad to be in one another's company. I cherished those brief moments when my mother slid her hand across the back seat and took mine in hers. I wanted to close my eyes and never let that moment end when she reached out to me, a simple gesture that we had not shared for quite some time.

The lunch ended much too quickly as we feigned an airplane to catch at two o'clock and drove them back to the cottage. It struck me that if all went as I hoped it would, this would be the last time I would see the little house filled with furniture, photographs, and treasures from my childhood. While the objects were still familiar to Mother, each time she told me about some trinket or picture, the story varied from something her cousin brought back from Thailand to a prize that Dad had won in a raffle. Nora would be so pleased that I listened to these tales with great interest and expressed wonder and joy over them as if it were indeed true that this was the only surviving vase from the Ming dynasty. Not too many months before when dementia and Alzheimer's were words spoken about someone else's mother, I would have vehemently corrected her and chided her for telling such stories.

How long this journey had seemed, but it was far from over. I was still not certain that Louisa would go through with plans for Mother to leave her home, and the legalities of how to make that happen were not clear to me. My research, and Mother's insistence that only a doctor could make her move, kept nagging at me. Louisa had not wanted to take the formal step of invoking a Power of Attorney or seeking Guardianship of Mother. Her reasoning had not been well articulated six months prior when Tom and I returned from San Angelo and stopped off to see her and her family. She had literally screamed at us and walked out of the room with tears streaming down her cheeks, which were flushed with emotion.

"Nora, she just kept screaming that it wasn't time, it wasn't time."

"That must have been awful, truly awful, to hear your sister yelling at you," Nora comforted.

"The worst part was that when Tom calmly suggested that a Guardianship would be appropriate for Mom, she angrily told him that she was tired of him sticking his nose into her family. This was *her* mother and he had no part in these decisions," I said somewhat angrily. "Matt defended her and told us to just let Mom grow old in peace."

The chocolate dessert in front of me suddenly became less appealing with the memory of the heated remarks aimed at my husband and our views on long term care. I stared off into empty space until Nora's soft voice brought me back to the conversation.

"Words spoken in the heat of a disagreement can sting and they can remain in the forefront of one's memory for a very long time," she wisely reminded me. "Each of you obviously had your own perspective on this, and they differed greatly. How did the discussion end? With your sister leaving the room?"

"She exited the room, leaving all of us sitting there in silence. I was very proud of Tom for holding his tongue. Later he told me that it would have served no purpose to enter into an argument with Louisa in her state of mind. He knew she was not only in physical pain, but was in emotional turmoil, as well," I said, vigorously pushing my spoon around in the chocolate mousse. "Louisa did not leave the room for long, though. She came back with a piece of paper - I don't even remember now what it was – and started to talk. I interrupted her from across the room where I was seated on the sofa and told her very calmly that I did not appreciate her excluding Tom from the conversation. He is a part of this family and decisions about any member of the family affect us all."

"Good for you," Nora exclaimed. She had long said she believed I was afraid of Louisa and applauded me for disagreeing with my sister in such a public forum.

I smiled weakly, finally admitting that I was ready to push Louisa's feelings aside in favor of my mother's well being; and certainly to defend my husband against the ravings of a person who was not completely in control of what she was saying.

Six months had passed since Louisa's outburst and we found ourselves no closer to a resolution to Mother's care than when we discussed it in the Butler' family room. Granted, in the interim Louisa had undergone life-changing surgery for scoliosis and was fighting a brave battle to regain her strength and composure, but Alzheimer's was not waiting. Mother had declined so much during that time that she truly did not know her friends from her cousins, or how to set the table, or what year it was.

Louisa had, no doubt, grown tired and frustrated at my constant pushing to see an attorney. Mother was beyond the point that we could easily guarantee her financial safety, mostly from her own actions and ill-advised decisions. At the height of her paranoia period, as if we could date the stages she moved through like some geological strata, she frantically moved money between banks and securities without giving anyone else in the family access to the funds. Mother was terrified that someone would steal her money and failed to recognize the need for flexibility as her medical needs intensified. Louisa stood staunchly behind her in these moves and praised her for making her own decisions regarding CDs and money markets, even the highly-risky one she purchased at a kiosk in the mall one day.

After our visit with Dr. Owens, however, Louisa could no longer argue the fact that Mother was not capable of managing her own medical and financial future. She had been operating on the assumption that Mother could make at least some wise decisions for herself, but that idea was now firmly laid to rest.

Chapter 16

*I*t sounded surreal to seek control of Mother's person like she was a piece of property, but it was painfully clear now to Louisa that our mother could no longer make decisions for herself. Her every action, every thought, every decision had to be guided, right down to the choice of appropriate clothing for the day. We tearfully said goodbye to her, and on the pretense of rushing to catch a flight back home, we drove away from the beautiful little cottage with the white picket fence around the front porch. There is forever in my mind an image of her standing slightly hunched forward, feet planted wide behind her walker, with one hand slightly raised and a forlorn and worried look on her face. Life was so uncertain for her now.

On the other hand, her daughters were certain of their need to meet with a family law attorney, and after a quick lunch, we headed downtown. Finding a handicap parking spot in front of the building was a God-send as Louisa could not travel far on the walker, and I could not tolerate the heat, already feeling fatigued and slightly dizzy from our day's busy itinerary. We made our way into the high-rise office building and were greeted by a very cordial receptionist who ushered us into a wood-paneled conference room to wait for Esther Carlisle.

She welcomed us with an easy going manner and invited us to "please call me Esther" before getting down to the purpose of our visit. Louisa had asked me in the elevator on the way up to act as the spokesperson because finding appropriate words to express herself often eluded her. I was glad to take on that role, for I wanted to quickly get to the primary reason for the consultation.

The attorney was not easily persuaded of the need to commit Mom, nor if a guardianship was the best route. We showed her the Durable Power of Attorney with Mother's selection of Option B, "This power shall become effective upon the declaration of incompetency by a physician." Esther bemoaned this choice because it necessitated the involvement of a physician and a judge to declare Mother incapable of handling her own affairs. Option A would have put the Power of Attorney into effect immediately upon execution of the document. However, I explained that at the time it was signed, she was deeply suspicious of others and refused to even consider someone else managing her affairs on her behalf.

We were quite surprised to learn that, even if the Power of Attorney could be invoked based on a physician's statement that Imogene Adams was no longer competent, she could at any time revoke the document and continue to carry out her own transactions and affairs.

"You mean to say that she could completely undo any actions that you took?" Nora was stunned to ask.

"Absolutely," I replied. "The attorney was startled when in unison we said that Mom had to be curtailed from making any decisions on her own. She was really sharp, Nora. The meeting was almost like a court proceeding in itself. We countered every objection she had for going forward with a guardianship until she finally seemed satisfied that we had considered all angles and had made the best decision."

Esther listened to our case and quizzed us thoroughly on all options – whether Louisa should file for guardianship, or whether I should. We discussed Mother's intention through the signed Designation of Guardian that Louisa should be appointed her guardian, and we further explained Mother's great fear and misgivings about me. Perhaps seeing Louisa in a body brace, wheeling herself along behind a walker, and sucking on a narcotic lollipop almost dissuaded the attorney from taking Louisa's petition seriously. She doubted that Louisa was capable of handling her client's affairs, but Louisa assured her that the brace and walker were only temporary and as the months rolled on that she would be more than able to tackle Mother's finances and medical care. I kept my mouth closed at that point, something for which my father would have applauded me. If Louisa faltered or found herself unable to meet the challenge, I was ready to be her back-up, just as

Mother had specified in the Designation of Guardian.   Belaboring that fact at this point was superfluous.   After half an hour of hearing our arguments, the very pedantic and methodical attorney was satisfied that a guardianship was the best route - the only route - to securing safety and health for Mother.   She was pleased that Dr. Owens was willing, if not eager, to provide any documentation needed to support Louisa's petition.

The final argument to present to Esther was how Louisa would care for Mother long distance. She had to be convinced that there was no intention to "take the money and run," as she so indelicately put it. Louisa and I had given this much thought, and I laid out a plan by which Mother would be admitted to the Alzheimer's unit at Waverly Place, where her every medical need would be seen to and her daily living skills would be supplemented as needed. A room had already been selected for her, and we knew how to transition her from the cottage into the Johnston Center, terminating the contract on the cottage, and moving her belongings out as she had already described in her last wishes. It was ironic that this would be carried out before she actually passed away, but the transition from independent living to a long-term care facility was a passing in some sense.

Esther countered with the suggestion that Mother should come live with or near one of us, and we were quick to point out that because of her feelings towards me, no matter how unfounded, living with Tom and me was not a comfortable option. Additionally, care facilities for the elderly in the Northeast cost three times what they do in the South – a sound reason for keeping her in place. Louisa was equally adamant that moving her closer to the Butlers was not a suitable arrangement because she is not physically or emotionally capable of being a caregiver when her own needs necessitated so much energy.

The ideal solution was to honor Mother's original wishes and move her into the most appropriate housing and care arrangement at Waverly Place – her intentions from the day she moved into the cottage. We showed Esther the letter which she had written some time ago outlining her desire to stay in the senior community she had chosen for herself.   Even years ago, she felt motivated to write one of her infamous letters - which brought the rolling of eyes when she presented it us in our Christmas stockings - but for which we are now grateful. Her own words reinforced the idea that the Johnston Center should become her new home.

Midway through the conference, Esther divulged that she was in possession of Mother's last will and testament which had been drawn up by Jacob Erly, a former attorney with the same law firm. We were startled to learn this fact and even more amazed that she had agreed to meet with us. Esther assured us that she had conducted her due diligence to discover any conflicts of interest. She stated that it was possible that she could not take on our case because Mother was essentially a client of the law firm by way of Jacob. Jacob had been a close friend of our family, having served as Dad's BSA council executive, the equivalent of the president of a board of directors for a non-profit. Mother trusted him implicitly and had sought out his help when she was determined to strike me from the family record books, and she dictated to Jacob what Esther referred to as the "strangest will I have ever seen."

I assured Esther that I was aware of the will and asked if it could be probated given Mother's condition at the time, implying that she was not of sound mind. Esther seemed startled that I knew about the will and asked if I had read it, to which Louisa quickly intervened stating that she had the original in a safe deposit box and that she had not shown it to me. For a few seconds the temptation to ask for permission to read the document stuck in my throat, but we were not there for the purpose of determining my eligibility as an heir to the small estate, which was grower smaller by the moment as the cost of around-the-clock care was quickly diminishing her funds.

In the seconds that followed, many thoughts ran through my mind before I heard myself say, "I have no interest in reading the ranting of my mother when she is so ill. We are not here to probate her will. We are here to facilitate her life."

My reply directed the three of us back to the matter at hand.

"The appearance of Mom's will written in the heat of anger caught me off guard, Nora," I admitted. "I knew of its existence, but here it was in a folder lying on the conference table not two feet from my hand. It had slipped my mind for a number of months as we focused on making changes in Mom's care and living arrangements. Esther brought it rushing back into my mind and I found myself once again having to fight back feelings of disgust and anger. It was very difficult to set those feelings aside and I had to imagine physically taking the folder, sealing it inside a box, and storing it on the top shelf on a dark closet. My mind knew the will was conceived out of fear and mistrust by someone other than my mother."

"How very wise of you to handle your feelings that way," Nora affirmed. "I pray that you can feel good about the way you dealt with it."

The smile on my face must have showed her that emotions, which once would have taken me weeks to work through, were in my thoughts for only moments before being stowed in their proper place as secondary to the lives of the two women I loved more than any other. I suddenly knew what Louisa meant when she said my acceptance of Mother's condition made things easier on the relationship between us. Lifting the burden of ill-feelings from my heart also lifted them from the shoulders of my sister.

Finally satisfied that a judge would not find fault with Louisa's long distance plan for care nor with her ability to serve as guardian, Esther asked that Dr. Owens's declaration of incompetency be sent over. Once she received his documentation, the whole process from filing to hearing would take only a few weeks. In order to keep the process moving along, we volunteered to pick up the papers from Dr. Owens's office and hand deliver them back to the attorney's office the next morning. We left her office feeling a certain amount of anxiety over having to take such drastic steps on Mother's behalf, yet elated that after two years, the process was finally under way.

Louisa called ahead to request the incompetency documents and Dr. Owens's nurse had the papers ready by the time we arrived. As we sat in the car under a shade tree in the parking lot, I opened the envelope to read his conclusions out loud. Very plainly and simply he stated that Mrs. Adams was not competent enough to handle her own affairs, and because she was in the severe stage of Alzheimer's, she should immediately be moved into a long-term care facility.

Louisa was completely silent, and I let her digest the hard

truth that was now in stark black and white. The only sound was that of the car engine and the air conditioner going full blast. Louisa leaned her head against the window. Finally she spoke.

"So it is Alzheimer's. I didn't think it was...and she is in the severe stage," she said, quoting the doctor's assessment.

I reached over to my sister and gave her arm a squeeze. There was little I could say to ease her pain.

"Nora, I felt badly on the one hand but elated on the other to read his diagnosis and recommendation," I confessed. "Any hesitancy on Louisa's part melted away in those few moments. My heart ached for her, for any shred of reversing Mom's journey was now gone. It was definite – Mother had severe Alzheimer's. Louisa could no longer deny nor change the direction we must go."

Nora sat back in the big brown leather booth and smiled. We both knew that our bi-weekly conversations would soon come to a close. She could sense the calm feeling of resolution that had come over me. My dear friend had listened and gently guided me through the tangle of emotions through which I had journeyed with hard, angry strides at times and with heavy, grieving steps at other times. The path was, indeed, beginning to level out and become more beautiful as we all walked more confidently toward the future. The future did not frighten me, although I am sure that it will be unsettling for my mother for quite some time. I held fast to Nora's promise that Mother's thoughts would become sweeter as time passed and that she would indeed reach a state of contentedness.

"So, what is the next step, Allison?"

"Mother will be served with papers indicating that a petition has been filed for a guardian to be established for her. A court-appointed attorney will meet with her to explain the proceedings and then we wait for a hearing date to be set. Louisa will travel to San Angelo and appear in court, at which time the physician's statement will be read. Louisa will explain how she plans to manage Mom's health care, living arrangements, and financial dealings while living hundreds of miles away, and the judge will make his ruling," I said, describing each step of the way.

"Is this difficult for you? We did not have to go to these extremes with Mommie. What you have to do just tears me apart. I am so pleased at your strength through all of this."

I laughed a bit before replying, "I have not felt strong at times. It is difficult to keep the goal in sight. It is still not achieved. The judge could very well rule against Louisa. We are several steps closer, though, and I believe we will prevail against whatever obstacles Mom may put up. I pray that I am not this much trouble when I reach her age. Tom tells me that I probably will be."

Nora and I chuckled as I continued to tell her of our progress in securing guardianship and a place for Mother in the Alzheimer's unit.

The brief plane trip back to Louisa's was uneventful except for the brief exchange of thoughts about the upcoming guardianship hearing. It troubled me that Louisa's appointment as guardian might be impeded by her physical handicaps, and that the judge would not be able to see beyond the brace, the walker, and the medicated lollipop she constantly kept between her lips. As the flight attendant handed out drinks, Louisa came to for a while and I took the opportunity to broach the subject with her. The words were difficult to find, but we had both reached a point where the honest sharing of thoughts was appreciated. Louisa was receptive to the suggestion that she wean herself off the brace in time for the hearing; and to my comfort, she took it a step further to say that she intended to be reliant only on a cane and to dispense with the walker. The next topic was not so easy to bring up, for I knew that Louisa's reliance on narcotics was a somewhat sensitive subject.

"Is it possible to time your lollipops on the day of the hearing so that you won't need one while you are in the courtroom?" I began. "There is a real possibility that the judge will not rule in your favor, and though your family understands the reason for the medication, the judge might not think it in Mom's best interest."

The purpose of the hearing was two-fold – to render a decision as to our parent's competency and, if deemed necessary, to assign a guardian to act on her behalf. Mother's incompetency would be easier to prove than Louisa's suitability as a guardian. My younger sister needed every opportunity to show the judge that she was able to handle another person's financial affairs and medical care.

My question hung as if suspended in the air, which seemed closer than usual in the plane...and then Louisa turned to me and nodded that she understood. Her eyes were moist, and I could only imagine how difficult this was for her. One never hopes to acknowledge that a relative is incapable of taking care of themselves, but to petition for the legal right to care for one's mother at the expense of her own self-will just seemed, well...wrong... necessary, but wrong.

As we were discussing courtroom strategy, Esther called Mother's caregiver to inform her that on Tuesday at ten o'clock the following week a courier would be hand delivering court documents to Mrs. Adams. Forewarned by Louisa, Elena was expecting the call and put the appointment on her mental calendar.

The day arrived and she made certain that her client was out of bed, had breakfast, and was fully dressed - quite a feat as Mrs. Adams usually fought her on early morning activities. Nevertheless, the impossible was accomplished and the doorbell promptly rang at ten o'clock. Mother jumped and let out a little yelp as the doorbell rang, and she anxiously asked who it was as Elena went to the door. The courier announced herself and explained that she had a delivery for Imogene Adams which must be placed directly in her hands. Mother did not move from the sofa, nor did she invite the woman in.

"What is it?" she asked, eyeing the envelope suspiciously.

"I do not know what is in the envelope," the courier replied. "My instructions are to place it in your hands and ask you to sign for it."

"I'm not signing anything until I know what it is. Open it and read it to me," was the surly response from the elderly woman, still firmly planted across the living room on the sofa.

"I am sorry, ma'am, but I am not allowed to open it."

"Elena, you do it."

"Ma'am, she is not allowed to. It has to be delivered directly to you."

"Why?" was Mother's gruff rebuttal.

"It is from the San Angelo County Court and you are required to sign for it."

"The courthouse! Oh, Elena, you have to read it to me."

The exchange went back and forth a few more times before the courier allowed Elena to take the envelope to Mrs. Adams, slit open the envelope, and slid the document out for her to see. The courier stood in the open doorway.

"Read it to me," Mom demanded, and Elena read the opening few paragraphs, which were written in legalese and served only to further confuse the issue.

"Ma'am, could you please sign the delivery acknowledgement, and I will be on my way," asked the courier from the doorway.

"No."

"But, Ma'am..." the courier sputtered.

Elena decided to intercede and gently explained in as few words and as simple sentences as possible that signing the delivery slip did not mean she agreed with the document, but just that she had received it. After several repetitions of this explanation, Mother, still sitting unmoved on the sofa, signed the delivery slip and ordered the courier away from her door step.

"Is this from Allison?" she asked fearfully, to which Elena explained again that it was from the court and that an attorney would be coming by to explain it to her.

Mother flipped through the pages and said, "Allison's name is not anywhere in here. This is good."

She nodded her head in approval and instructed Elena to put the papers on the dining room table and continued sitting in the, the same position on the sofa, completely unmoving.

When Louisa relayed the story to me, I did not know whether to sigh or to laugh. My name was, indeed, sprinkled throughout the document as the alternate in the event that Louisa became incapacitated. We were saddened to have proof that Mother could no longer read.

Louisa was also frustrated with Mother because she had lied in order to cover up the fact that she did not understand the papers that had been served. It was painfully obvious to Louisa that the fog which shrouded Mother's mind had only deepened. She chose not to accuse her of lying about it, for chastisements only drove Mother further into the fog. Rather, Louisa praised her for taking this important step to have her legally declared as guardian.

Already under the impression that Louisa had been her custodian for some time, Mother showed no real comprehension of the legal proceedings that were about to occur on her behalf.

The court-appointed attorney arrived the next day to discuss the case. Because of client-attorney privilege he asked Elena to go into the garage, but to leave the door open in case Mrs. Adams called out for her. She could not hear the attorney's explanations or questions, but the conference took what seemed to be an agonizingly long time as Elena stood in the hot garage with one ear closely cocked toward the door. The only words that reached her ears were loud protests, "No, I don't want to live in the Big House. No."

After the attorney's departure, Elena sat down beside Mrs. Adams and listened to her distressed cries. Mother rocked back and forth in the dining room chair as the kind caregiver held her close. She slowly gained control of her emotions again, and sitting up straight in the chair with chin held high, said with renewed confidence, "My attorney said he would do everything he could to keep me in my house."

Her confidence was short lived and the next two days she went without sleeping, ate very little, and was frightened by every sound that reached her ears and every shadow of the birds flying by her window. She hid in her bedroom under the sheets. By Thursday afternoon Mother was so distraught and weak that her attorney decided that she should not appear in court the next day. The psychiatrist concurred and ordered a prescription for an even stronger sedative than the one he had already prescribed, in the hope of abating his patient's hysteria. Louisa had flown to San Angelo that morning, accompanied by Matt's mother, Jill, and the two of them were unable to calm her and reluctantly left her in the hands of the woman who had cared for her for the past two-and-a-half years. Elena gently took her hand and sat down beside the bed to watch over her frightened client.

The hearing on Friday afternoon was preceded by a meeting between Louisa and Esther Carlisle in which they reviewed all the details of the past few years, as well as the timely declaration of incompetency. Esther quizzed Louisa on the line of questioning she was likely to encounter from the judge. Neither believed that

Mother's attorney would contest anything they offered in the way of a long-term care plan, nor for the management of her estate.

"When Louisa and I talked on the phone the night before, I told her how proud I was of her. At one time she had been the consummate professional standing in front of high level executives, teaching and guiding them. If anyone could take the witness stand with full confidence and poise, it would be Louisa. I told her so, and she shakily thanked me. Speaking in front of a classroom about effective leadership, however, is a bit different than taking the stand to revoke all of your mother's rights."

"I don't know that I could do that," Nora said. "You know that so many prayers were with all of you that day, though. Someone from the Prayer Lift at church asks me almost on a daily basis how the three of you are doing."

"We know that we do not walk this path alone," I said with assurance.

The court hearing began on time, and Louisa took the stand supported only by a cane. Her hands and mouth were free of any evidence of a lollipop and her mind was clear. Although Mother was not present in the courtroom, which we came to understand was not unusual and actually played to the petitioner's advantage, the judge was quick to evaluate the psychiatrist's assessment of her condition and with very few questions for her attorney, declared Mrs. Adams incompetent.

The process of assigning a guardian took a bit longer, as he was concerned about how a long distance caregiver would most effectively give Mrs. Adams the care she needed. Thanks to the expert coaching by her attorney, Louisa's well thought out plan was readily approved. The judge set the guidelines and conditions for the custodial care of the Mrs. Adams, and Louisa received instructions on the documentation of her medical care and the accounting for every penny of the estate that was spent on her behalf.

"Nora, the hearing went very well," I said enthusiastically when we talked briefly on the phone the day afterwards. "It is done. Mother is safe from herself... or at least her financial matters are safe. We still can't move her because of the judge's order that Louisa has to post a bond."

"A bond - whatever for?" asked Nora, puzzled over the stipulation by the judge.

"Apparently, this is standard," I explained. "She is required to post a bond of some three hundred dollars or so with the county clerk that she will not remove all of her mother's money and skip town with it, as Esther so eloquently phrased it. Court did not let out in time for Louisa to post the bond on Friday, so the attorney will post it for her on Monday. Once that is done, Louisa can move Mom over to the Johnston Center."

I paused before going on, "We had talked about how Louisa and Elena could just drive up to the center and walk Mom in with the help of the admissions nurse, but the requirement of posting the bond means the move will have to be delayed until next weekend. She isn't telling Mom, of course, and we decided that it would probably be a good idea for me to continue to remain silent."

Nora was quick to understand and as the one who was always concerned about my welfare asked, "Are you alright with that? I would think it is terribly difficult not to reach out to your mother right now."

One of the things I loved about Nora is that she hears between the lines the emotions that I don't even know I am feeling. Once again, she knew I was, in fact, troubled by the edict of silence that was imposed upon me. Granted, I had agreed with Louisa that it was best for Mother to remain as calm and unruffled as possible. It was, therefore, in Mother's best interest for me to remove myself from her world for just a little while - which made my heart ache for her all the more.

Unbeknownst to Mother, Louisa and her family were to return to San Angelo the next weekend to move her from the little cottage into the Alzheimer's unit. Louisa called me several times that week to share ideas on the gentlest way to bring about the transition.

"She won't go over to the Johnston Center on her own accord," I had pointed out. "She just won't do it. We have to think of a way to get her into that part of the building in such a way that it will not arouse her suspicions."

"We can just show up on her doorstep and ask her to take us on a tour," Louisa had suggested.

"Louisa, she won't do it. Do you recall that she always had someone else take us on tours over there, simply because she would not step foot in the place?" I reminded her. "I truly don't think she has ever been in the Johnston Center. I think she has always been afraid – afraid not necessarily of the place, but afraid of the residents. You know how she speaks about them in very pitying terms and is so condescending about their behaviors."

Reluctantly, Louisa agreed that she could not just show up at Mother's and expect her to willingly cross that threshold, either physically or figuratively. Symbolically, if nothing else, it meant the death of life as she knew it, and the beginning of a journey to the end surrounded by people she pitied, even sneered at. To go through that doorway meant that she had become one of them, and that thought terrified her.

"What about telling Mom that her Thursday hair appointment could not be scheduled and they would have to go to the beauty salon on Saturday, the day you plan on arriving there," I suggested, and a plan began to emerge. "She and Elena would walk over to the salon next to the center where you and your family would be waiting, along with the admissions nurse."

"That's a great idea," Louisa said and conferenced Elena into the call to explain the plan.

Elena was used to our plans. For two years we had been coming up with secretive means to make Mother's life easier and safer in order to preserve her self-esteem and dignity. In most cases we had succeeded - Louisa and Elena more so than I. Mother had responded well to our backhanded manipulations, little suspecting that changes were slowly being made to keep her from harm. The disappearance of the phone, magazine subscriptions, and most notably, the car, were all carefully orchestrated to cause her the least amount of pain.

At first she accused Elena of stealing the newspapers and magazines or hiding the car keys, but eventually did not even remember that she had subscribed to the newspaper or *Ladies Home Journal*, while the car soon became a distant memory. Louisa was quite skilled at working with Mother and strove very hard to maintain her dignity as an adult and parent. I was not so forgiving, and quite literally wanted to tell Mother to be realistic and to just get over it. I hadn't the patience to guide and redirect and ameliorate; but moving Mother out of the little house into a place that she truly dreaded would require all of those skills.

Saturday morning arrived, and Elena and Mother set out to the administrative building which housed the front offices. Slowly making their way past the chapel, the dining room, beauty salon, sauna, and pharmacy they rounded a corner which led to a ramped hallway adjoining the infirmary, the rest home, the assisted living unit... and the Alzheimer's center. Elena had used her brilliant and practiced art of bending the truth at just the right moment for just the right purpose and told Mom they had to go over to the administration building to give blood on Saturday at ten in the morning. The beauty salon ruse had not worked because the hairdresser, unaware of the real reason for changing the appointment, had chirped that she did not work on Saturdays. So, Elena came up with the Red Cross blood drive for the victims of the floods in Alabama, and always one to perform her civic duty, Mom agreed that was a good thing to do.

"Nora, Mom never thought to question why the Red Cross wanted the blood of an eighty-year-old on more medications than one could count. She just dutifully followed Elena into the hallway toward the beauty salon... and toward the Johnston Center."

Mother's head was down as she concentrated on the downward slope of the ramped hallway. Upon turning the corner at the bottom, she lifted her head and suddenly recognized Matt standing with a group of people at the end of the short hallway.

"Elena, I think that is Matt," she exclaimed, and her pace quickened ever so slightly.

"*Matt,*" Louisa whispered as her husband took a step forward. *"Don't go to her. She has to come to us."*

They were standing only yards from the center's entrance and dared not move in her direction for fear that she would venture no further. She paused before continuing the short distance between them where they enthusiastically greeted her. It was a day that would be filled with surprises - some joyful, some full of anguish – and Louisa let the joy of the moment linger on as long as possible before saying, "Mom, I have something to tell you. Let's go in here."

Louisa gently took her arm and guided her into a room filled with comfortable upholstered chairs circled around a beautifully polished mahogany table. The room was decorated as a family dining room might be and they all sat down around the table before Louisa continued.

"Nora, I don't know the exact words that Louisa used, but I know they were delivered as gently and straight to the point as Louisa could manage. She told her that one of the conditions for Louisa officially becoming her guardian was that Mom move out of the cottage into a place that could take care of her, and that the doctor and the judge mandated that it was not safe for her to be in her house anymore."

Nora listened intently as I described Mother's reaction to the words she hoped would never come.

"We had no idea what might run through her head or what she might say or do. They were fully prepared to let the admissions nurse sedate her, if necessary, a thought that just made all of us cringe," I said to Nora.

My friend's face showed compassion and understanding. The journey that she and I had begun so many months before was almost at a close.

Acknowledging her support, I continued, "From some source of strength deep inside herself, Mom found that gracious and mature person that had continued to live behind the fog and simply said, 'That attorney lied to me, didn't he?... Well, if that is the way it has to be, I will go.'"

My voice faltered and my lips quivered as a sense of pride swept over me. My mother had risen to the fullest sense of self and, overcoming the dread and anxiety of the moment she knew would eventually come upon her, she took my sister's hand and squeezed it as if to say that it would be alright. Louisa tells me that she cried a little, but only a little, before they all rose from the table, shuffled their dueling walkers back out into the hallway and turned toward the Alzheimer's entrance. The admissions nurse took Mrs. Adams's arm and with a grandchild on either side they began the longest journey of the past two-and-a-half years, yet only twenty short steps into Grandmother's new home and new life. The nurse took up the call and talked without stopping, explaining and pointing out the cozy surroundings and the beautiful faces on the residents. The two ladies with a cat sitting across their laps waved at her; the gentleman tapping his knee to the beat of a lively guitar concert in the main living area smiled at her; and a cheerful charge nurse approached them with a stack of snow-white towels in her arms.

Louisa and the grandchildren helped her settle into the room and pointed out that some of her clothes were already hanging in the armoire. A bouquet of fresh flowers with the card that read, "From Your Family" sat on the bedside table. It was several weeks before anyone ventured to tell her that the bedspread, lace curtains, and flowers had all been sent to her room by Tom and me, but by that time she was in love with the room and pleased that even long distance we cared for her. Initially, she thought the bedspread was from a previous vintage, the occupant of the room before her, and told Charlotte to take it off the bed and throw it on the floor in a corner, an order which her granddaughter dutifully obeyed. Louisa was furious when she saw the spread crumpled in the corner, and after a very trying day, began to cry.

"Mom, we bought that bedspread especially for you. If you don't like it we will take it back and exchange it," she sobbed. "We just want you to be happy and thought it would make your room pretty."

Remembering her manners, Mother took Louisa in her arms and apologized until her youngest daughter's tears quit flowing, and then she remorsefully asked Charlotte to retrieve the spread and put it back on the bed. In weeks to come she would brag about how pretty it was to the neighbors that wandered into her room.

Residents are free to walk wherever they want to go - except through the alarmed doors leading to the outside world. Most seemed content to explore each other's rooms and one such lady wandered into the room while Charlotte was helping her grandmother unpack. Playing the role of gracious hostess in reverse, Grandmother told the unwelcome guest in very sweet tones that her family was visiting and she would need to come back another time.

Charlotte was appalled that the bewildered visitor responded with a resounding, "No! I'm staying."

The gracious Southern tones in Mom's voice turned into

bellows, "You will leave my room."

The petite lady fainted and Charlotte rang for a nurse while Mother stood defiantly with two hands firmly holding onto her walker ready to defend her new home. A nurse came in and calmly lifted the little lady to her feet with the gentle chastisement, "Oh, you are just faking. Let's go back to the living room."

Peace and calm returned to the room, and Mother smiled with satisfaction that she had firmly claimed ownership of Room 401.

"My family got this bedspread for me," she later told Elena, beaming with pride.

Louisa wisely orchestrated the move into hourly rotations so that each of her family spent time alone with Mother urging her to make her own decisions about where she wanted the paintings hung or where she wished to place her sweaters in the dresser drawers. The dresser was the only piece of furniture that made the journey with her from the cottage. Matt and Charlie brought it over and set it into place along the wall directly opposite her bed. Mother placed family pictures and other personal items on the dresser, and as the day progressed and the room gradually came to life with things that were familiar to her, she began to feel that the Johnston Center was home.

When Louisa left with her family the following afternoon, Mother was seated at a table having lunch with a group of people busily engaged in a conversation. Louisa just smiled over at her and quietly walked out the door, waving her security card at the alarm. Mother was at peace, if only for that moment, but she was safe and at peace.

"Mom loves her new apartment, Nora. I call it an apartment even though it is only one room, but it has its own shower and bathroom. None of the other rooms do. Hers is the only one. Isn't that wonderful? She can have that privacy she covets so dearly."

Nora and I were having our last dinner together as care giver and care receiver. The journey alongside my mother had been rough, filled with many stumbling blocks which often seemed impassable. At times my mother and I had walked arm in arm, and at others I could only stand to one side, trying to remove obstacles in her way. Nora understood this journey, and I was grateful that she had been there to hold me up, to keep me going, and to redirect me when my path seemed to veer away. She had been my mentor in a sense, and always would be, for I admired her sincere and sweet qualities. We laughed together over our meal, this time with the deep and satisfying laughter of a joyful ending, and we knew that there would be many more dinners as steadfast friends.

Although Nora and I had reached the end of our walk together, Mother's journey was far from its end. I hoped that she would be making her way around the Johnston Center, making friends with all the men and women, and establishing her territory.

"There were fresh flowers in her room the first time she saw it, and some of her favorite paintings and pictures were already on the walls. Louisa and Matt bought her a new armchair where she sits and stares out the window between fresh new lace curtains. Elena says her face lights up when she sits there to study the trees outside. She needs to wear a diaper all the time now, and a nurse has to help her dress. They get her up when it's time to go to breakfast with all the other residents in the dining room where she carries on a lively conversation about how her husband built Waverly Place and her daughter, who is twenty-seven, will come sing for them. The staff takes her on walks outside where they explore the various kinds of plant life in the rock garden. One of her favorite places to visit is the vending machine where the nurse and she giggle over all the choices. The nurses love her, and Louisa and I just shake our heads and wonder where the mean and abusive woman she had been for the last two years suddenly went. But, we don't dwell on that for too long, because she seems content, and has even told us that this is a good place to be."

"Nora, I had an epiphany this week," I exclaimed as we settled deeper into the high backed leather booth to enjoy our cups of coffee and tea. "I have placed certain expectations on my mother. I expect her to know not just my name, but to remember that I don't like green beans and am afraid of elevators. I expect her to continue to share the same love of traveling, but she is not even certain where Paris is or what the seashore looks like. I expect her to speak kindly of others, even when she can't recall their relationship. I expect her to remember our birthdays and to act like a lady... when she is doing well to wear matching shoes and to remember what a fork is for. I expect her to want to go to worship services and to be among God's people when she doesn't remember that she needs Him."

"Nora, I was very young when I first heard about Alzheimer's and never dreamed that it could be part of my family's life," I said.

She smiled, "Youth has a blessed naiveté that does not always serve us well in later life. Growing old is a gift."

I returned her warm smile and told her about my first experience with Alzheimer's many years ago. I was serving as director of music ministries for a church back in Texas and knew most of the members of the congregation whose faces smiled back at me every Sunday morning. For the longest time the sweetest smiles were on the faces of two elderly women – sisters - who faithfully attended services every week. Gradually over a few months their smiles began to flatten and turn down and their eyes became empty and expressionless. Their feet slowed to a shuffle along the sidewalk and sometimes these two darling women could call others by name, and sometimes not.

One Sunday, Shirley was not in her usual spot next to Mildred on the aisle in the third row of pews, and I learned in staff meeting the next day that she had been moved out of her home of fifty-six years into a nursing home. The nursing home was a familiar place, as my hand bell choir had performed there on several occasions, and I decided to stop by to see her. I soon found my friend sitting on a bench in the hallway between two residential wings and sat down next to her. Her face was troubled as she slowly turned and met my gaze. There was a lack of recognition in her eyes, and she did not answer when I asked her how she was doing and that we had missed her in church. Bewilderment crossed her face because the words "church" and "church family" no longer had meaning for her. I left the nursing home more troubled than when I had entered. In staff meeting the next day, we were told that Shirley's family had requested that we not visit her because it upset her too much when she did not recognize people she was certain that she should know. It was then that the ugly truth of Alzheimer's was introduced to me.

"Over the next few years, Nora, I slowly began losing friends, and parents of friends..., and now I am losing my own parent."

I did go back to the nursing home on a regular basis, but instead of pressing my name and the name of the church upon Shirley, I simply sat with her and anyone else who looked lonely and talked to them about their pretty blue dress, walked with them outside in the garden, or read the next chapter of a book out loud. In spite of the fact that Shirley could barely respond with a smile, there was still an innate beauty in her spirit. We laughed and sang and did little jigs in the sunshine and it did not matter that her memories were buried beneath a layer of cobwebs. In thinking back on those special times with Shirley, I realize that Mother is becoming more and more like her.

Nora put her elbows on the table and cradled her chin in her hands, leaning forward to listen intently to the stirrings in my heart. She always knows when to sit still and just listen and when to jump in with "ah-ha" or "hmm."

"I expect too much from my mother. The pressure I have placed on her to continue to perform with the sound mindset of a mature adult is unfair. I have been unrealistic in expecting, even demanding that she remain a fully functioning adult. She is a Shirley. I just need to tell her that she looks pretty in her new dress, read her a chapter out of her favorite book, comb her hair, and tuck her in at night. She will smile back at me and reach up to touch my face before she falls contentedly asleep."

Rather than thinking of her life as diminishing or fading away, my mother's inner beauty still prevails; and when all the outer layers of unrealistic expectations are peeled away, the pure light of who she really is will still shine. My mother is a child of God. She is making her way through a dark place, but I must believe that her journey does not stop here and that she will keep moving forward toward joy.

Afterword

*F*riends will traverse many obstacles to be near each other. Mother could no longer go to her friends, but they came flocking to her; and the day that Louisa and I had dreaded turned into a day of renewed possibilities and hope for new kinds of friendships that transcend the mind's ability to remember and holds true to the feeling that one is indeed loved.

There was a feeling of rightness in giving the furniture to friends who loved the pieces and could truly use them in their own homes. As the day wore on, several of Mother's acquaintances, who knew nothing about her transition into the Alzheimer's unit, serendipitously dropped by the cottage, fully expecting to greet their dear friend, but instead finding her family there. Each received something precious from her belongings and left promising to visit her often, a testament to the strong ties friendship that Mother had created over the years.

Word spread quickly throughout her circle of friends. Pastor Art rejoiced to hear that she had made the transition to the center and that my sister had been appointed guardian. Art was a regular visitor to Waverly Place's nursing home and the Alzheimer's unit, and he promised to check in on Mother as often as possible. Her church had been, and would continue to be faithful to her in spite of the many times she claimed they had forgotten about her.

Sylvia was among the first to hear about the move and drove right over to wish Mother well in her new home. She privately told Louisa how much she missed her old friend, and that the travel group, which Sylvia has resurrected, would not be the same without Imogene. She found it hard to believe that Mother's needs had become so acute, but having experienced it firsthand while staying with her in the hospital, Sylvia was relieved to know that she would be properly cared for in the very place that Imogene had handpicked some years ago. Judy, Art, and Sylvia became a frequent visitor, and on some days Mother knew who her visitors were, and on some days not.

Christmas will be celebrated at our house this year. Louisa's family will make the trip north, but this time it will be without Mother. We will unpack her porcelain Nativity Scene and place it in the center of a candlelit window, and one of us will place the Christ Child in her stead. The gathering around the Christmas table will be a bittersweet time of joy, relief, and sadness as Mother's absence will be deeply felt.

Our thoughts and prayers will be with her, though, for even while she does not remember who we are, nothing can change the fact that she remains our beloved mother and grandmother.

"God bless you, Mom," I quietly whispered as we all settled down to watch a movie with bowls of popcorn on our laps and Granddog at our feet.

Made in the USA
San Bernardino, CA
28 November 2012